Controversies in Female Pelvic Reconstruction

Guest Editors

ROGER R. DMOCHOWSKI, MD
MICKEY KARRAM, MD

UROLOGIC CLINICS OF NORTH AMERICA

www.urologic.theclinics.com

Consulting Editor
SAMIR S. TANEJA, MD

August 2012 • Volume 39 • Number 3

SAUNDERS an imprint of ELSEVIER, Inc.

W.B. SAUNDERS COMPANY
A Division of Elsevier Inc.

1600 John F. Kennedy Blvd. • Suite 1800 • Philadelphia, PA 19103-2899

http://www.theclinics.com

UROLOGIC CLINICS OF NORTH AMERICA Volume 39, Number 3
August 2012 ISSN 0094-0143, ISBN-13: 978-1-4557-4902-7

Editor: Stephanie Donley

Urologic Clinics of North America (ISSN 0094-0143) is published quarterly by Elsevier Inc., 360 Park Avenue South, New York, NY 10010-1710. Months of issue are February, May, August, and November. Business and Editorial Offices: 1600 John F. Kennedy Blvd., Suite 1800, Philadelphia, PA 19103-2899. Periodicals postage paid at New York, NY and additional mailing offices. Subscription prices are $339.00 per year (US individuals), $561.00 per year (US institutions), $396.00 per year (Canadian individuals), $687.00 per year (Canadian institutions), $492.00 per year (foreign individuals), and $687.00 per year (foreign institutions). Foreign air speed delivery is included in all *Clinics* subscription prices. All prices are subject to change without notice. **POSTMASTER:** Send address changes to *Urologic Clinics of North America*, Elsevier Health Sciences Division, Subscription Customer Service, 3251 Riverport Lane, Maryland Heights, MO 63043. Customer Service: 1-800-654-2452 (US). From outside the United States, call 1-314-447-8871. Fax: 1-314-447-8029. E-mail: JournalsCustomerServiceusa@elsevier.com (for print support) and JournalsOnlineSupport-usa@elsevier.com (for online support).

Reprints. For copies of 100 or more, of articles in this publication, please contact the Commercial Reprints Department, Elsevier Inc., 360 Park Avenue South, New York, New York 10010-1710. Tel.: 212-633-3813; Fax: 212-462-1935; E-mail: reprints@elsevier.com.

Urologic Clinics of North America is covered in MEDLINE/PubMed (*Index Medicus*), *Excerpta Medica, Current Contents/Clinical Medicine, Science Citation Index,* and *ISI/BIOMED*.

Printed and bound by CPI Group (UK) Ltd, Croydon, CR0 4YY

Transferred to Digital Print 2012

Contributors

CONSULTING EDITOR

SAMIR S. TANEJA, MD
The James M. and Janet Riha Neissa Professor of Urologic Oncology; Professor of Urology and Radiology; Director, Division of Urologic Oncology, Department of Urology, New York University Langone Medical Center, New York University Cancer Institute; Program Leader, Genitourinary Oncology Program, New York University Cancer Institute, New York, New York

GUEST EDITORS

ROGER R. DMOCHOWSKI, MD, FACS
Professor, Department of Urologic Surgery, Vanderbilt University Medical Center, Nashville, Tennessee

MICKEY KARRAM, MD, FACOG
Director of Urogynecology, The Christ Hospital; Clinical Professor of Ob/Gyn and Urogynecology, Department of Obstetrics and Gynecology, Division of Female Pelvic Medicine and Reconstructive Surgery, The Christ Hospital/University of Cincinnati, Cincinnati, Ohio

AUTHORS

MATTHEW D. BARBER, MD, MHS
Professor of Surgery and Vice Chair for Clinical Research, Center for Urogynecology and Pelvic Reconstructive Surgery, Obstetrics, Gynecology and Women's Health Institute, Cleveland Clinic, Cleveland, Ohio

BENJAMIN M. BRUCKER, MD
Assistant Professor of Urology, Department of Urology, New York University, New York, New York

KIMBERLY L. BURGESS, MD
Instructor of Urology, Department of Urology, Mayo Clinic, Rochester, Minnesota

CHARLES W. BUTRICK, MD
Director, The Urogynecology Center, Overland Park, Kansas

ANITA CHEN, MD
Department of Gynecologic Surgery, Mayo Clinic Florida, Jacksonville, Florida

BENJAMIN E. DILLON, MD
Department of Urology, University of Texas Southwestern Medical Center, Dallas, Texas

ROGER R. DMOCHOWSKI, MD, FACS
Professor, Department of Urologic Surgery, Vanderbilt University Medical Center, Nashville, Tennessee

CHRISTOPHER S. ELLIOT, MD, PhD
Fellow in Female Pelvic Medicine and
Reconstruction Surgery, Division of
Urogynecology and Pelvic Reconstructive
Surgery, Stanford University School of
Medicine, Palo Alto, California

DANIEL S. ELLIOTT, MD
Assistant Professor of Urology, Department of
Urology, Mayo Clinic, Rochester, Minnesota

DEBORAH R. ERICKSON, MD
Professor of Surgery, Division of Urology,
Department of Surgery, University of Kentucky
College of Medicine, Lexington, Kentucky

MATTHEW FULTON, MD
Urology Resident, Department of Urology,
Oakland University William Beaumont School
of Medicine, Royal Oak, Michigan

HOWARD B. GOLDMAN, MD
Center for Female Pelvic Medicine and
Reconstructive Surgery, Glickman Urological
and Kidney Institute, Cleveland Clinic, Lerner
College of Medicine, Cleveland, Ohio

ALEX GOMELSKY, MD
Associate Professor of Clinical Urology,
Department of Urology, Louisiana State
University Health Sciences Center –
Shreveport, Shreveport, Louisiana

MICKEY KARRAM, MD, FACOG
Director of Urogynecology, The Christ
Hospital; Clinical Professor of Ob/Gyn and
Urogynecology, Department of Obstetrics and
Gynecology, Division of Female Pelvic
Medicine and Reconstructive Surgery,
The Christ Hospital/University of Cincinnati,
Cincinnati, Ohio

MELISSA R. KAUFMAN, MD, PhD
Assistant Professor, Department of Urologic
Surgery, Vanderbilt University, Nashville,
Tennessee

KIMBERLY KENTON, MD, MS
Professor & Division Director, Division of
Female Pelvic Medicine & Reconstructive
Surgery, Department of Obstetrics &
Gynecology; Department of Urology, Stritch
School of Medicine, Loyola University Chicago,
Maywood, Illinois

DOMINIC LEE, MD
Department of Urology, University of Texas
Southwestern Medical Center, Dallas, Texas

EUGENE LEE, MD
Clinical Instructor of Urology, Department
of Urology, New York University, New York,
New York

GARY E. LEMACK, MD
Department of Urology, University of Texas
Southwestern Medical Center, Dallas, Texas

VINCENT LUCENTE, MD
Chief Medical Officer, The Institute for Female
Pelvic Medicine & Reconstructive Surgery;
Chief, Gynecology, St. Luke's University Health
Network, Allentown; Clinical Professor of
Obstetrics and Gynecology, Temple University
College of Medicine, Philadelphia,
Pennsylvania

BRIAN K. MARKS, MD
Center for Female Pelvic Medicine and
Reconstructive Surgery, Glickman Urological
and Kidney Institute, Cleveland Clinic, Lerner
College of Medicine, Cleveland, Ohio

MILES MURPHY, MD, MSPH
Associate Medical Director, The Institute
for Female Pelvic Medicine & Reconstructive
Surgery, Allentown; Clinical Assistant
Professor, Department of Obstetrics and
Gynecology, Temple University School of
Medicine, Philadelphia, Pennsylvania

VICTOR W. NITTI, MD
Professor of Urology, Department of Urology,
New York University, New York, New York

KENNETH M. PETERS, MD
Peter and Florine Distinguished Chair of
Urology, Department of Urology, Beaumont
Hospital; Professor and Chairman of Urology,
Department of Urology, Oakland University
William Beaumont School of Medicine,
Royal Oak, Michigan

PAUL D.M. PETTIT, MD
Department of Gynecologic Surgery, Mayo
Clinic Florida, Jacksonville, Florida

RENEE B. QUILLIN, MD
Division of Urology, Department of Surgery,
University of Kentucky College of Medicine,
Lexington, Kentucky

OLGA RAMM, MD, MS
Division of Female Pelvic Medicine &
Reconstructive Surgery, Department of
Obstetrics & Gynecology; Department of
Urology, Stritch School of Medicine, Loyola
University Chicago, Maywood, Illinois

W. STUART REYNOLDS, MD, MPH
Assistant Professor, Department of Urologic
Surgery, Vanderbilt University Medical Center,
Nashville, Tennessee

MONICA L. RICHARDSON, MD, MPH
Fellow in Female Pelvic Medicine and
Reconstruction Surgery, Division of
Urogynecology and Pelvic Reconstructive
Surgery, Stanford University School of
Medicine, Palo Alto, California

BERI RIDGEWAY, MD
Assistant Professor of Surgery, Center for
Urogynecology and Pelvic Reconstructive
Surgery, Obstetrics, Gynecology and Women's
Health Institute, Cleveland Clinic, Cleveland,
Ohio

CRISTINA SAIZ, MD
The Institute for Female Pelvic Medicine &
Reconstructive Surgery; Fellow, St Luke's
University Health Network, Allentown,
Pennsylvania

ERIC R. SOKOL, MD
Assistant Professor of Obstetrics and
Gynecology, Co-Director of Division of
Urogynecology and Pelvic Reconstructive
Surgery, Stanford University School of
Medicine, Palo Alto, California

JAMES L. WHITESIDE, MD, MA, FACOG
Associate Professor, Department of Obstetrics
and Gynecology, Division of Female Pelvic
Medicine and Reconstructive Surgery,
Dartmouth Medical School, Dartmouth-
Hitchcock Medical Center, Lebanon,
New Hampshire

DANI ZOOROB, MD
Urogynecology Fellow, Department of
Obstetrics and Gynecology, Division of Female
Pelvic Medicine and Reconstructive Surgery,
The Christ Hospital/University of Cincinnati,
Cincinnati, Ohio

Contents

results are disappointing and retreatment is often necessary. Proper patient selection and management of patient expectations are paramount to successful application of UBT.

Stress urinary incontinence (SUI), the involuntary leakage of urine associated with an increase in intraabdominal pressure (coughing, laughing, and sneezing), affects 12.8% to 46.0% of women. SUI is the most common type of urinary incontinence in women younger than 60 years and accounts for at least half of incontinence in all women. Retropubic and transobturator midurethral sling procedures are safe and effective treatments for stress urinary incontinence but have different complication profiles. History, examination, and additional testing may assist in choosing the correct sling type. Appropriate counseling and managing patient expectation are necessary to optimize patient satisfaction.

The midurethral sling (MUS) is now the most commonly performed surgical treatment for stress urinary incontinence (SUI), and is considered the gold standard for patients with genuine SUI. This article examines the use of the MUS to treat all forms of SUI, with an emphasis on the nonindex patient (ie, intrinsic sphincter deficiency, lack of urethral hypermobility, mixed incontinence, failed MUS, concomitant prolapse, obesity, and elderly). The efficacy and safety of the MUS to treat SUI is assessed in these specific populations. Based on the available evidence, the discussion attempts to identify populations in whom MUS may not be appropriate.

The concept of the autologous pubovaginal sling involves supporting the proximal urethra and bladder neck with a piece of graft material, achieving continence either by providing a direct compressive force on the urethra/bladder outlet or by reestablishing a reinforcing platform or hammock against which the urethra is compressed during transmission of increased abdominal pressure. Pubovaginal slings using a biological sling material (whether autologous, allograft, or xenograft) can be used successfully to manage primary or recurrent stress incontinence. This article addresses the indications for the use of an autologous bladder-neck sling, describes the surgical techniques, and discusses outcomes and technical considerations.

Fascial slings remain a successful and durable option for treatment of female stress urinary incontinence (SUI). With limited risk of disease transmission, extrusion, or complications associated with mesh, use of autologous fascia is an attractive option, particularly for complex reconstructive cases. With generally robust outcomes, pubovaginal slings also continue to be a viable option for treatment of primary SUI after appropriate patient counseling regarding risks of bladder outlet obstruction and de novo urgency symptoms.

compartment prolapse can present with bulge symptoms as well as defecatory dysfunction, including constipation, tenesmus, splinting, and fecal incontinence. The diagnosis can successfully be made on clinical examination. Treatment of posterior prolapse includes pessaries and surgery. Both traditional colporrhaphy and site-specific defect repair have excellent success rates. Complications from surgery can include sexual dysfunction, de novo dyspareunia, and defecatory dysfunction. Compared with native tissue repair, biological and synthetic grafting has not improved overall anatomic and subjective outcomes.

The prevalence of posterior-compartment prolapse (rectocele) is not known. The authors have found that operative repair symptomatically improved a majority of patients with impaired defecation associated with a large rectocele, but this improvement was likely related at least in part to factors other than the size of the rectocele. Multiple surgical techniques are available for rectocele repair, and the literature is not clear regarding indications for each type of surgical intervention. This article reviews the literature regarding various types of posterior-compartment repair, and draws conclusions regarding their absolute efficacy and relative efficacy in comparison with one another.

Our understanding of interstitial cystitis/painful bladder syndrome (IC/BPS) has evolved with the advancements in our understanding of visceral pain syndromes. The concept of IC/BPS as a visceral pain disorder is used as a model to base a targeted approach to the management of patients with IC/BPS. Guidelines for the treatment of both the bladder and nonbladder pain disorders are reviewed.

Management of interstitial cystitis/bladder pain syndrome (IC/BPS) is individualized for each patient. All patients benefit from education and self-care advice. Patients with Hunner lesions usually respond well to fulguration or triamcinolone injection, which can be repeated when the symptoms and lesions recur. For patients without Hunner lesions, numerous treatment options are available. The tiers of the American Urological Association Guidelines present these options in an orderly progression, balancing the benefits, risks, and burdens. Along with specific IC/BPS treatments, it is also important to have resources for stress reduction, pain management, and treatment of comorbid conditions.

Implantable sacral nerve stimulation is a minimally invasive, durable, and reversible procedure for patients with urinary urge and fecal incontinence who are refractory to conservative therapy. The therapy is safe compared with other surgical options. An intact external or internal rectal sphincter is not a prerequisite for success in patients with fecal incontinence.

Neuromodulation is an effective, minimally invasive technique for the management of urinary urgency and frequency, urgency incontinence, nonobstructive urinary retention, and fecal incontinence. This article reviews the physiology of neuromodulation, indications, implantation methods, and outcomes.

Once thought of as a long-term solution to pelvic organ prolapse, currently synthetic mesh augmentation is regarded as a dark area that is being critically assessed by surgeons, hospitals, industry, and most importantly the Food and Drug Administration. The development of midurethral sling kits has revolutionized the surgical treatment of stress incontinence. These systems, however, were not rigorously tested but instead marketed after being cleared by the Food and Drug Administration through a simple regulatory process using a previously approved predescent material. This article reviews the management of mesh complications of synthetic slings and mesh used to augment prolapse repair.

Since the introduction of the synthetic midurethral sling, several transvaginal mesh delivery systems have been developed for treating stress incontinence and pelvic organ prolapse. Widespread use of these "kits" has introduced a new dilemma of mesh-specific complications that female pelvic surgeons must manage. Differing treatment techniques have been described and controversy exists as to which method is preferred for vaginal mesh extrusion, mesh perforations, pelvic pain, and dyspareunia. This article addresses the differing management strategies for mesh complications after reconstructive surgery and highlights the available literature on the success of each option.

GOAL STATEMENT

The goal of *Urologic Clinics of North America* is to keep practicing urologists and urology residents up to date with current clinical practice in urology by providing timely articles reviewing the state of the art in patient care.

ACCREDITATION

The *Urologic Clinics of North America* is planned and implemented in accordance with the Essential Areas and Policies of the Accreditation Council for Continuing Medical Education (ACCME) through the joint sponsorship of the University of Virginia School of Medicine and Elsevier. The University of Virginia School of Medicine is accredited by the ACCME to provide continuing medical education for physicians.

The University of Virginia School of Medicine designates this enduring material activity for a maximum of 15 *AMA PRA Category 1 Credit*(s)™ for each issue, 60 credits per year. Physicians should claim only the credit commensurate with the extent of their participation in the activity.

The American Medical Association has determined that physicians not licensed in the US who participate in this CME enduring material activity are eligible for a maximum of 15 *AMA PRA Category 1 Credit*(s)™ for each issue, 60 credits per year.

Credit can be earned by reading the text material, taking the CME examination online at http://www.theclinics.com/home/cme, and completing the evaluation. After taking the test, you will be required to review any and all incorrect answers. Following completion of the test and evaluation, your credit will be awarded and you may print your certificate.

FACULTY DISCLOSURE/CONFLICT OF INTEREST

The University of Virginia School of Medicine, as an ACCME accredited provider, endorses and strives to comply with the Accreditation Council for Continuing Medical Education (ACCME) Standards of Commercial Support, Commonwealth of Virginia statutes, University of Virginia policies and procedures, and associated federal and private regulations and guidelines on the need for disclosure and monitoring of proprietary and financial interests that may affect the scientific integrity and balance of content delivered in continuing medical education activities under our auspices.

The University of Virginia School of Medicine requires that all CME activities accredited through this institution be developed independently and be scientifically rigorous, balanced and objective in the presentation/discussion of its content, theories and practices.

All authors/editors participating in an accredited CME activity are expected to disclose to the readers relevant financial relationships with commercial entities occurring within the past 12 months (such as grants or research support, employee, consultant, stock holder, member of speakers bureau, etc.). The University of Virginia School of Medicine will employ appropriate mechanisms to resolve potential conflicts of interest to maintain the standards of fair and balanced education to the reader. Questions about specific strategies can be directed to the Office of Continuing Medical Education, University of Virginia School of Medicine, Charlottesville, Virginia.

The faculty and staff of the University of Virginia Office of Continuing Medical Education have no financial affiliations to disclose.

The authors/editors listed below have identified no professional or financial affiliations for themselves or their spouse/partner:
Matthew D. Barber, MD, MHS; Benjamin M. Brucker, MD; Kimberly L. Burgess, MD; Benjamin E. Dillon, MD; Stephanie Donley, (Acquisitions Editor); Christopher S. Elliot, MD, PhD; Daniel S. Elliott, MD; Matthew Fulton, MD; Alex Gomelsky, MD; Kimbery Kenton, MD, MS; Dominic Lee, MD; Eugene Lee, MD; Brian K. Marks, MD; Renee B. Quillin, MD; Olga Ramm, MD, MS; W. Stuart Reynolds, MD, MPH; Monica L. Richardson, MD, MPH; Beri Ridgeway, MD; Cristina Saiz, MD; and Dani Zoorob, MD.

The authors/editors listed below identified the following professional or financial affiliations for themselves or their spouse/partner:
Charles W. Butrick, MD receives research support from Boston Scientific, and is on the Speakers' Bureau for Astellas and Medtronic, Inc.
Roger R. Dmochowski, MD (Guest Editor) is on the Advisory Board for Merck, J&J, and Allergan.
Deborah R. Erickson, MD is a consultant for Trillium Therapeutics.
Howard B. Goldman, MD is a consultant and is on the Speakers' Bureau for Ethicon.
Mickey Karram, MD (Guest Editor) is a consultant for AMS and Astellas Pharma, is on the Speakers' Bureau for AMS and Astellas Pharma, receives research support from Astellas Pharma and Allergan, and owns stock in EMEDS CO.
Melissa R. Kaufman, MD is on the Speakers' Bureau for Astellas and Allergan.
Gary E. Lemack, MD receives research support from Allergan and NIDDK, and is on the Speakers' Bureau for Allergan, Astellas, and Pfizer, Inc.
Vincent Lucente, MD receives research support from and is a consultant and is on the Spreakers' Bureau for AMS, Bard, Coloplast, and Ethicon.
Miles Murphy, MD, MSPH is a consultant for Ethicon/Gynecare and Coloplast, and receives research support from AMS.
Victor W. Nitti, MD receives research support from Allergan, AMS, and Astellas; is on the Speakers' Bureau and Advisory Board for Allergan; is a consultant for AMS; and is on the Advirsory Board for Astellas and Medtronic.
Kenneth M. Peters, MD receives research support from Pfizer, Inc., Cook Myosite, AMS, and Allergan; is a consultant and is on the Advisory Board for Medtronic; and is a consultant for Trillium Therapeutics/Uroplasty.
Eric R. Sokol, MD owns stock in Pelvilon, and receives research support from Contura.
William Steers, MD (Test Author) is employed by the American Urologic Association, is a reviewer and consultant for NIH, and is an investigator for Allergan.
Samir S. Taneja, MD (Consulting Editor) is a consultant for Eigen, Gtx, and Steba Biotech, is an industry funded research/investigator for Gtx and Steba Biotech, and is on the Speakers' Bureau for Janssen.
James L. Whiteside, MD, MA is on the Advisory Board for the International Academy Pelvic Surgery.

Disclosure of Discussion of Non-FDA Approved Uses for Pharmaceutical Products and/or Medical Devices.
The University of Virginia School of Medicine, as an ACCME provider, requires that all faculty presenters identify and disclose any off-label uses for pharmaceutical and medical device products. The University of Virginia School of Medicine recommends that each physician fully review all the available data on new products or procedures prior to clinical use.

TO ENROLL

To enroll in the Urologic Clinics of North America Continuing Medical Education program, call customer service at 1-800-654-2452 or visit us online at www.theclinics.com/home/cme. The CME program is available to subscribers for an additional fee of $207.00.

UROLOGIC CLINICS OF NORTH AMERICA

DOWNLOAD
Free App!

Review Articles
THE CLINICS

NOW AVAILABLE FOR YOUR iPhone and iPad

Preface

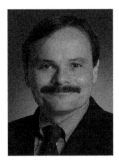 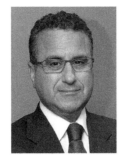

Roger R. Dmochowski, MD   Mickey Karram, MD
Guest Editors

The subspecialty of Female Pelvic Medicine has undergone substantial evolution and development over the last several decades. The recent American Board of Medical Specialties recognition of pelvic medicine as a stand-alone subspecialty within the shared domains of urology and gynecology further underscores this evolutionary and developmental process. The intent of this collection of articles is to review a variety of areas of controversy within the domain of female pelvic medicine in order that updated evaluation and management strategies can be reviewed and, where differences exist in the management of these conditions between specialties, the reasons can be elaborated and explained. For many of the conditions addressed in this edition, several different management strategies may provide reasonable outcomes and successful resolution of the condition, associated patient bother, and overall improvement of the quality of life of the woman who presents with these complaints. Parallel to the development of female pelvic medicine has been an emphasis on improved outcomes reporting. Where appropriate, outcomes of importance have been underscored and emphasized so as to focus the proceduralist on the importance of these for both objective outcomes reporting and informed consent. Inherent to the improvement of outcomes for pelvic floor procedures is an emphasis on decreasing variability of care and standardization of process. Care variability has consistently been shown to lead to outcomes variability and inherent increases in resource expenditures;

therefore, process standardization as it applies to interventions for pelvic floor conditions must continue apace, increasing consumer demand for these services. The term "process" used here is not meant to reference only the actual procedure but also the preparation for, perioperative management of, and the postoperative oversight that surrounds the intervention event. A motivated, informed, and engaged patient is critical to an optimization of outcomes and management of less than optimal results. No proceduralist in fact operates alone, and our interventions are byproducts of the team that delivers care, the dedicated professionals that also deliver care alongside of us (nurses, nurse practitioners, physician assistants, and therapists, just to mention a few). It is incumbent on us to recognize them and include them in the care delivery process in a collegial, respectful, and mutually appreciative manner. This edition recognizes them and applauds their role in the care of our patients.

A special emphasis of this edition is focused on addressing controversies surrounding new technologies. Special emphasis has been placed on robotics, mesh use (incontinence and prolapse), and bulking agents, as all represent added inherent expense to an overtaxed health care system. Technological evolution is critical to continued advancement of care; however, the informed and graded adoption of technologies represents the most thoughtful inclusion of these advancements into care. Indeed, some new technologies bring with them new issues and associated concerns and these

Urol Clin N Am 39 (2012) xv–xvi
http://dx.doi.org/10.1016/j.ucl.2012.07.001

must be recognized, understood, and managed with utmost diligence to protect our patients and to control the consumption of health care finances.

It is our hope that this collection of articles will provide the interested reader with a state-of-the-art snapshot of current best practice while also emphasizing areas that as of yet are not managed in a consensus fashion. This edition attempts to address areas of variability and care with the ultimate goal that practitioners in this domain will continue to standardize care delivery while integrating new technologies and new developments in the understanding of the underlying pathophysiology and causations of the included conditions.

Roger R. Dmochowski, MD
Department of Urologic Surgery
Vanderbilt University Medical Center
A1302 Medical Center North
Nashville, TN 37232-2765, USA

Mickey Karram, MD
The Christ Hospital
2123 Auburn Avenue, Suite 307
Cincinnati, OH 45219, USA

E-mail addresses:
roger.dmochowski@vanderbilt.edu
(R.R. Dmochowski)
Mickey.karram@thechristhospital.com
(M. Karram)

Making Sense of Urodynamic Studies for Women with Urinary Incontinence and Pelvic Organ Prolapse
A Urogynecology Perspective

James L. Whiteside, MD, MA

KEYWORDS

- Urodynamics • Urinary incontinence • Pelvic organ prolapse • Testing

KEY POINTS

- Support for routine urodynamic testing in the management of women presenting with urinary incontinence is eroding.
- The clinical features of urodynamic testing and its diagnostic and prognostic precision and accuracy are all problematic with growing evidence urodynamic test results do not meaningfully improve clinical outcomes.
- Precise understanding of lower urinary tract dysfunction remains elusive and contributes to the limitations of testing.

INTRODUCTION

Much has been published regarding when and if multichannel urodynamic studies (UDS) should be done in the settings of female urinary incontinence and pelvic organ prolapse. Controversy exists over whether routine urodynamic testing in this context renders a net patient benefit. The net benefit of a test is the product of several variables related to the test and the condition it seeks to identify. These variables include the following: (1) the test's pretest and posttest probabilities in predicting a given condition; (2) the rate probability differences for the condition change recommended treatment interventions; (3) the difference between the benefits and harms of treatment; and (4) the potential harm caused by a test. These variables have all, to varying degrees, been addressed for UDS testing. In what follows, these factors are considered stepwise hoping to arrive at some conclusions regarding the net *patient* benefit of *routine* UDS in the settings of female urinary incontinence and pelvic organ prolapse. How physicians benefit from UDS testing will also be considered because this too can influence how the medical community regards the utility of a test.

Predicting Disease Probability?

Several organizations have tempered their enthusiasm for routine UDS testing. As early as 1996, the former Agency for Health Care Policy and Research (now called the Agency for Healthcare Research and Quality) proposed that some women did not need UDS testing before surgical treatment.[1] In 2006, the British National Institute for Health and Clinical Excellence (NICE) discouraged UDS testing before any conservative therapy and stated that, in select populations, this testing was not routinely recommended before stress incontinence surgery.[2] In

Department of Obstetrics and Gynecology, Division of Female Pelvic Medicine and Reconstructive Surgery, Dartmouth Medical School, Dartmouth-Hitchcock Medical Center, One Medical Center Drive, Lebanon, NH 03756, USA
E-mail address: James.L.Whiteside@Hitchcock.org

Urol Clin N Am 39 (2012) 257–263
http://dx.doi.org/10.1016/j.ucl.2012.06.001
0094-0143/12/$ – see front matter © 2012 Elsevier Inc. All rights reserved.

2005 and reaffirmed in 2011, the American College of Obstetrician Gynecologist practice bulletin on urinary incontinence in women stated: "limited data support the need for cystometric testing in the routine or basic evaluation of urinary incontinence."[3] Most recently, the Cochrane Collaboration summary on UDS testing for the management of urinary incontinence in children and adults concluded that although testing may change clinical decision making, there is insufficient evidence to show that the outcomes of these decisions render better clinical outcomes.[4] These summary conclusions reflect the diagnostic and therapeutic challenges of managing female lower urinary tract disease.

The precise causes of the various forms of lower urinary tract dysfunction are not clearly understood; correspondingly, the diagnostic criteria of lower urinary tract diseases are many times fuzzy. For example, female stress urinary incontinence could be regarded as one area of success both in our understanding of pathophysiology and in our directed treatments. Yet it remains unclear whether female stress urinary incontinence stems from a lack of anatomic support or of intrinsic urethral function; conceivably, a sling may work by providing a backboard or by correcting neuromuscular function.[5] This sort of fundamental lack of understanding compounds across the translational spectrum from theory to clinical practice. The International Continence Society (ICS) posits on expert opinion that the role of UDS testing is to reproduce the lower urinary tract symptom in controlled conditions so that the cause of the symptom can be determined and objective information rendered to the clinician.[6] Echoing the conclusions of the Cochrane Collaboration, objective information may, indeed, be rendered with UDS testing but it is not clear that this information improves clinical outcomes. Furthermore, given the aforementioned problem of the compounding error that begins with our incomplete understanding of lower urinary tract diseases, the hope that patients' symptoms could be reproduced with UDS testing is illusory.

Test characteristics are often described in terms of accuracy and precision. The distinctions between these 2 concepts are well defined when discussing a game of darts but less so in respect to most medical contexts. Generally, an accurate test is better than a precise test because, in the former case, there is at least the possibility that what is measured reflects some reference. In defining a test's net benefit, that reference should point to some useful understanding of reality. A test with poor precision renders uncertainty that the result has approximated the reference; the

more uncertain, the less useful the test becomes. In the case of UDS testing, both accuracy and precision are problematic.

The ICS states that there is diagnostic agreement between different observers over urodynamic traces in about 80% of cases.[6] This finding is a misrepresentation of the study cited for that estimate. Logically and experimentally, the reliability and agreement of urodynamic interpretations vary with the diagnosis.[7] As expected, physician evaluators agree more often with themselves than with colleagues but, except for stress incontinence, the reliability and agreement estimates for urodynamic interpretations are moderate at best (at best 38% interobserver agreement for detrusor overactivity with incontinence).[7] The lack of clear quantitative referents leads to the precision problems identified for urodynamic interpretations. The lack of such referents only highlights the diagnostic problems of lower urinary tract diseases and, even if these referents existed, they may have no clinical value.

The accuracy of UDS testing is unknowable. Should estimates of lower urinary tract function rely on the results of UDS testing or the patient's symptoms? Patient history in predicting urodynamic findings is variable. Patient history has a positive predictive value of identifying urodynamic stress incontinence that ranges between 52% and 100%. Still, detrusor overactivity (DO) is identified in 11% to 16% of women with pure stress incontinence symptoms.[8] Conversely, 22% of women with urgency symptoms are found to have urodynamic stress incontinence.[9] Symptoms may suggest some urodynamic findings but clearly not all and not all the time. Overall, the correlation between the clinical and urodynamic diagnosis in classifying urinary incontinence diagnoses is poor, and to assume the urodynamic observations are the referent standard is unwise based on the current evidence.[10]

Pelvic floor problems are contextualized diseases and decision making by patients and physicians is never exclusively summarized by symptom inventory or testing results. This feature alone should give pause to any practice of routine urodynamic testing. The patients' therapeutic goal should drive the ascertainment of diagnostic information. The focus on how UDS testing impacts clinical outcomes is the subject of at least 2 forthcoming randomized trials: the Value of Urodynamics prior to Stress Incontinence Surgery (VUSIS)[11] and Value of Urodynamic Evaluation (ValUE)[12] trials. The results of the Stress Incontinence Surgical Treatment Efficacy Trial (SISTEr trial) in comparing the efficacy of the Burch urethropexy and pubovaginal sling did not demonstrate that urodynamic testing predicted the treatment outcome or postoperative voiding dysfunction.[13,14] Yet women with Valsalva leak point pressures or maximum urethral closure pressures in the lowest quartile were nearly 2-fold likely to experience recurrent urine leakage 1 year after an obturator or retropubic midurethral sling.[15] This sort of prognostic information poses a metaphysical problem. Assuming these findings are reproducible in routine clinical practice, how much is prognosis worth? This sort of question cannot be answered without engaging patients.

In the case of pelvic organ prolapse, UDS testing is hoped to clarify who might have lower urinary tract dysfunction following repair. Pelvic organ prolapse does impact lower urinary tract function, yet it is unclear that UDS testing adds much additional diagnostic or prognostic information. The Colpopexy and Urinary Reduction trial (CARE trial) showed that urine leakage with preoperative prolapse reduction, although variable with technique, predicted a higher risk for postoperative stress incontinence at 3 months; yet this same trial recommended prophylactic incontinence surgery in all women undergoing a sacrocolpopexy.[16] Following this logic, a woman's preoperative continence could be seen as having no diagnostic value in the choice to perform a concurrent incontinence procedure. Indeed, the mean risk of developing postoperative stress incontinence following the surgical repair of vaginal prolapse is around 15% regardless of the preoperative clinical symptoms if a concurrent incontinence procedure is performed.[17] That mean risk jumps to between 59% and 65% without concurrent incontinence surgery in the settings of either positive occult testing in a woman without clinical symptoms of stress incontinence or positive clinical symptoms.[17] Reduction testing to identify occult incontinence is not an effective method to guide surgeon decision making.[17] The use of urodynamic testing with occult testing does not seem to improve on clinical judgment. The decision to perform an incontinence surgery concurrent with any repair of vaginal prolapse is largely without evidenced guidance and, as such, patient choice should prevail.

Common Treatments for Different Problems?

When 2 or more diseases possess the same treatment, the value of any testing that makes these distinctions is dubious. Conservative treatments such as physical therapy, behavior modification, medications, or pessary, can address a variety of lower urinary tract symptoms. For interested patients, these options could be pursued without a precise diagnosis, and the results of any therapeutic trial may render diagnostic information

more useful than that discoverable from UDS testing. There are, however, other settings whereby the information gathered from UDS testing makes distinctions without differences. The distinction between types I and II stress urinary incontinence and type III has been based on the urodynamic measure of Valsalva leak point pressure. For years, this distinction drove differential stress incontinence treatment: a Burch urethropexy for types I and II and a pubovaginal sling for type III. The SISTEr trial did not confirm the utility of this distinction.

Digesu and colleagues[18] conducted a large study of 4500 women with symptoms suggestive of overactive bladder (OAB). A postvoid residual urine of more than 100 mL was identified in 8% of women.[18] A third of the patients had DO on UDS testing, with only 28% having OAB symptoms.[18] The investigators argued that without UDS testing, some women could have been treated with anticholinergic medications and made worse and other asymptomatic women would have been denied treatment. An opposite conclusion seems equally reasonable. Besides documenting the poor correlation between DO and OAB, to initiate anticholinergic medications only on urodynamic evidence of DO delays care and denies many symptomatic women of a medication they may find helpful. Hashim and Abrams'[19] study of patients with OAB found 30% of women with no OAB symptoms had DO on testing. In women with OAB symptoms and no DO, it is unknowable if the test or the diagnosis failed. Treatment considerations, however, necessarily prioritize the symptom, thus, undermining the value of UDS testing. For urinary urgency and frequency, the distinction between OAB and DO does not seem to render a rational difference in the treatment approach.

Per the most recent Cochrane Collaboration review, clinical decision making may be altered by UDS testing, but clinical outcomes do not seem to be altered.[4] Specifically, there is no difference in the number of women with posttreatment urinary incontinence if they did or did not undergo pretreatment UDS testing.[4] The rate at which probability differences in UDS diagnoses will result in meaningful changes in intervention seems to be low and, correspondingly, factors negatively in rendering a positive net patient benefit to routine UDS testing.

Benefit versus Harm of Treatments?

The benefit of treatment in the context of lower urinary tract dysfunction is the restoration of normal bladder function. This restoration would include painless urine storage and efficient and painless voiding. The physical harm of any treatment would threaten one of these basic functions.

There are, however, nonphysical harms in treatment, such as inconvenience or financial cost. Harm is any cost that subtracts from the benefit of an action (eg, treatment), and the first law of thermodynamics tells us that no action is without some cost. There is a probability range for the possible costs associated with a given action. A risk is ordinarily understood as a cost with low probability but that can subtract more greatly from the actions benefits. Patients can best balance nonphysical costs because the factors that influence them are often unknown to the clinician. Physical costs of treatment, however, are often well known by clinicians, yet their relative valuation by patients still remains unknown and perhaps unknowable. Taken together, with respect to the matter of any testing, if the net treatment costs exceeds benefits, then the value of testing is undermined.

Physical-therapy treatments for lower urinary tract dysfunctions possess little cost beyond financial cost and inconvenience. Over the long run, these nonphysical costs can be significant enough to lead to discontinuation,[20] hence, the long-term net benefit seems to be low for many women. Medical treatments for urinary incontinence have variable effects on lower urinary tract dysfunction; although the benefits may be meager,[3] the physical costs by way of side effects are common. These side effects include dry mouth, constipation, and dizziness, among others. Although some individual responses may tilt toward net treatment benefit, for many women, medications taken to treat lower urinary tract dysfunction seem to be a wash, with nearly 60% discontinuing the medications at 6 months.[21] The financial costs of anticholinergic medications can be an important barrier to continued use and age impacts the severity of side effects. A small net treatment benefit potentially compromises the net benefit of testing if other factors dominate, such as the harms of testing. Given that the patient valuation of benefits from nonsurgical therapies are difficult to estimate, routine UDS testing before such therapies seems unwise.

Surgical interventions for lower urinary tract dysfunction face the same challenges in restoring lower urinary tract dysfunction. The harms of surgical treatment could be understood in terms of immediate operative and postoperative complications as well as longer-term problems. Operative complications include injury to the lower urinary tract, hemorrhage, bowel injury, wound complications, and infection. Postoperative complications include voiding problems, voiding urgency, altered bladder sensation, and altered sexual function among others. As has been already noted earlier,

bladder problems are contextualized diseases. Environmental buffers and barriers alter how a given lower urinary tract problem manifests in the life of an individual. For example, postsurgical alterations in sexual function may not be an adverse effect in a nun. Although long-term results (>4 years) of any incontinence surgery are often reported to be greater than 80%, the SISTEr trial documents an alternative reality. The Kaplan-Meier curves for the success of surgical treatment of urinary incontinence never plateau, with the 2-year outcomes for the 2 surgical approaches around 50%.[22] In this same trial, patient satisfaction from surgery was generally high (73%), but the only baseline predictor of lower satisfaction was greater-urge incontinence symptoms.[23] Given that patients undergoing stress incontinence surgery expect not only the resolution of urine leakage but also urgency and frequency symptoms[24] and given that these symptoms are among those that baseline predict postsurgery dissatisfaction, what role does UDS testing have in clarifying the presurgery net treatment benefit? What is in view here is trying to understand the net benefit of surgery in treating urinary incontinence; there are, indeed, objective and subjective outcomes that document patient benefit but there are also various personalized costs. In neither case are these benefits or costs necessarily clarified by UDS testing.

What about sacral nerve stimulation? Following the recommended basic assessment of any woman presenting with lower urinary tract complaints, a diary of bladder function will have been obtained. That diary documents, at a minimum, the criteria used to judge the efficacy of sacral nerve testing. As has already been stated earlier, there is a disconnection between OAB symptoms and DO, yet for obvious reasons, the OAB symptom is the priority in treatment decisions. Given that office sacral nerve testing is a feasible strategy for testing this therapy option, there is the potential for significant net treatment benefit. For appropriate patients, why add the costs of UDS testing?

What about pelvic organ prolapse surgery? As has already been mentioned, the role of UDS testing in the setting of pending pelvic organ prolapse surgery repair is unclear. Barrier testing may have some predictive role in elucidating which patients will leak following vaginal prolapse repair but this does not require UDS testing. Predicting voiding problems following vaginal prolapse surgery is hampered by the lack of poor definitional referents and the multiple overlapping factors that contribute to voiding problems in this population (eg, medications, age, infection, and so forth). Taken together, there are benefits to surgical and nonsurgical treatments of vaginal prolapse but there are also costs and UDS testing does little to clarify either.

The Harm of Testing?

There is little patient risk in undergoing multi-channel urodynamic testing. One randomized double-blind study of antibiotic prophylaxis following UDS showed a 23% infection rate among controls.[25] This rate was not significantly less with antibiotic prophylaxis (18%); however, both rates seem higher than common experience.[25] A systematic review on this topic, although citing poor study methodology among the 8 trials reviewed, reported that 13 individuals would need antibiotic prophylaxis to prevent 1 significant bacteriuria of unknown clinical significance.[26] Beyond infection risk, there are patient discomforts associated with the test, yet one study found 81% of women would repeat UDS testing.[27] This Asian survey study of men and women undergoing UDS testing showed that among pain, physical burden, and embarrassment, all were rated low. Embarrassment rated highest, although a male clinician performing the testing among female patients may have biased this outcome.[27] These subjective ratings may also vary between cultures. Nevertheless, the risk of infection and the reported subjective pain and embarrassment of UDS testing seems to be low.

Although the immediate individual harms of UDS testing seem to be low, there are other contexts to understand the harm of testing. Testing could alter clinical decision making away from the best therapy whereby best could be defined not only in terms of clinical outcomes but the costs to achieve a given clinical outcome. Testing also carries costs to the health care system. Within the British National Health System, the financial resources devoted to health care are fixed, meaning that any money spent on one health expense takes it from others. Within such a system, the net societal benefit determines how health resources are used. Understandably, reducing any testing without a clear benefit is imperative in these systems. The NICE position on UDS testing reflects this thinking. Although such a system has not arrived on US shores, it is clear that the era of limitless health spending is drawing to an end. The interest in capitated health care financing will put powerful pressures on any testing that does not render a clear benefit in clinical decision making.

The Physician Benefit

Never do surgery on an unstudied bladder. So goes the refrain heard among physicians who insist on performing urodynamic testing in all women seen for a pelvic floor disorder. When asked about the diagnostic yield of such testing, the refrain is repeated, which suggests that obeisance to authorities as much as anything else compels testing. There is also the sense that the performance of UDS is self-actualizing to a clinician's subspecialty medical focus that may render a referral benefit. It should also not go unnoticed that there are powerful financial reasons to do urodynamic testing. Medicare reimbursement for multichannel urodynamic testing can exceed $1000 and private insurers would be expected to reimburse much more than that amount. For comparison, Medicare professional reimbursement for an office cystoscopy is less than $200. It would be profoundly naïve to think that financial incentives do not influence how physicians think about urodynamic testing.

There are efficiency considerations for performing UDS testing. For example, Nager and Jasmine[17] note in surgical planning to correct vaginal prolapse, clinical or urodynamic testing can be done to detect occult urinary incontinence. Clinical testing would seem easier for most patients and physicians, yet it is conceivable that UDS testing may offer the most efficient way to identify the relevant information necessary to make a clinical decision acknowledging that in many cases that decision will be no better than had it been made without the results of UDS testing.

It is useful to distinguish between puzzles and mysteries. Mysteries are not clarified with more information, whereas puzzles are only solved with it. For example, Malcolm Gladwell thinks the Enron debacle was a mystery; the trouble was not because Enron's management did not reveal enough information but rather it was that analysts failed to make sense of the data that were supplied.[28] Judgment is needed to navigate a mystery because additional information may only make things less clear. Female bladder dysfunction is a mystery. What medical progress has meant for the problem of female bladder dysfunction (and for many other settings in medicine) is the transformation of a puzzle into a mystery. Although in the past UDS testing may have rendered information that quickly resolved a puzzle, today, amidst all that we know (and do not know) about bladder dysfunction and its management, judgment is what is most needed by patients and clinicians. Knowledge of patients' therapeutic goals, a careful history and physical examination, simple office testing, and awareness of what the individual surgeon can and cannot deliver renders sufficient data to base good judgment in many cases of female lower urinary tract dysfunction.

SUMMARY

No organization has called for completely abandon-
ing UDS testing. At the same time, increasingly
organizations and academics are hesitant to
endorse routine UDS testing in women presenting
with lower urinary tract dysfunction. The mollifica-
tion of historic enthusiasm to performed UDS
testing is largely based on growing evidence that it
renders little additional information over basic office
assessment. The decision to pursue conservative
therapy or even in some settings when surgery
might be appropriate, is not significantly altered by
the information gathered from UDS testing.

Despite an abundance of articles touching on
the questions surrounding UDS testing, few are
of good quality. What has been presented so far
has been admittedly slanted against UDS testing,
but then the aim of this presentation was to
dissuade routine use. Clearly, there are medical
conditions that can impact bladder function (eg,
diabetes, multiple sclerosis, stroke, and so forth)
whereby UDS could inform surgical and medical
care. Judgment will find such settings whereby
UDS testing will render a net patient benefit, yet
for the careful observer, these settings may
become increasingly uncommon. The approach
taken in this discussion has been to consider those
variables that impact the calculus of determining
the net patient benefit of a medical test. These
variables are not static; each changes with patient
and clinician potentially altering the equation. It is
again a call for judgment to carefully consider
each of these variables in trying to make sense
of UDS in women with urinary incontinence and
pelvic organ prolapse.

EDITOR'S COMMENTS

The role of urodynamics in pelvic reconstruction (and the management of prolapse and urinary incontinence) is again undergoing serious discussion and re-consideration. There is evidence to suggest that
urodynamics is not beneficial in women with pure stress urinary incontinence and that there is little
outcome predictive value of this testing modality in this circumstance. However it remains, at the
current time, the choice of the individual surgeon as to the importance of performing urodynamics
in the previously un-operated patient with subjective symptomatic pure stress urinary incontinence.
Less debatable is the role of urodynamics in patients who require repeat surgery or who have developed
de novo symptoms after surgical intervention. Urodynamics remains the only method that currently
exists to evaluate bladder storage pressures and the appropriateness of bladder evacuation in a dynamic
way (as opposed to post void residual volume which is a static and poorly reproducibly measure). Urodynamics also provides critical information regarding bladder sensory function and offers predictive
capabilities in the management of the neurogenic patient who may have high storage pressures or
high pressures related to detrusor overactivity. Additionally, the addition of fluoroscopy to urodynamics
provides a method with which bladder storage criteria can be linked to vesico-ureteral function and may
provide early prediction of impending functional renal compromise. Both of the editors use urodynamics as a critical aspect of their reconstructive practice for purposes of defining patient baseline symptoms
in an objective way and also for purposes of counseling when urodynamic abnormalities are identified.

Roger R. Dmochowski, MD
Mickey Karram, MD

REFERENCES

1. Fantl JA, Newman DK, Colling J. Urinary incontinence in adults: acute and chronic management,
in AHCPR clinical practice guidelines, No. 2. U.S.
Department of Health and Human Services, Agency
for Health Care Policy and Research; 1996.
2. NICE. Urinary incontinence. The management of
urinary incontinence in women. UK: National Institute of Clinical Excellence; 2006.
3. Urinary incontinence in women. ACOG practice
bulletin; no. 63. Washington, DC: American College of
Obstetricians and Gynecologists (ACOG); 2005.
4. Glazener CM, Lapitan MC. Urodynamic studies for
management of urinary incontinence in children
and adults. Cochrane Database Syst Rev 2012;1:
CD003195.
5. Chai TC. Coining a new term-Urovesicology:
advancing towards a mechanistic understanding
of bladder symptoms. Transl Androl Urol 2012;1:50–7.
6. Hosker G, Rosier P, Gajewski J, et al. Committee 6:
dynamic Testing. In: Abrams P, Cardozo L, Khoury S,
et al, editors. Incontinence. Paris: Health Publications
Ltd; 2009. p. 413. Available at: http://www.icsoffice.
org/Publications/ICI_4/files-book/Comite-6.pdf. Accessed June 6, 2012.
7. Whiteside JL, Hijaz A, Imrey PB, et al. Reliability and
agreement of urodynamics interpretations in a female
pelvic medicine center. Obstet Gynecol 2006;108(2):
315–23.
8. James M, Jackson S, Shepherd A, et al. Pure stress
leakage symptomatology: is it safe to discount detrusor instability? Br J Obstet Gynaecol 1999;
106(12):1255–8.

9. Jarvis GJ, Hall S, Stamp S, et al. An assessment of urodynamic examination in incontinent women. Br J Obstet Gynaecol 1980;87(10):893–6.

10. van Leijsen SA, Hoogstad-van Evert JS, Mol BW, et al. The correlation between clinical and urodynamic diagnosis in classifying the type of urinary incontinence in women. A systematic review of the literature. Neurourol Urodyn 2011;30(4):495–502.

11. van Leijsen SA, Kluivers KB, Mol BW, et al. Protocol for the value of urodynamics prior to stress incontinence surgery (VUSIS) study: a multicenter randomized controlled trial to assess the cost effectiveness of urodynamics in women with symptoms of stress urinary incontinence in whom surgical treatment is considered. BMC Womens Health 2009;9:22.

12. Nager CW, Brubaker L, Daneshgari F, et al. Design of the value of urodynamic evaluation (value) trial: a non-inferiority randomized trial of preoperative urodynamic investigations. Contemp Clin Trials 2009; 30(6):531–9.

13. Nager CW, FitzGerald M, Kraus SR, et al. Urodynamic measures do not predict stress continence outcomes after surgery for stress urinary incontinence in selected women. J Urol 2008;179(4):1470–4.

14. Lemack GE, Krauss S, Litman H, et al. Normal preoperative urodynamic testing does not predict voiding dysfunction after Burch colposuspension versus pubovaginal sling. J Urol 2008;180(5):2076–80.

15. Nager CW, Sirls L, Litman HJ, et al. Baseline urodynamic predictors of treatment failure 1 year after mid urethral sling surgery. J Urol 2011;186(2):597–603.

16. Visco AG, Brubaker L, Nygaard I, et al. The role of preoperative urodynamic testing in stress-continent women undergoing sacrocolpopexy: the Colpopexy and Urinary Reduction Efforts (CARE) randomized surgical trial. Int Urogynecol J Pelvic Floor Dysfunct 2008;19(5):607–14.

17. Nager CW, Jasmine TK. Pelvic organ prolapse and stress urinary incontinence in women: combined surgical treatment. In: Brubaker L, editor. UpToDate. Waltham (MA): UpToDate; 2012. Available at: http://www.uptodate.com/contents/pelvic-organ-prolapse-and-stress-urinary-incontinence-in-women-combined-surgical-treatment. Accessed June 6, 2012.

18. Digesu GA, Khullar V, Cardozo L, et al. Overactive bladder symptoms: do we need urodynamics? Neurourol Urodyn 2003;22(2):105–8.

19. Hashim H, Abrams P. Is the bladder a reliable witness for predicting detrusor overactivity? J Urol 2006;175(1):191–4 [discussion: 194–5].

20. Borello-France D, Burgio KL, Goode PS, et al. Adherence to behavioral interventions for urge incontinence when combined with drug therapy: adherence rates, barriers, and predictors. Phys Ther 2010;90(10):1493–505.

21. Gopal M, Haynes K, Bellamy SL, et al. Discontinuation rates of anticholinergic medications used for the treatment of lower urinary tract symptoms. Obstet Gynecol 2008;112(6):1311–8.

22. Albo ME, Richter HE, Brubaker L, et al. Burch colposuspension versus fascial sling to reduce urinary stress incontinence. N Engl J Med 2007;356(21): 2143–55.

23. Burgio KL, Brubaker L, Richter HE, et al. Patient satisfaction with stress incontinence surgery. Neurourol Urodyn 2010;29(8):1403–9.

24. Mallett VT, Brubaker L, Stoddard AM, et al. The expectations of patients who undergo surgery for stress incontinence. Am J Obstet Gynecol 2008; 198(3):308.e1–6.

25. Siracusano S, Knez R, Tiberio A, et al. The usefulness of antibiotic prophylaxis in invasive urodynamics in postmenopausal female subjects. Int Urogynecol J Pelvic Floor Dysfunct 2008;19(7):939–42.

26. Latthe PM, Foon R, Toozs-Hobson P. Prophylactic antibiotics in urodynamics: a systematic review of effectiveness and safety. Neurourol Urodyn 2008; 27(3):167–73.

27. Yokoyama T, Nozaki K, Nose H, et al. Tolerability and morbidity of urodynamic testing: a questionnaire-based study. Urology 2005;66(1):74–6.

28. Gladwell M. Open secret: Enron, intelligence, and the perils of too much information. New York: New Yorker; 2007.

Urodynamics
Role in Incontinence and Prolapse: A Urology Perspective

Benjamin E. Dillon, MD, Dominic Lee, MD,
Gary E. Lemack, MD*

KEYWORDS

- Urodynamics • Pelvic organ prolapse • Stress urinary incontinence • Burch colposuspension

KEY POINTS

- Parameters to assess urethral dysfunction have been disappointing.
- It appears to be the consensus that UDS is not necessary in all cases of uncomplicated SUI.
- UDS can be beneficial in unmasking SUI in patients presenting with prolapse.
- UDS should be used judiciously with a clear understanding as to why the test is being performed.

INTRODUCTION

Changes in pelvic floor as well as urethral anatomy and function occur with aging, which can result in prolapse and urinary incontinence. With more than 10,000 baby boomers turning 65 each day for the next 18 years, our health care system will be flooded with women presenting with pelvic floor prolapse and incontinence for years to come.[1] Rates of incontinence and pelvic organ prolapse (POP) in women of this age demographic is estimated to be 30% to 94%, and 1 in 8 women may require surgical repair for POP or incontinence by their eighth decade, with a reoperation rate of 30%.[2] Similarly, rates of stress urinary incontinence (SUI) range from 30% to 50% in the same age demographic.[3] Urinary incontinence is reported to alter the quality of life (QOL) in 15% to 35% of adult American women.[4,5] Aside from the socially debilitating impact incontinence has on patient's lives, it also comes at a significant cost to health care systems. Urinary incontinence is thought to be responsible for at least 12.4 billion dollars of health care spending with about 400 million dollars attributable to urodynamics (UDS), at a cost of approximately 1000 US dollars per

study.[5–7] For many, UDS has become part of the standard workup for a woman presenting with incontinence although it is often not clear that the information gleaned from the study will contribute to determining treatment options, assist in patient counseling, or help predict outcomes. This article reviews the role of UDS in the evaluation of urinary incontinence and POP.

HISTORICAL BACKGROUND

In 1999, as an initiative of the National Institute of Diabetes and Digestive and Kidney Diseases and the National Institute of Child Health and Human Development, the Urinary Incontinence Treatment Network (UITN) was formed. The UITN is a group of 9 independent sites comprising Urologists and Urogynecologists at each site with a single coordinating center. The primary task of the UITN was to develop trials to evaluate treatment of urinary incontinence in women, with the major focus being on surgical treatment. Emerging from the UITN were 3 level-I randomized controlled trials dedicated to the treatment of SUI; the SISTEr trial (Stress Incontinence Surgical Treatment Efficacy Trial), TOMUS (The Trial Of Mid-Urethral Slings),

Department of Urology, University of Texas Southwestern Medical Center, 5323 Harry Hines Boulevard, Dallas, TX 75390-9110, USA
* Corresponding author.
E-mail address: Gary.Lemack@utsouthwestern.edu

Urol Clin N Am 39 (2012) 265–272
http://dx.doi.org/10.1016/j.ucl.2012.05.001

and the ValUE (Value of Urodynamic Evaluation) trial. The primary aim of the SISTEr trial was to assess the efficacy of the Burch colposuspension (BC) compared with that of the pubovaginal sling (PVS), whereas TOMUS, designed as an equivalence study, compares the efficacy and safety of 2 minimally invasive midurethral slings: the retropubic transvaginal tape (RMUS) and the transobturator tape (TMUS). The ValUE trial was designed to examine the role of preoperative UDS in women undergoing anti-incontinence procedures. These trials are, today, among the most solid data available to urologists in the diagnosis and treatment of SUI and that is why their importance is stressed in this review although other critical articles in this arena are also equally emphasized.

THE ROLE OF UDS IN THE PREDICTION OF SUI SEVERITY

Aside from using history and clinical examination to determine the presence of SUI, clinicians rely heavily on UDS to help in not only determining the presence of SUI but also attempting to quantify its severity. Urethral dysfunction has been traditionally assessed with urethral pressure profile (UPP) (with maximal urethral closure pressure [MUCP] being the most common measure of UPP) and more recently by valsalva leak point pressure (VLPP). UPP may be a technically difficult parameter to measure consistently.[8,9] VLPP may be easier to measure clinically; however, there is a lack of standardization of the types of provocative maneuvers used and the timing of VLPP assessment. In addition to the acknowledged technical difficulties in performing VLPP and MUCP, there have been concerns regarding their reliability and correlation with symptom severity. VLPP has only modest correlations at best with several incontinence questionnaires and with voiding diaries.[10]

Data from the SISTEr trial indicated that VLPP did not correlate with several presumed (physical examination) indices of SUI severity, such as POP-Quantified stage, POP-Quantified Aa measurement, Qtip angle at rest and strain, and change in angle. Also, VLPP failed to correlate with UDS parameters (volume of first leakage, volume at first sensation, presence of detrusor overactivity [DO], maximum cystometric capacity [MCC], maximum flow rate [Q_{max}], and detrusor pressure at maximum flow rate [$pdet.Q_{max}$]).[11] However, lower VLPP was associated with higher Q_{max} suggesting that although VLPP does not measure symptom severity, it may accurately assess urethral function. In this same study, higher body mass index was associated with a higher VLPP, thereby suggesting that over time, more patients who are obese may have compensated by strengthening their pelvic floor.

The supine empty bladder stress test (SEBST), which indicates a low threshold for leakage in the supine position and with an empty bladder, was expected to correlate with more severe forms of incontinence, lower VLPP, and MUCP. In 2010, data from TOMUS demonstrated that VLPP and MUCP showed only a moderate correlation to each other ($r = 0.36$, $P<.001$), and little to no correlation to the SEBST.[12] Overall, the majority of the available data suggest that the ability of urodynamic urethral function tests to predict incontinence symptom severity must be questioned.

URODYNAMIC PREDICTORS OF SUI OUTCOME

MUCP and VLPP may not reliably predict SUI severity; however, their usefulness in predicting outcomes after treatment of SUI has been suggested for years. Historically, lower preoperative MUCP has been associated with higher failure rates, specifically when vaginal bladder neck suspensions or BC are performed.[13,14] However, in a prospective randomized trial comparing the results of a modified BC with PVS for the treatment of SUI in women with urethral hypermobility and low pressure urethra (MUCP <20 cm H_2O), Sand and colleagues[15] reported that MUCP does no affect the success of a PVS or modified BC, and overall, the 2 procedures had equivalent outcomes at 3 months. Similarly, MUCP testing was not found to predict treatment outcome in a randomized study of 60 women undergoing tension-free vaginal tape (TVT) or PVS procedures.[16]

There is conflicting data regarding the role of VLPP in predicting stress-specific success of incontinence procedures, be it a vaginal suspension, PVS, or synthetic midurethral slings (MUS). For example, Chaiken and colleagues[17] reported that VLPP findings were of little prognostic significance in predicting the surgical success of PVS (using VLPP to differentiate between intrinsic sphincteric deficiency [ISD] and urethral hypermobility). Rodriquez and colleagues[18] investigated the ability of VLPP to predict outcomes after a distal urethral sling procedure. The questionnaire-based outcomes revealed similar success, bother, and symptoms regardless of preoperative VLPP. Conversely, other studies have shown that women with very low VLPP (<60 cm H_2O) were less likely to have a successful outcome after a MUS procedure compared with those with higher VLPP.

In the SISTEr trial, the impact of the presence of urodynamic SUI and VLPP on surgical success was studied. Patients with urodynamic SUI (which represented about 89% of patients) were 2 times more likely to have overall success compared with those who did not; however, this difference did not reach statistical significance.[7] For both treatment groups (BC and PVS), there was no difference between mean VLPP values between surgical successes and failures, demonstrating that lower VLPP values did not portend worse overall outcomes.[7] This finding is in contrast to results from TOMUS in which patients with more severe urethral dysfunction, as determined by lower VLPP, were more likely to have treatment failure following either TMUS or RMUS.[19,20] Overall, women with a VLPP or MUCP in the lowest quartile were 2 fold more likely to have SUI 1 year after TMUS or RMUS procedures.[21]

Although both VLPP and MUCP did seem to be predictive of treatment success, their role in determining which MUS procedure to recommend was not clarified in TOMUS. Rechberger and colleagues[22] compared the efficacy of the RMUS with that of TMUS for SUI, specifically investigating the influence of preoperative VLPP on outcome. Using the Stamey incontinence questionnaire, the investigators reported that the efficacy of the 2 procedures is comparable; however, at 18 months, patients who have ISD, defined as a VLPP of up to 60 cm H_2O, fared better with an RMUS compared with a TMUS. Thus, although the role of urethral function testing remains somewhat speculative about determining which incontinence operation to recommend for SUI, credible available data suggest that patients with more severe sphincteric function seem to fare worse after MUS procedures.

Several investigators have studied the ability of pressure-flow studies (PFS) to predict the outcome after surgery for SUI. Wang and Chen[23] conducted a study on 79 women undergoing TVT for SUI and concluded that women with normal preoperative PFS were more likely to have better QOL and pad test results compared with those with abnormal PFS as determined by Q_{max} less than 12 mL/sec and pdet.Q_{max} of 20 cm H_2O or more. This finding is in contrast to the findings of the UITN in which, among 280 women with PFS before BC or PVS procedures, opening detrusor pressure, pdet.Q_{max}, and closing detrusor pressures had no impact on improvement in SUI after surgery.[24]

The presence of DO on preoperative UDS may affect surgical planning and preoperative counseling. Some investigators have reported that patients having both DO and SUI on preoperative UDS had a lower success rate (69% vs 97%) than those with only SUI following TVT.[25] In contrast, Duckett and Tamilselvi[26] also reported outcomes of patients undergoing TVT who had DO and SUI and found that both subjective and objective cure rates were similar to cure rates found in patients with SUI only. The investigators concluded that the presence of preoperative DO does not negatively affect efficacy. Similarly, in the SISTEr trial and TOMUS, baseline DO did not predict stress-specific treatment failure.[27,28] As with most aspects of the field, the definition of success varied greatly between studies, making comparisons between studies quite difficult. Although conflicting data exist, the majority of evidence seems to suggest that, regarding SUI outcomes, the presence of preoperative DO does not predict treatment failure.

UDS PREDICTORS OF RETENTION AND VOIDING DYSFUNCTION

One of the most disappointing outcomes of anti-incontinence procedures is the development of postoperative urinary retention and/or voiding dysfunction. Miller and associates[29] sought to predict patients who would develop urinary retention after PVS for SUI. They found that 19% of patients who voided without a detrusor contraction developed urinary retention, compared with 0% of those who had a contraction preoperatively. Of the 655 participants in the SISTEr trial, 57 participants (8 BC and 49 PVS) developed voiding dysfunction (defined as the need for surgical revision to facilitate bladder emptying or the use of any type of catheter after the 6-week visit), with 19 (all PVS) requiring surgical intervention. There were no preoperative UDS findings that were associated with an increased risk of voiding dysfunction. In particular, preoperative voiding pressures and degree of abdominal straining were not associated with postoperative voiding dysfunction.[30] Results from TOMUS showed a statistically significant difference in the development of voiding dysfunction between treatment groups at both the 12- and 24-month time points. At 12 months, patients who underwent RMUS procedure had a higher incidence of voiding dysfunction compared with those who underwent a TMUS procedure (2.7% vs 0%, $P = .004$). This disparity became even greater at 24 months with 3% of patients in the RMUS group reporting voiding dysfunction requiring surgical intervention compared with 0% of patients in the TMUS group ($P = .002$).[27,31] To date, no data have been published from TOMUS regarding preoperative UDS predictors of voiding dysfunction. Others have noted that patients with abnormal, preoperative noninvasive PFS (Q_{max} <15 mL/sec) and abnormal flow pattern can predict voiding dysfunction after TVT.[32]

URODYNAMIC PREDICTORS OF DE NOVO OR PERSISTENT URGE URINARY INCONTINENCE

Another disheartening outcome of anti-incontinence surgery is the development of urge de novo urinary incontinence. Panayi and colleagues[33] found that opening pressure may play a role in the development of postoperative DO after TVT. The investigators found that median preoperative opening detrusor pressure was higher in women who developed postoperative DO. Alperin and colleagues[34] studied clinical and UDS parameters of 200 women undergoing MUS procedure for treating SUI. In the final analysis, including 92 patients, 56% of patients with filling pdet greater than 15 cm H_2O (indicating abnormal compliance) developed de novo urge incontinence compared with 21% in patients whose pressure was lesser than 15 cm H_2O (odds ratio [OR] 4.6). The investigators concluded that preoperative UDS is necessary because it might identify those patients who have altered compliance and therefore, might be at increased risk of developing de novo urge incontinence after a MUS procedure. A secondary analysis from the SISTEr trial reported on the risk of urge urinary incontinence (UUI) after surgery for SUI. Overall, the presence of preoperative DO increased the odds of developing UUI. Specifically, patients with preoperative DO had an OR of 2.20 (P = .030) of developing symptoms of UUI and an OR of 2.41 (P = .008) of requiring treatment of those symptoms.[35] Duckett and Tamilselvi[26] reported that in patients undergoing TVT, an objective cure (as determined by cystometry) of DO was achieved in 47%, whereas a subjective cure of urgency symptoms was achieved in 63%, based on King's Quality of Life Questionnaire in women with MUI who underwent TVT.

URODYNAMIC CHANGES AFTER SUI SURGERY

A discussion of the role of UDS in SUI surgery would be incomplete without mentioning the UDS changes seen after SUI surgery. Although the exact mechanism by which anti-incontinence surgery works is still in question, the 2 leading theories are that urethral outlet resistance is increased[36] and/or the proximal urethra is displaced to a more intra-abdominal location optimizing the pressure transmission to the proximal urethra and bladder neck.[37] Recently, the UITN reported on the changes in UDS 2 years after the SISTEr trial. Both the BC and PVS procedures seemed to increase outlet resistance, with the PVS possibly being more obstructive in nature. Average flow rates decreased in both groups, with a greater decrease observed in the PVS group (2.4 mL/sec vs 3.8 mL/sec, P = .039). Furthermore, a significant increase of 11.4 cm H_2O in pdet.Q_{max} was seen after the sling procedure, whereas the BC group only saw an increase in 1.7 cm H_2O, a value which did not reach clinical significance.[38,39] In a companion paper, surgical success depended, to some extent on changes in UDS parameters. Patients successfully treated had a greater increase in pdet.Q_{max} (11.06 cm H_2O, P<.001) than those who failed (3.15 cm H_2O, P = .009).[38]

These findings were similar to prior studies that saw an increase in outlet resistance with both BC and PVS. Klutke and colleagues[36] used PFS as a measure of success 1 year after undergoing BC and found that in patients who had a successful outcome, a decrease in pdet.Q_{max} and Q_{max} was seen. A decrease in noninvasive flow rates have also been seen in patients undergoing PVS, in addition to elevated post-void residuals, an increase in pdet.Q_{max}, and decreased Q_{max}.[40,41]

More modest changes in UDS parameters are also seen after MUS. After MUS, average flow rate and Q_{max} were decreased at 12 months after procedure. Q_{max} for RMUS decreased from 22 mL/sec preoperatively to 20 mL/sec postoperatively (P<.005), whereas TMUS showed a similar reduction from 22 mL/sec to 19 mL/sec (P<.001). In addition, there was an increase in pdet.Q_{max}, from 18 to 21 cm H_2O (P = .01) for RMUS and 18 to 23 cm H_2O (P<.001) for TMUS.[31] Overall, UDS changes after MUS seem to vary with some studies reporting no change in pdet.Q_{max} after MUS, whereas others, such as TOMUS, showed a subtle increase in pdet.Q_{max}.[42,43]

THE ROLE OF UDS IN PROLAPSE

The role of UDS in assessing and predicting incontinence in women undergoing surgery for POP has been debated for years. Borstad and Rud[44] examined risk factors that may contribute to the development of SUI following surgery for POP. In a retrospective study of 102 women presenting for POP, 73 were continent before undergoing a Manchester procedure for POP, with UDS being performed both before and after surgery. Postoperative SUI developed in 22% of patients. When preoperative UDS parameters were investigated, women who developed SUI had lower mean closing pressure (53.3 vs 43.2 cm water P = .04).[44] Roovers and colleagues[45] published results from a retrospective study of 76 women undergoing vaginal prolapse (anterior colphorraphy and/or posterior colphorraphy, and/or vaginal hysterectomy) surgery, all of whom had UDS (without reduction) before procedure.

The investigators found that preoperative UDS, (specifically DO, urodynamic SUI, MCC, and MUCP) only poorly predicted postoperative SUI (likelihood ratio of 1.2).

Jha and colleagues[46] reported that preoperative UDS changed the surgical management at prolapse in a significant number of patients. In a retrospective study, the investigators examined 72 patients who underwent prolapse (anterior repair and/or vaginal hysterectomy) surgery. Sixty percent of the subjects had preoperative UDS (both with and without prolapse reduction), of which 53% demonstrated abnormal results with prolapse reduction. Pure urodynamic SUI was seen in 19% of patients, compared with 30% with DO, with or without urinary incontinence. The surgical management was altered in 7% (2 patients underwent TVT and 1 SPT for voiding dysfunction) of patients following preoperative UDS with prolapse reduction.

In 2008, the CARE (Colpopexy and Urinary Reduction Efforts) trial was published by the Pelvic Floor Dysfunction Network. One goal of the CARE trial was to assess the importance of prolapse reduction in predicting SUI following sacrocolpopexy. Preoperative UDS was performed with clinicians blinded to results. At the time of sacrocolpopexy, patients were randomized to BC or no BC group. The study ended early because the BC group had a significantly lower rate of SUI than the no BC group. In the trial, 5 different methods of reduction were used (Pessary, Manual, Swab, Forceps, and Speculum). SUI without prolapse reduction was uncommon, being seen in only 3.7% of women (all with advanced prolapse). Overall, there was a 19% incidence of urodynamic SUI with prolapse reduction, with speculum reduction having the highest incidence of SUI at 30% and pessary with the lowest rate at 6%. Furthermore, women who demonstrated SUI on prolapse reduction were more likely to report postoperative SUI at 3 months.[47]

Although prolapse reduction during UDS may be beneficial in predicting patients who will demonstrate SUI in the postoperative setting, reducing the prolapse at the time of the study has little bearing on most other UDS parameters. Mueller and colleagues[48] confirmed this in a study of 31 women with prolapse undergoing UDS. They examined MCC, voided volume, Q_{max}, pdet.Q_{max}, time to Q_{max}, and MUCP in the reduced and nonreduced states. The investigators did not find any significant difference in UDS parameters after prolapse reduction, with the exception of MUCP (58 vs 40 cm H_2O, $P = .001$).

Ballert and colleagues[49] examined the role of preoperative UDS in determining the need for MUS at the time of prolapse repair. One hundred and forty patients had UDS performed without prolapse reduction. If SUI was not documented, prolapse was reduced and UDS repeated with pessary reduction. Patients were then categorized as having urodynamic SUI (SUI without prolapse reduction), occult SUI (SUI only after prolapse reduction), or no SUI (with or without prolapse reduction). At the time of surgery, patients with either urodynamic SUI or occult SUI had MUS placed during prolapse repair. The investigators found that the risk of later intervention for SUI due to obstruction from MUS was similar to the risk of intervention in patients who developed SUI but did not demonstrate it on preoperative evaluation (8.5% vs 8.3%). Furthermore, the risk of intervention in patients who demonstrated clinical SUI only (no occult or UDS SUI) and did not receive MUS at the time of prolapse repair was 30%. The investigators concluded that based on their protocol, in patients who demonstrate clinical SUI (by report), UDS may not be necessary before undergoing surgery for POP.

Most recently, Elser and colleagues[50] reported on the use of preoperative UDS to determine the need for anti-incontinence procedure at the time of abdominal sacrocolpopexy. In a retrospective review, 463 patients were categorized into 2 groups. 204 (46.3%) women were categorized into group 1 (consisting of patients demonstrating any evidence of SUI on UDS, including occult SUI), with 122 (59.8%) overall having urodynamic SUI (with or without reduction) and 82 (40.2%) having occult SUI only. The remaining 53.7% (group 2) of patients did not have SUI. All patients who demonstrated preoperative SUI underwent MUS placement. At 6 weeks postoperatively, significantly more women from group 2 reported being dry compared with group 1 (92.8% vs 87.3%, $P = .049$). The investigators subsequently reported that preoperative UDS is valuable before surgery for POP. Specifically, in women who don't report SUI preoperatively, there is no benefit in performing a concomitant anti-incontinence procedure at time of sacrocolpopexy.

At present, the debate continues between those in favor of prophylactic SUI treatment at time of prolapse repair and others who worry about the potential risks of performing a surgical procedure that may never have been needed. For now, patient counseling remains essential to minimize postoperative dissatisfaction, with the precise role of urodynamic testing being unclear. The presence of urodynamic SUI suggests that a concomitant anti-incontinence procedure may be recommended, at the time of POP repair, although it can't be stated with certainty that UDS is indicated before any prolapse repair.

SUMMARY

Since its inception, UDS has evolved both technically and from an interpretation standpoint. Some of the initial parameters, such as MUCP and VLPP, used to assess urethral dysfunction and thereby the severity of SUI have produced disappointing results. However, MUCP and VLPP may help counsel patients before MUS, as these studies may help predict SUI outcomes after surgery. The evolving consensus is that UDS is not necessary in all cases of uncomplicated SUI.[51] Until more definitive studies are published about the use of UDS in women, it should be used judiciously, with a clear understanding as to why UDS is being performed and what clinically relevant information may be gleaned from it.

EDITOR'S COMMENTS

The role of urodynamics in pelvic reconstruction (and the management of prolapse and urinary incontinence) is again undergoing serious discussion and re-consideration. There is evidence to suggest that urodynamics is not beneficial in women with pure stress urinary incontinence and that there is little outcome predictive value of this testing modality in this circumstance. However it remains, at the current time, the choice of the individual surgeon as to the importance of performing urodynamics in the previously un-operated patient with subjective symptomatic pure stress urinary incontinence. Less debatable is the role of urodynamics in patients who require repeat surgery or who have developed de novo symptoms after surgical intervention. Urodynamics remains the only method that currently exists to evaluate bladder storage pressures and the appropriateness of bladder evacuation in a dynamic way (as opposed to post void residual volume which is a static and poorly reproducibly measure). Urodynamics also provides critical information regarding bladder sensory function and offers predictive capabilities in the management of the neurogenic patient who may have high storage pressures or high pressures related to detrusor overactivity. Additionally, the addition of fluoroscopy to urodynamics provides a method with which bladder storage criteria can be linked to vesico-ureteral function and may provide early prediction of impending functional renal compromise. Both of the editors use urodynamics as a critical aspect of their reconstructive practice for purposes of defining patient baseline symptoms in an objective way and also for purposes of counseling when urodynamic abnormalities are identified.

Roger R. Dmochowski, MD
Mickey Karram, MD

REFERENCES

1. In 2011 the baby boomers start to turn 65: 16 statistics about the coming retirement crisis that will drop your jaw. The American Dream. 2011 [online].
2. Olsen AL, Smith VJ, Bergstrom JO, et al. Epidemiology of surgically managed pelvic organ prolapse and urinary incontinence. Obstet Gynecol 1997; 89(4):501–6.
3. Lee J, Dwyer PL. Age-related trends in female stress urinary incontinence surgery in Australia–Medicare data for 1994–2009. Aust N Z J Obstet Gynaecol 2010;50:543.
4. Klutke C, Siegel S, Carlin B, et al. Urinary retention after tension-free vaginal tape procedure: incidence and treatment. Urology 2001;58:697.
5. Ward RM, Hampton BS, Blume JD, et al. The impact of multichannel urodynamics upon treatment recommendations for female urinary incontinence. Int Urogynecol J Pelvic Floor Dysfunct 2008;19:1235.
6. Nager CW, Brubaker L, Daneshgari F, et al. Design of the Value of Urodynamic Evaluation (ValUE) trial: a non-inferiority randomized trial of preoperative urodynamic investigations. Contemp Clin Trials 2009;30:531.
7. Nager CW, FitzGerald M, Kraus SR, et al. Urodynamic measures do not predict stress continence outcomes after surgery for stress urinary incontinence in selected women. J Urol 2008;179:1470.
8. Kuhn A, Nager CW, Hawkins E, et al. A comparative study of water perfusion catheters and microtip transducer catheters for urethral pressure measurements. Int Urogynecol J Pelvic Floor Dysfunct 2007; 18:931.
9. Weber AM. Is urethral pressure profilometry a useful diagnostic test for stress urinary incontinence? Obstet Gynecol Surv 2001;56:720.
10. Albo M, Wruck L, Baker J, et al. The relationships among measures of incontinence severity in women undergoing surgery for stress urinary incontinence. J Urol 2007;177:1810.
11. Lemack GE, Xu Y, Brubaker L, et al. Clinical and demographic factors associated with valsalva leak point pressure among women undergoing burch bladder neck suspension or autologous rectus fascial sling procedures. Neurourol Urodyn 2007; 26:392.
12. Nager CW, Kraus SR, Kenton K, et al. Urodynamics, the supine empty bladder stress test, and incontinence severity. Neurourol Urodyn 2010;29:1306.

13. Bergman A, Koonings PP, Ballard CA. Proposed management of low urethral pressure type of genuine stress urinary incontinence. Gynecol Obstet Invest 1989;27:155.

14. Koonings PP, Bergman A, Ballard CA. Low urethral pressure and stress urinary incontinence in women: risk factor for failed retropubic surgical procedure. Urology 1990;36:245.

15. Sand PK, Winkler H, Blackhurst DW, et al. A prospective randomized study comparing modified Burch retropubic urethropexy and suburethral sling for treatment of genuine stress incontinence with low-pressure urethra. Am J Obstet Gynecol 2000;182:30.

16. Wadie BS, El-Hefnawy AS. Urethral pressure measurement in stress incontinence: does it help? Int Urol Nephrol 2009;41:491.

17. Chaikin DC, Rosenthal J, Blaivas JG. Pubovaginal fascial sling for all types of stress urinary incontinence: long-term analysis. J Urol 1998;160:1312.

18. Rodriguez LV, de Almeida F, Dorey F, et al. Does valsalva leak point pressure predict outcome after the distal urethral polypropylene sling? Role of urodynamics in the sling era. J Urol 2004;172:210.

19. Barber MD, Kleeman S, Karram MM, et al. Risk factors associated with failure 1 year after retropubic or transobturator midurethral slings. Am J Obstet Gynecol 2008;199:666.e1.

20. Costantini E, Lazzeri M, Giannantoni A, et al. Preoperative MUCP and VLPP did not predict long-term (4-Year) outcome after transobturator mid-urethral sling. Urol Int 2009;83:392.

21. Nager CW, Sirls L, Litman HJ, et al. Baseline urodynamic predictors of treatment failure 1 year after mid urethral sling surgery. J Urol 2011;186:597.

22. Rechberger T, Futyma K, Jankiewicz K, et al. The clinical effectiveness of retropubic (IVS-02) and transobturator (IVS-04) midurethral slings: randomized trial. Eur Urol 2009;56:24.

23. Wang AC, Chen MC. The correlation between preoperative voiding mechanism and surgical outcome of the tension-free vaginal tape procedure, with reference to quality of life. BJU Int 2003;91:502.

24. Kirby AC, Nager CW, Litman HJ, et al. Preoperative voiding detrusor pressures do not predict stress incontinence surgery outcomes. Int Urogynecol J 2011;22:657.

25. Bunyavejchevin S. Can pre-operative urodynamic study predict the successful outcome of tension free vaginal tape (TVT) operation in Thai women with stress urinary incontinence? J Med Assoc Thai 2005;88:1493.

26. Duckett JR, Tamilselvi A. Effect of tension-free vaginal tape in women with a urodynamic diagnosis of idiopathic detrusor overactivity and stress incontinence. BJOG 2006;113:30.

27. Albo ME. The trial of mid-urethral slings (TOMUS): design and methodology. J Applied Res 2008;8:1.

28. Albo ME, Richter HE, Brubaker L, et al. Burch colposuspension versus fascial sling to reduce urinary stress incontinence. N Engl J Med 2007;356: 2143.

29. Miller EA, Amundsen CL, Toh KL, et al. Preoperative urodynamic evaluation may predict voiding dysfunction in women undergoing pubovaginal sling. J Urol 2003;169:2234.

30. Lemack GE, Krauss S, Litman H, et al. Normal preoperative urodynamic testing does not predict voiding dysfunction after Burch colposuspension versus pubovaginal sling. J Urol 2008;180:2076.

31. Kraus S. Urodynamic changes 12 months after retropubic and transobturator midurethral slings. In: AUA Annual Meeting Washington, DC, May, 2011.

32. Wang KH, Neimark M, Davila GW. Voiding dysfunction following TVT procedure. Int Urogynecol J Pelvic Floor Dysfunct 2002;13:353.

33. Panayi DC, Duckett J, Digesu GA, et al. Preoperative opening detrusor pressure is predictive of detrusor overactivity following TVT in patients with pre-operative mixed urinary incontinence. Neurourol Urodyn 2009;28:82.

34. Alperin M, Abrahams-Gessel S, Wakamatsu MM. Development of de novo urge incontinence in women post sling: the role of preoperative urodynamics in assessing the risk. Neurourol Urodyn 2008;27:407.

35. Kenton K, Richter H, Litman H, et al. Risk factors associated with urge incontinence after continence surgery. J Urol 2009;182:2805.

36. Klutke JJ, Klutke CG, Bergman J, et al. Urodynamics changes in voiding after anti-incontinence surgery: an insight into the mechanism of cure. Urology 1999;54:1003.

37. Belair G, Tessier J, Bertrand PE, et al. Retropubic cystourethropexy: is it an obstructive procedure? J Urol 1997;158:533.

38. Kraus SR, Lemack GE, Richter HE, et al. Changes in urodynamic measures two years after Burch colposuspension or autologous sling surgery. Urology 2011;78:1263.

39. Kraus SR, Lemack GE, Sirls LT, et al. Urodynamic changes associated with successful stress urinary incontinence surgery: is a little tension a good thing? Urology 2011;78:1257.

40. Fulford SC, Flynn R, Barrington J, et al. An assessment of the surgical outcome and urodynamic effects of the pubovaginal sling for stress incontinence and the associated urge syndrome. J Urol 1999;162:135.

41. Mitsui T, Tanaka H, Moriya K, et al. Clinical and urodynamic outcomes of pubovaginal sling procedure with autologous rectus fascia for stress urinary incontinence. Int J Urol 2007;14:1076.

42. Lukacz ES, Luber KM, Nager CW. The effects of the tension-free vaginal tape on voiding function:

a prospective evaluation. Int Urogynecol J Pelvic Floor Dysfunct 2004;15:32.

43. Sander P, Sorensen F, Lose G. Does the tension-free vaginal tape procedure (TVT) affect the voiding function over time? Pressure-flow studies 1 year and 3(1/2) years after TVT. Neurourol Urodyn 2007;26:995.

44. Borstad E, Rud T. The risk of developing urinary stress-incontinence after vaginal repair in continent women. A clinical and urodynamic follow-up study. Acta Obstet Gynecol Scand 1989;68:545.

45. Roovers JP, van Laar JO, Loffeld C, et al. Does urodynamic investigation improve outcome in patients undergoing prolapse surgery? Neurourol Urodyn 2007;26:170.

46. Jha S, Toozs-Hobson P, Parsons M, et al. Does preoperative urodynamics change the management of prolapse? J Obstet Gynaecol 2008;28:320.

47. Visco AG, Brubaker L, Nygaard I, et al. The role of preoperative urodynamic testing in stress-continent women undergoing sacrocolpopexy: the Colpopexy and Urinary Reduction Efforts (CARE) randomized surgical trial. Int Urogynecol J Pelvic Floor Dysfunct 2008;19:607.

48. Mueller ER, Kenton K, Mahajan S, et al. Urodynamic prolapse reduction alters urethral pressure but not filling or pressure flow parameters. J Urol 2007; 177:600.

49. Ballert KN, Biggs GY, Isenalumhe A Jr, et al. Managing the urethra at transvaginal pelvic organ prolapse repair: a urodynamic approach. J Urol 2009;181:679.

50. Elser DM, Moen MD, Stanford EJ, et al. Abdominal sacrocolpopexy and urinary incontinence: surgical planning based on urodynamics. Am J Obstet Gynecol 2010;202:375.e1.

51. Nager CW, Brubaker L, Litman HJ, et al. A randomized trial of urodynamic testing before stress-incontinence surgery. N Engl J Med 2012;366:1987.

Bulking Agents
A Urogynecology Perspective

Dani Zoorob, MD[a], Mickey Karram, MD[a,b],*

KEYWORDS

- Bulking agent • Contigen • Durasphere • Coaptite • Bulkamid

KEY POINTS

- Numerous bulking agents are currently FDA approved.
- Contigen (cross-linked bovine collagen) has been studied the most; however, recently its production has ceased.
- Lack of long-term durability continues to be the major reason bulking is rarely a first-line therapy in women who suffer from stress incontinence.

INTRODUCTION

A bulking agent is a material injected into the wall of the urethra to improve urethral coaptation in women suffering from stress incontinence. The concept was initially described in the 1930s when sodium morrhuate and paraffin[1] were used to augment urethral resistance. Sclerosing agents were also used for inducing permanent urethral scaring to improve urinary leakage. Eventually, collagen, Teflon, and autologous fat were found to be efficacious, and only collagen demonstrated proven safety and endured extensive testing, becoming the gold standard for injectable agents. Since then, multiple other products have been developed by industry, each with its particular success rates and complications.

Although the cause of stress incontinence remains unknown, the most accepted theory divides patients into 3 groups. Group 1 includes patients who have urethral mobility with an intact urethral sphincter. Historically, these patients are thought not to be good candidates for injection of a bulking agent because outcomes of suspension procedures or slings have been very good. Group 2 includes patients with a mobile urethra who are thought to have a deficient urethral sphincter and group 3 includes women who have a well-supported urethra with a deficient sphincter (intrinsic sphincter deficiency [ISD]). ISD was defined in 1992 as the damage to the urethral sphincteric system regardless of the cause.[2] The goal of using bulking agents is to maintain urethral coaptation during the storage phase and control during transient abdominal pressure variations while permitting voiding as needed.[3] Injecting a material into the proximal urethra provides bulk and mucosal resistance, resulting in resistance to passive urine flow.[4] Success with the use of bulking agents is reported to occur when the functional length of the urethra increases, which results in an increase in the efficiency of pressure transmission in the proximal quarter of the urethra. This process resists bladder neck opening during increases in intraabdominal pressure as would happen with stress urinary incontinence (SUI).[5] Klarskov reported that certain bulking agents actually increase the strength of the sphincter, possibly by increasing the volume of the muscle cell and thereby its ability to contract and generate power.[6]

INDICATIONS

Bulking agents are used to manage stress incontinence in women, with the main indication being ISD. This indication, however, includes the need for touchup or rescue urinary control after the patients with incontinence have had meager outcomes with alternative incontinence techniques such as slings. Other indications include the need

[a] Department of Obstetrics and Gynecology, Division of Female Pelvic Medicine and Reconstructive Surgery, The Christ Hospital/University of Cincinnati, 231 Albert Sabin Way, Cincinnati, OH 45267, USA; [b] The Christ Hospital, 2123 Auburn Avenue, Suite 307, Cincinnati, OH 45219, USA
* Corresponding author. The Christ Hospital, 2123 Auburn Avenue, Suite 307, Cincinnati, OH 45219.
E-mail address: Mickey.karram@thechristhospital.com

Urol Clin N Am 39 (2012) 273–277
http://dx.doi.org/10.1016/j.ucl.2012.06.012
0094-0143/12/$ – see front matter © 2012 Elsevier Inc. All rights reserved.

to operate under local or no anesthesia, such as in patients who are medically fragile or unstable. Being elderly with the inability to succumb to the postoperative discomfort and subsequent immobility is yet another indication. Because of the way urethral coaptation works, bulking may be used in patients who have poor bladder emptying with concurrent sphincter weakness. Other potential indications are in patients who are still interested in child bearing, patients whose anticoagulation cannot be reversed long enough to allow for alternative incontinence surgical management, and patients who refuse to undergo a more invasive surgical procedure such as a sling or suspension.

INJECTABLE AGENTS

The success of any material implanted refers to its efficacy over time while maintaining a low–side-effect profile.[3] Successful use of bulking agents depends on the nature of the material injected, ease of administration of the material, and the host milieu including integrity of the paraurethral tissue and fascia.[7] Material biocompatibility, including low host reactivity, low carcinogenesis potential, and low risk of migration, is also important. Historically, sodium morrhuate and paraffin as well as sclerosing agents were used with questionable outcomes. Autologous fat injections were also used, with poor outcomes and complication rates reaching 32%.[8] Teflon (polytetrafluoroethylene), marketed as Polytef (DuPont, USA), was also tested but was not approved by the Food and Drug Administration (FDA) because of particle migration. Two products with high potential were Tegress (CR Bard, Inc, Covington, GA, USA) and Deflux (Q-Med, Uppsala, Sweden). Deflux, made of dextranomer/hyaluronic acid, was proven to have high efficacy in vesicoureteral reflux, but trials did not prove its efficacy in the treatment of SUI. Deflux was also associated with the formation of sterile pseudoabscesses in 16% of the patients.[9] Tegress, also marketed as Uryx (Genyx Medical, Inc, Aliso Viejo, CA, USA), was made of a copolymer of ethylene vinyl alcohol, which was highly efficacious in the treatment of SUI, but urethral erosions (up to 37% of patients) precluded its use and was withdrawn from the market in 2006.[10,11] Contigen (CR Bard, Covington, GA, USA), made of glutaraldehyde cross-linked bovine collagen, has been studied the most and is used as a reference for testing newer agents. However, in 2011, its production ceased.

Zuidex (Q-Med AB, Uppsala, Sweden), made of hyaluronic acid with dextronomer, was highly effective in controlling reflux in the pediatric population but was withdrawn from the market because of high rates of erosion.[12]

These agents can be injected submucosally by either a transurethral or a periurethral technique. In the transurethral technique, the agent is injected under direct guidance using a needle introduced through the operative channel of a cystoscope. In the periurethral technique, the needle is introduced lateral to the urethral meatus and positioned submucosally. Administering a dye before injecting the bulking agent can help localize the tip of the needle. Schultz and colleagues[13] in a prospective randomized trial showed no difference in the long-term outcomes between the 2 techniques, although immediate postoperative urinary retention was slightly higher in the patients undergoing periurethral technique.

In 2008, Kuhn and colleagues[14] randomized 30 patients to either a midurethral or bladder neck injection site. The study showed no difference in outcomes, with slightly higher patient satisfaction in the midurethral group. In a similar study by Lightner and colleagues,[12] proximal injections of Contigen were associated with better outcomes (84% vs 65%) compared with midurethral injections of Zuidex. However, conclusions from this study are not possible because it compared different products at different injection sites.[12]

The following is a detailed discussion of the various bulking agents currently in use.

Durasphere

Durasphere (Boston Scientific, Natick, MA, USA) comprises zirconium beads (250–300 μm in diameter) suspended in a water-based carrier. Durasphere is considered inert and was approved by the FDA in 1999 for the treatment of incontinence in patients with ISD. The large bead size reduces migration, but a case report has revealed its migration into the lymphatics.[15] Durasphere is available in 1- or 3-mL prefilled syringes.

Implantation involves the use of a standard cytoscopic equipment and proprietary 18-gauge needle setup. Modifications of the basic needle exist, with one having a bent tip to facilitate localization and injection. Infrequent clogging of the needle and subsequent increased resistance have been reported, which resulted in the reformulation of the product (called Durasphere EXP) in 2006 to facilitate use.

In 2001, a multicenter RCT showed 80.3% improvement of 1 continence grade in the Durasphere group versus 69.1% in the collagen group.[16] In a study with extended follow-up, Chrouser and colleagues[17] showed that 33% and 21% of patients reported persistence of effective treatment after 24 and 36 months, respectively.

Complications in patients using this system were few. Periurethral mass formation has been reported in 2.9% of patients[18,19]; urethral prolapse (with Durasphere material in the prolapsed tissue) has also been reported.

Bulkamid

Bulkamid (Contura International, Soeborg, Denmark) is a nonresorbable polyacrylamide hydrogel made of cross-linked polyacrylamide and water. Bulkamid contains no solid particles (crystals or particulates), theoretically abolishing the risk of migration. Clinical trials are being conducted using Bulkamid in the United States. In Europe, it is marketed as Aquamid and has been used as a facial filler for many years in plastic reconstructive surgery.[20] Being a gel, it can be injected through the operative channel of a regular cystoscope using a special 23-gauge needle or the Bulkamid Urethral Bulking System—a specially designed endoscopic instrument that facilitates injection.

In 2006, a prospective study showed 38% of patients subjectively dry with an additional 43% reporting improvement. Objectively, 93% decrease in overall 24-hour leakage and 87% decrease in incontinence episodes were reported.[6] In 2010, another study by the same researcher showed subjective improvement in 60% of patients, with equal efficacy in SUI and mixed urinary incontinence groups over 12 months.[21] The study did report a reinjection rate of up to 35%. In 2012, a study which followed 135 women over 2 years showed good maintenance of the durability of success with 64% subjective cure rate at 2 years compared with 67% at 1 year.[22]

Coaptite

Coaptite (Boston Scientific, Natick, MA, USA) is made of 75- to 125-μm diameter calcium hydroxyapatite particles suspended in an aqueous gel. Hydroxyapatite is naturally found in teeth and bones of humans and usually well tolerated when injected. The FDA approved Coaptite as a bulking agent in 2005. The gel, carrying the particles, is designed to provide the initial postoperative bulking, but as it gets resorbed, it allows for tissue ingrowth around the calcium hydroxyapatite particles. Coaptite is radio-opaque and can be easily identified during imaging. A specialized 21-gauge needle with side-injecting or end-injecting capability is used for injecting Coaptite. The side-injecting needle is called the Sidekick needle. In a multicenter RCT, Mayer and colleagues[23] compared the efficacy of Coaptite with that of Contigen and reported an improvement on the Stamey incontinence scale in 63.4% and 57.0% of patients, respectively. Complications in the study were vaginal erosion

of the Coaptite and the subtrigonal placement. Similar to Durasphere, urethral prolapse has been reported with the use of Coaptite.[24]

Macroplastique

Macroplastique (Uroplasty Inc, Minneapolis, MN, USA) is a nonbiodegradable hydrogel containing a polydimethylsiloxane (silicone) elastomer suspended in a water-soluble gel[25] with the silicone particles measuring between 50 and 400 μm (25% of the particles <50 μm, which has raised concerns for migration).[26] Injection is done using a proprietary transurethral injection device called the Macroplastique Implantation Device (Uroplasty Inc, Minneapolis, MN, USA), which has a multi-channeled needle-positioning device with 3 needle entry points at the 2 and 10 o'clock positions allowing for 1.5-mL injections each and at the 6 o'clock position allowing for a 2.5-mL injection. Macroplastique may also be injected using a standard cystoscope through an 18-gauge Uroplasty rigid endoscopic needle.

In 2009, Ghoniem and colleagues[27] reported that 61.5% of patients treated with Macroplastique reported a significant clinical improvement and 36.9% reported a dry/cure effect compared with 48% and 24.8%, respectively, in the group treated with Contigen. This randomized study had a 12-month follow-up period, and the results were statistically significant. In 2010, Ghoniem and colleagues[28] reported a multicenter study with 24-month follow-up showing 84% of patients with sustained success at 12 months with 67% reporting a completely dry effect. Of those dry patients, 87% maintained cure at 24 months.

In 2005, Maher and colleagues[29] compared Macroplastique and pubovaginal slings and found that objective cure rates were significantly better with slings reaching 81%, but that symptomatic and subjective cure rates were similar between the 2 modalities. Follow-up at 62 months showed 62% and 21% continence success rates as well as 69% and 29% satisfaction rates for pubovaginal slings and Macroplastique, respectively.

Permacol

Permacol (Tissue Science Laboratories, Aldershot, UK) is a dermal implant made from nonreconstituted porcine dermal collagen. When implanted, it allows the ingrowth of new tissue, which can potentially be permanent.

In 2005, Bano and colleagues[30] compared the efficacy of Permacol and Macroplastique in a prospective cohort of patients and reported 64% and 46% improvement in Stamey incontinence stage, respectively. At 6 months postoperatively, only the results of the Permacol seemed to be sustained.

SUMMARY

Despite the many studies available, the Cochrane review published in 2012 reports insufficiency of data to provide a basis for practice citing a lack of well-designed RCTs that assess bulking agents.

At present, a lack of long-term durability of success with these agents continues to be the major reason bulking is rarely a first-line therapy in women who suffer from stress incontinence.

EDITOR'S COMMENTS

Bulking therapy continues to be an under-utilized component in the armamentarium for the management of stress urinary incontinence. As greater cost containment strategies enter into the algorithmic approach to the management of stress incontinence it would bear to reason that bulking may assume a greater role as an option for the management of stress urinary incontinence. Bulking therapy has historically been considered to be less effective than surgery, however, it is to be noted that published bulking trials were done under strict regulatory criteria, whereas, many of the historical surgery trials were done under less stringent criteria and therefore direct comparisons of efficacy rates are certainly problematic.

Critical to the success of bulking, is careful patient selection. Ideally, the patient should manifest hypermobility of the proximal urethra and bladder neck of less than 30 degrees. There should be evidence of adequate urethral mucosal blood supply and estrogen effect. Anatomic pathology such as urethral diverticula and intraurethral foreign body should also be excluded prior to the consideration of the option of bulking.

Also critical to the success of bulking is injection technique. It is absolutely crucial to avoid over injection (minimized volume and chose appropriate localization of bulking material (mid and proximal urethra). The goal of bulking is not to "coapt" the urethral mucosa but to obtain static increase in resistance in urethral outlet. Although not absolutely obstructive, the effect of bulking is presumed to be an augmentation effect which lends an element of resistance to a poorly functional urethral sphincter. The authors present their vision of their mutual approaches to bulking in a thorough and complete way and the interested pelvic reconstructionist is urged to consider this as a part of his/her armamentarium.

Roger R. Dmochowski, MD
Mickey Karram, MD

REFERENCES

1. Quackels R. Two cases of incontinence after adenomectomy cured by paraffin injection into the perineum. Acta Urol Belg 1955;23(3):259–62 [in French].

2. Agency for Health Care Policy and Research. U.S. Department of Health Care and Human Resources publication 92-0038. Rockville, MD: Agency for Health Care Policy and Research; 1996. Urinary incontinence in adults: clinical practice guidelines.

3. Kerr LA. Bulking agents in the treatment of stress urinary incontinence: history, outcomes, patient populations, and reimbursement profile. Rev Urol 2005; 7(Suppl 1):S3–11.

4. Smith DN, Appell RA, Winters JC, et al. Collagen injection therapy for female intrinsic sphincteric deficiency. J Urol 1997;157(4):1275–8.

5. Monga AK, Stanton SL. Urodynamics: prediction, outcome and analysis of mechanism for cure of stress incontinence by periurethral collagen. Br J Obstet Gynaecol 1997;104(2):158–62.

6. Klarskov N, Lose G. Urethral injection therapy: what is the mechanism of action? Neurourol Urodyn 2008; 27(8):789–92.

7. Appell RA, Dmochowski RR, Herschorn S. Urethral injections for female stress incontinence [review]. BJU Int 2006;98(Suppl 1):27–30 [discussion: 31].

8. Lee PE, Kung RC, Drutz HP. Periurethral autologous fat injection as treatment for female stress urinary incontinence: a randomized double-blind controlled trial. J Urol 2001;165(1):153–8.

9. Lightner DJ, Fox J, Klingele C. Cystoscopic injections of dextranomer hyaluronic acid into proximal urethra for urethral incompetence: efficacy and adverse outcomes. Urology 2010;75(6):1310–4.

10. Hurtado E, McCrery R, Appell R. The safety and efficacy of ethylene vinyl alcohol copolymer as an intraurethral bulking agent in women with intrinsic urethral deficiency. Int Urogynecol J Pelvic Floor Dysfunct 2007;18(8):869–73.

11. Hurtado EA, Appell RA. Complications of Tegress injections. Int Urogynecol J Pelvic Floor Dysfunct 2009;20(1):127 [author reply: 129].

12. Lightner D, Rovner E, Corcos J, et al. Zuidex Study Group. Randomized controlled multisite trial of injected bulking agents for women with intrinsic sphincter deficiency: mid-urethral injection of Zuidex via the Implacer

versus proximal urethral injection of Contigen cysto-scopically. Urology 2009;74(4):771–5.

13. Schulz JA, Nager CW, Stanton SL, et al. Bulking agents for stress urinary incontinence: short-term results and complications in a randomized comparison of periurethral and transurethral injections. Int Urogynecol J Pelvic Floor Dysfunct 2004;15(4): 261–5.

14. Kuhn A, Stadlmayr W, Lengsfeld D, et al. Where should bulking agents for female urodynamic stress incontinence be injected? Int Urogynecol J Pelvic Floor Dysfunct 2008;19(6):817–21.

15. Pannek J, Brands FH, Senge T. Particle migration after transurethral injection of carbon coated beads for stress urinary incontinence. J Urol 2001;166(4): 1350–3.

16. Lightner D, Calvosa C, Andersen R, et al. A new injectable bulking agent for treatment of stress urinary incontinence: results of a multicenter, randomized, controlled, double-blind study of Durasphere. Urology 2001;58(1):12–5.

17. Chrouser KL, Fick F, Goel A, et al. Carbon coated zirconium beads in beta-glucan gel and bovine glutaraldehyde cross-linked collagen injections for intrinsic sphincter deficiency: continence and satisfaction after extended followup. J Urol 2004;171(3): 1152–5.

18. Madjar S, Sharma AK, Waltzer WC, et al. Periurethral mass formations following bulking agent injection for the treatment of urinary incontinence. J Urol 2006; 175(4):1408–10.

19. Ghoniem GM, Khater U. Urethral prolapse after Durasphere injection. Int Urogynecol J Pelvic Floor Dysfunct 2006;17(3):297–8.

20. von Buelow S, Pallua N. Efficacy and safety of poly-acrylamide hydrogel for facial soft-tissue augmentation in a 2-year follow-up: a prospective multicenter study for evaluation of safety and aesthetic results in 101 patients. Plast Reconstr Surg 2006; 118(Suppl 3):85S–91S.

21. Lose G, Sørensen HC, Axelsen SM, et al. An open multicenter study of polyacrylamide hydrogel (Bulkamid®) for female stress and mixed urinary incontinence. Int Urogynecol J 2010;21(12):1471–7.

22. Toozs-Hobson P, Al-Singary W, Fynes M, et al. Two-year follow-up of an open-label multicenter study of polyacrylamide hydrogel (Bulkamid®) for female stress and stress-predominant mixed incontinence. Int Urogynecol J Pelvic Floor Dysfunct 2012, in press.

23. Mayer RD, Dmochowski RR, Appell RA, et al. Multicenter prospective randomized 52-week trial of calcium hydroxylapatite versus bovine dermal collagen for treatment of stress urinary incontinence. Urology 2007;69(5):876–80.

24. Palma PC, Riccetto CL, Martins MH, et al. Massive prolapse of the urethral mucosa following periurethral injection of calcium hydroxylapatite for stress urinary incontinence. Int Urogynecol J Pelvic Floor Dysfunct 2006;17(6):670–1.

25. Radley SC, Chapple CR, Lee JA. Transurethral implantation of silicone polymer for stress incontinence: evaluation of a porcine model and mechanism of action in vivo. BJU Int 2000;85(6):646–50.

26. Dmochowski R, Appell RA. Advancements in minimally invasive treatments for female stress urinary incontinence: radiofrequency and bulking agents [review]. Curr Urol Rep 2003;4(5):350–5.

27. Ghoniem G, Corcos J, Comiter C, et al. Cross-linked polydimethylsiloxane injection for female stress urinary incontinence: results of a multicenter, randomized, controlled, single-blind study. J Urol 2009;181(1):204–10.

28. Ghoniem G, Corcos J, Comiter C, et al. Durability of urethral bulking agent injection for female stress urinary incontinence: 2-year multicenter study results. J Urol 2010;183(4):1444–9.

29. Maher CF, O'Reilly BA, Dwyer PL, et al. Pubovaginal sling versus transurethral Macroplastique for stress urinary incontinence and intrinsic sphincter deficiency: a prospective randomised controlled trial. BJOG 2005;112(6):797–801.

30. Bano F, Barrington JW, Dyer R. Comparison between porcine dermal implant(Permacol) and silicone injection (Macroplastique) for urodynamic stress incontinence. Int Urogynecol J Pelvic Floor Dysfunct 2005;16(2):147–50 [discussion: 150].

Urethral Bulking
A Urology Perspective

W. Stuart Reynolds, MD, MPH*, Roger R. Dmochowski, MD

KEYWORDS

- Urinary incontinence • Intrinsic sphincter deficiency (ISD) • Stress urinary incontinence
- Urethral bulking • Urethral injection

KEY POINTS

- Proper patient selection is important for successful urethral bulking therapy (UBT): it is most appropriate for patients who are poor surgical candidates, must continue anticoagulation therapy, elderly, desire nonsurgical therapy for stress urinary incontinence (SUI), of child-bearing age, have persistent SUI after an anti-incontinence procedure, or have poor bladder emptying and may be at higher risk for urinary retention.
- Several synthetic agents are available for UBT with similar efficacy but unique biophysical properties, including silicone particles, carbon beads, calcium hydroxylapatite, and polyacrylamide hydrogel. Collagen is no longer available for use.
- Most clinical studies report modest efficacy over short durations of up to 75% cure/improvement, although long-term (12 months or greater) results are substantially less.
- UBT can be performed safely in the office with local anesthetic, either through a periurethral or a transurethral (ie, cystoscopic) approach.

INTRODUCTION

Urethral bulking therapy (UBT) is a procedural treatment of urinary incontinence that involves injecting material around the urethra to bulk the submucosal tissue layer and promote mucosal coaptation and hence continence. Although first described in 1938, widespread use of UBT increased with the introduction of collagen as an implant material in 1993, and its popularity peaked in the mid-1990s to the early-2000s. In 1998, UBT was the most commonly performed anti-incontinence procedure for female Medicare beneficiaries, at a rate of 3649 procedures per 100,000 women.[1]

Because of mediocre clinical results, especially long-term results, as well as the increase in popularity of alternative treatment options, interest in UBT has waned. Some have questioned the clinical usefulness of UBT in the era of minimally invasive surgical techniques for stress urinary incontinence (SUI) (eg, midurethral slings).[2] However, UBT may still have a role in SUI treatment, because it is minimally invasive, well tolerated, and beneficial, especially in the short term. Appropriate patient selection is paramount, because it cannot be used indiscriminately in all patients. In the right patient, UBT can play an important role.[3,4]

Patient Selection

UBT has traditionally been reserved for patients with isolated intrinsic sphincter deficiency (ISD) (ie, urodynamically proven low abdominal leak point pressure [ALPP] <100 cm H_2O), limited urethral mobility, and absence of detrusor instability.[5] However, a broader range of patients with all types of SUI has been treated with UBT.[6]

Department of Urologic Surgery, Vanderbilt University Medical Center, A1302 Medical Center North, Nashville, TN 37232-2765, USA
* Corresponding author.
E-mail address: william.stuart.reynolds@vanderbilt.edu

Urol Clin N Am 39 (2012) 279–287
http://dx.doi.org/10.1016/j.ucl.2012.05.002

In general, good candidates for UBT include those who[3]:

- Are poor surgical candidates
- Are elderly and at greatest risk of retention after a sling procedure
- Must continue anticoagulation therapy at all times
- Desire nonsurgical therapy using only local anesthesia
- Are unable to follow postoperative activity limitations required after anti-incontinence procedures
- Are young and desire more children in the future
- Have mild persistent SUI after an anti-incontinence procedure
- Have SUI and poor bladder emptying
- Have mild SUI associated with exercise.

In addition, UBT may be an adjuvant treatment after an incomplete response to more definitive treatment. Durable responses of 80% have been reported in patients treated with collagen injection for persistent SUI after failed suspension procedure or urethral surgery.[7] In other series, previous incontinence or prolapse surgery has not affected the success of subsequent UBT.[8,9]

Managing patient expectations is important. Almost all women have expectations that their urine leakage will be eliminated by anti-incontinence surgery.[2] Patients need to understand that injection therapy should be viewed as a process rather than a single intervention, and multiple injections may be required to achieve continence.[3]

Mechanism of Action

The mechanism of action of UBT is unclear. The goal of injecting bulking agents into the urethra is to obtain coaptation of the urethra during the storage phase and maintenance of that coaptation during periods of increased abdominal pressure.[10] Some investigators have proposed that collagen injection causes cephalad elongation of the urethra at the bladder neck that results in increased abdominal pressure transmission to the first quarter of the urethra.[11] This is shown by an increased ALPP, which has been correlated with successful urethral injection outcomes. As opposed to surgical procedures that may create a functional obstruction, injectable agents restore continence by increasing urethral resistance only at rest and allow the urethra to funnel and open during micturition.[12] This results in low urethral resistance during micturition and thus avoids a compensatory increase in detrusor pressure to overcome an increased urethral resistance

resulting from surgical incontinence procedures, which may contribute to overactive bladder symptoms and/or upper tract damage.

Technical Aspects of UBT

The 2 most accepted techniques for injection of bulking agents are retrograde suburothelial approaches. In the transurethral technique, the bulking agent is injected submucosally via a needle inserted through a conventional cystourethroscope under direct visual guidance. In the periurethral technique, the material is injected with a needle or specialty injector device placed percutaneously from a perimeatal injection site. The needle is localized and positioned submucosally under direct endoscopic vision in the urethra. The target of implantation via either technique is placement of the material in the wall of the urethra at the level of the bladder neck or proximal urethra.

Most patients can be injected under local anesthesia, with either topical lidocaine jelly in the urethra or periurethral infiltration with injectable lidocaine. The patient is placed in the lithotomy position and prepared in a typical sterile fashion as for a cystoscopic procedure. In the transurethral technique, the cystoscope is positioned in the midurethra and the injection needle inserted through the urethral wall into the proximal urethra so the bulking material can be deployed at the bladder neck and proximal urethra. With most agents on the market today, the material is inserted at different locations (eg, 3 and 9 o'clock; 12, 4, and 8 o'clock) such that coaptation, either horizontal or concentric, of the urethral mucosa is achieved with material injection. Care must be taken to inject slowly enough that the tissue can accommodate the material without extrusion of the material either from a new rent in the mucosa or from the needle puncture site after the needle is withdrawn. In general, enough material is injected until complete coaptation is achieved.

In the periurethral technique, the injection needle or device is inserted just lateral to the urethral meatus at the 4 and 8 o'clock positions and advanced within the wall of the urethra through the lamina propria to the proximal urethra/bladder neck area. Localization of the needle is performed with cystoscopic guidance. Gentle rocking of the injection needle can help to localize the needle tip and confirm the proper location of injection site. Submucosal instillation of methylene blue can assist in needle localization.[13] The use of a 15° angled injection needle (the so-called bent-needle technique) can also facilitate needle localization as well as ease of injection (ie, under lower pressure).[14] Care must be taken to avoid any puncture of the mucosa or extrusion of the injected material will occur. The material is injected in a similar fashion to the transurethral technique, with the appearance of raised mounds of mucosa until apposition is achieved from both sides. If extrusion of material develops, the needle can be repositioned more anteriorly and injection resumed. Once coaptation is achieved, then the procedure is completed and the needle and cystoscope are removed.

In female patients, either injection technique can be performed. Theoretic benefits of the periurethral approach are the avoidance of mucosal leakage and less local trauma and bleeding, although benefits of the transurethral approach include a direct visualization of the needle with more precise localization of the material.[15] Both techniques seem to be reasonably efficacious and safe.[15–17]

In addition to these 2 techniques, an antegrade, transvesical technique has been described for use in men.[18] In addition, injection with ultrasound guidance has been used, both transvaginally[19] and transurethrally.[20] Several proprietary, agent-specific techniques and devices have emerged in an attempt to simplify and standardize administration, often without the need for visual guidance. The Macroplastic Implantation System (MIS) (Uroplasty Inc, Minneapolis, MN, USA)[21] and the Implacer (Q-Med, Uppsala, Sweden)[22] are 2 such devices. Both devices rely on blind placement and localization of the device within the urethra, with designated injection sites to direct the material into the proximal urethral/bladder neck. This technique theoretically helps to simplify the procedure by not requiring cystoscopic equipment and thus can be performed in a standard outpatient clinic. However, neither of these devices is approved for use in the United States.

INJECTION AGENTS

Many different agents have been investigated as bulking materials (**Box 1**). The success of a particular agent depends on several factors, including the composition of the material, the usability of the material (ease of preparation and implantation), and the host environment where it is implanted (optimized hormonal environment, integrity of urethral mural components, and intact periurethral fascia).[23] The ideal bulking agent should be nonimmunogenic; permanent; nonmigratory; nonerosive; noninflammatory; easily stored, handled, and injected; painless; have no long-term side effects; and possess a high safety profile.[24] However, no existing agent satisfies all these requirements, and the search continues for improved materials and delivery methods.

Box 1
Past and current injection agents for UBT

Biologic agents

Nonautologous

    Collagen (Contigen)[a,b]

Autologous agents

    Autologous fat[b]

    Chondrocytes

Synthetic agents

Historical agents (sodium morrhuate, paraffin wax, sclerosing materials)[b]

Polytetrafluoroethylene (PTFE; Teflon)[b]

Ethylene vinyl alcohol copolymer (Tegress)[a,b]

Dextranomer/hyaluronic acid (Deflux, Zuidex)[b]

Silicone particles (Macroplastique)[a]

Carbon beads (Durasphere)[a]

Calcium hydroxylapatite (Coaptite)[a]

Polyacrylamide hydrogel (Aquamid, Bulkamid)[c]

[a] Food and Drug Administration approved for urethral injection therapy.
[b] Use no longer recommended or agent unavailable for urethral injection.
[c] Currently in clinical trials in the United States.

Historical Agents

The original report of UBT for the treatment of SUI described the use of sodium morrhuate in 1938.[25] Additional materials used historically include paraffin wax[26] and various sclerosing agents.[27] In the 1970s and 1980s, polytetrafluoroethylene (PTFE; Teflon) was used extensively,[28] but was never approved for use in the United States because of safety concerns of distant particulate migration.[23,29] Autologous fat also showed poor clinical results[30,31] with safety concerns[32] and is not recommended for UBT.

Ethylene vinyl alcohol (EVA) copolymer (Tegress, CR Bard, Inc., Covington, GA, USA) is an injectable solution of EVA dissolved in a dimethyl sulfoxide (DMSO) carrier that allows ease of injection and subsequent precipitation of EVA into a mass within the urethral submucosa. Clinical experience with Tegress showed equivalence in outcomes with collagen[5,33] and objective and subjective cure rates of 45% and 55%, respectively.[34] However, unacceptable rates of treatment-related complications, including a 37% urethral erosion rate, have been reported,[35] and the manufacturer voluntarily withdrew Tegress from the market in 2007.

Dextronomer/hyaluronic acid (Dx/HA) (Deflux, Zuidex, Q-Med, Uppsala, Sweden) is a copolymer of dextranomer microspheres and nonanimal stabilized hyaluronic acid (NASHA) gel. Deflux is commonly used for endoscopic treatment of vesicoureteral reflux with great efficacy.[36] However, for UBT, clinical results were disappointing. A multicenter US clinical trial of Zuidex was not able to achieve equivalency with transurethral collagen injection in 344 randomized women with ISD.[37] Furthermore, an unacceptably high complication rate occurred, particularly for sterile pseudoabscesses (up to 16%),[38] and efforts to obtain US Food and Drug Administration (FDA) approval were abandoned.

The best-studied urethral bulking agent is glutaraldehyde cross-linked bovine collagen (Contigen, CR Bard, Covington, GA, USA), which has been considered the gold standard of urethral bulking materials and the FDA required direct comparison with collagen for any new bulking agent in clinical trials.[23] However, despite a long track record, albeit with mediocre results, collagen for urethral injection is no longer available as of August 2011, because the manufacturer (Allergan, Inc, Irvine, CA, USA) ceased production.[39]

Silicone Particles (Macroplastique)

Macroplastique (Uroplasty Inc, Minneapolis, MN, USA) is a nonbiodegradable hydrogel composed of vulcanized polydimethylsiloxane (silicone) elastomer suspended in a water-soluble carrier gel (polyvinylpyrrolidone) that also serves as a lubricant for the injection system.[40] The elastomer is a particulate of various shapes and configurations, with marked variability in particle size: particles range from less than 50 μm to 400 μm in largest dimension, with 25% of the particles less than 50 μm,[23] raising some concern for potential particulate migration. Histologic examination in porcine injection models reveals the particles to be organized in collagen-encapsulated, firm nodules with evidence of fibroblast and small-vessel in-growth, and no evidence of loss of volume at 6 weeks.[40]

Macroplastique requires no preadministration hypersensitivity testing, and the material does not require refrigeration or special handling. It is supplied in preloaded 2.5-mL syringes. Silicone injection can be performed using standard cystoscopic equipment, with an 18-gauge Uroplasty rigid endoscopic needle, or using a proprietary, nonendoscopic transurethral injection device, the MIS (Uroplasty Inc, Minneapolis, MN, USA). The MIS consists of a multichanneled needle positioning device with 3 angled needle entry ports orientated at the 6, 2, and 10 o'clock positions

for injections of 2.5 mL, 1.5 mL, and 1.5 mL of material, respectively. Ease of use and operator satisfaction with the device has been objectively reported with acceptable 3-month safety and efficacy,[21] although this is not currently available in the United States. The recommended endoscopic Macroplastique injection technique, similarly to the MIS, involves injection at the 6, 2, and 10 o'clock positions with 2.5 mL, 1.5 mL, and 1.5 mL of material, respectively.

General concerns regarding implantation of permanent silicone material in patients have tempered enthusiasm for Macroplastique in the United States,[23] whereas its use in Europe has been more widespread. Recently, a North American trial of 12 sites in the United States and Canada has been reported, randomizing 247 patients with ISD to transurethral injection of either Macroplastique or Contigen.[41] With 12 months' follow-up, the investigators reported statistically significant clinical improvement and dry/cure rates in 61.5% and 36.9% of patients treated with Macroplastique, respectively, and in 48% and 24.8% of patients treated with Contigen, respectively. Safety profiles and adverse events were similar between the 2 groups, with no serious treatment-related complications occurring with Macroplastique. Tamanini and colleagues[42] reported on 15 patients (out of the original 21-patient observational cohort) with 60 months' follow-up and showed subjective success rates of 80%, and statistically significant decreases in daily pad usage, pad weight, and Valsalva leak point pressure. In another study with 60 months' follow-up, Zullo and colleagues[43] reported on 61 patients with ISD with cure rates of 18% and improvement rates of 39%. In a systematic review, a wide variety of cure and improvement rates (0%–66% and 0%–37%, respectively) have been reported with follow-up time periods of 3 to 36 months.[44]

Adverse events are reported with Macroplastique and include short-lived, self-limited dysuria, frequency, and hematuria in many patients[44,45] and transient urinary retention in 6% to 10% of patients.[41,44,45]

Carbon Beads (Durasphere)

Durasphere (Boston Scientific, Natick, MA, USA) is composed of pyrolytic carbon-coated zirconium beads (ranging in diameter from 251 to 300 μm) suspended in a water-based carrier gel composed of 2.8% glucan (a simple polysaccharide). It is considered a sterile, nonpyrogenic, nonreactive, injectable bulking agent that gained FDA approval for use in patients with ISD in 1999. Because of safety concerns of particle migration with other injectable agents, Durasphere was designed with larger-caliber particles (>80 μm) to prevent migration[46]; however, asymptomatic local lymphatic and periurethral carbon bead migration has been reported.[47]

Durasphere requires no special storage or handling precautions and is injected using standard endoscopic instruments and a proprietary 18-gauge injection needle device. In addition, a bent needle is available (18 or 20 gauge) for periurethral injection. The system comes with 1-mL or 3-mL filled syringes and transurethral injection of the material can be performed under local anesthesia. Technical difficulty injecting Durasphere has been encountered, with the carbon beads clogging the injection needle, resulting in increased resistance with higher pressures required to inject the material. Madjar and colleagues[48] proposed a modified injection technique to overcome this difficulty by using submucosal hydrodissection with 1.5 mL of 1% lidocaine before Durasphere injection. In addition, the manufacturer has reformulated the carbon bead size and carrier gel to allow more efficacious injection (Durasphere EXP) via a customized, side-firing 18-gauge or 20-gauge injection needle.

The use of carbon beads has met with moderate clinical success. In a randomized controlled study of 355 women with ISD comparing bovine collagen injection with Durasphere, no significant difference was noted between Durasphere and collagen: 80.3% treated with Durasphere and 69% treated with collagen were improved by 1 or more continence grade at 12 months.[46] Similar results were seen in a trial comparing 52 patients treated either with Durasphere or Contigen in which 80% and 62% of women improved greater than 1 incontinence grade at 2.6 years' follow-up, respectively. Forty percent of patients receiving Durasphere and 14% of patients receiving Contigen were reported as dry.[48]

As is the case with many injectable agents, long-term follow-up shows a reduction in clinical success. Chrouser and colleagues[49] reported on 56 patients treated with Durasphere, with clinical efficacy of 33% and 21% at 24 and 36 months of follow-up, respectively. Nevertheless, a third of patients thought that treatment was a success.

In addition to adverse effects common to urethral injection therapy (eg, dysuria, hematuria), noninfectious periurethral abscess and urethral prolapse have been described in a few cases.[48,50]

Calcium Hydroxylapatite (Coaptite)

Coaptite (Boston Scientific, Natick, MA, USA) is an injectable material that is nonpyrogenic, composed of particles of calcium hydroxylapatite (CaHA) ranging in diameter from 75 to 125 μm (mean 100 μm) suspended in an aqueous gel carrier composed of sodium carboxymethylcellulose and glycerin. The gel carrier facilitates injection and provides the initial bulk mass of the treatment; it is designed to degrade over time, allowing in-growth of tissue around the CaHA particles. CaHA is identical to constituents of bone and teeth and has been used in orthopedic and dentistry procedures with excellent biocompatibility.[5] Coaptite does not require refrigeration or special handling precautions and is dispensed in 1-mL prefilled syringes. A preprocedure skin test for hypersensitivity is not required.

Injection is performed via standard endoscopic instruments with a supplied 21-gauge rigid injection needle with either end-firing or side-firing capability (Sidekick needle). The material is injected at the proximal urethra at multiple sites until circumferential coaptation is achieved, and approximately 2 to 4 mL of material is required. Because CaHA is radiopaque, the material can be visualized on radiographic studies, facilitating accurate localization and placement.[51]

In a pilot study, Mayer and colleagues[52] injected 10 patients with a mean of 4 mL of Coaptite and reported that 7 of the 10 patients noted substantial improvement in pad use or cure (3 patients) at 1 year. The daily mean pad use decreased from 2.59 to 1.64 and the mean 24-hour pad weight declined 90%. The investigators reported that the agent was well tolerated with no significant safety issues.

In the first large, multicenter clinical trial of Coaptite, Mayer and colleagues[53] randomized 296 women with ISD to either CaHA or cross-linked collagen. At 12 months' follow-up, 63.4% of patients treated with CaHA and 57% of patients treated with collagen reported improvement of 1 Stamey incontinence grade or more (no statistical difference). Fewer patients required repeat or multiple injections with CaHA compared with collagen (62% vs 74%, respectively) with a significantly smaller volume of injected material required for CaHA. Patient tolerability was equivalent for the 2 injection materials; however, 2 patients undergoing CaHA injection had technical complications, with improper placement of the material resulting in vaginal erosion in 1 and subtrigonal placement of another. No long-term sequelae of these 2 events were noted.

Urethral prolapse after CaHA injection has been reported in 2 patients.[54,55] Both were treated with local excision with resolution of persistent voiding complaints.

Polyacrylamide Hydrogel (Aquamid, Bulkamid)

Bulkamid (Contura International, Soeborg, Denmark) is a polyacrylamide hydrogel (PAHG) composed of nonpyrogenic water and cross-linked polyacrylamide. It is biocompatible, nonresorbable, and nonallergenic, and, because of its hydrogel nature, it contains no solid particles (ie, microspheres or microcrystals), thereby eliminating any risk of particle migration. PAHG (Aquamid, Contura International, Soeborg, Denmark) has been extensively used clinically in Europe as a soft-tissue filler in aesthetic enhancement and reconstructive procedures.[56]

Bulkamid requires no special handling or refrigeration and is supplied in a 1-mL preloaded sterile syringe. It can be injected transurethrally using a 23-gauge needle and standard endoscopic equipment or using a proprietary endoscopic system, the Bulkamid Urethral Bulking System (Contura International, Soeborg, Denmark). This system is a specially designed endoscopic instrument, with an 11-cm female urethra urethroscope and a disposable rotatable sheath that includes a working channel for the needle, a 2.7-mm lumen for an endoscopic lens, and water flow tubing (in and out). The rotatable sheath allows 360° rotation of the working channel. Approximately 0.5 mL of material is injected each at the 3, 6, and 9 o'clock positions to achieve full coaptation.

Bulkamid (and its predecessor Aquamid) has been used clinically for endoscopic treatment of SUI. Lose and colleagues[57] injected 25 women with SUI with Aquamid. At 12 months' follow-up, 38% and 43% of patients were subjectively dry or improved after 1 or 2 injections. At 12 months, urine leakage (by 24-hour pad test) was objectively decreased by 93% (from a baseline of 56 g to 4 g) and the number of incontinence episodes (by voiding diary) by 87% (from a baseline of 4.6/24 hours to 0.6/24 hours). Adverse events included UTI (10 patients), transient urinary retention (5 patients), and transient de novo urgency and urge incontinence (3 patients).

In another study by this group investigating the effects of urethral injection therapy on urethral pressure reflectometry measurements, 15 women with SUI were injected with polyacrylamide hydrogel and followed for 3 months after surgery.[58] Ten patients were considered cured/improved and showed improvements in urethral pressure measurements compared with baseline. In a recently published case series, two-thirds of 135 women reported being cured or improved after 12 months' follow-up, with significant reductions in incontinence episodes per 24 hours and pad weight testing.[59]

Bulkamid and Aquamid are not presently available in the United States; however, clinical trials are currently ongoing.

SUMMARY

UBT provides a minimally invasive, low-risk treatment alternative for SUI in appropriately selected patients. Although many agents have been used and are available for UBT, research and development of new materials continue in attempts to find the perfect agent.

EDITOR'S COMMENTS

Bulking therapy continues to be an under-utilized component in the armamentarium for the management of stress urinary incontinence. As greater cost containment strategies enter into the algorithmic approach to the management of stress incontinence it would bear to reason that bulking may assume a greater role as an option for the management of stress urinary incontinence. Bulking therapy has historically been considered to be less effective than surgery, however, it is to be noted that published bulking trials were done under strict regulatory criteria, whereas, many of the historical surgery trials were done under less stringent criteria and therefore direct comparisons of efficacy rates are certainly problematic.

Critical to the success of bulking, is careful patient selection. Ideally, the patient should manifest hypermobility of the proximal urethra and bladder neck of less than 30 degrees. There should be evidence of adequate urethral mucosal blood supply and estrogen effect. Anatomic pathology such as urethral diverticula and intraurethral foreign body should also be excluded prior to the consideration of the option of bulking.

Also critical to the success of bulking is injection technique. It is absolutely crucial to avoid over injection (minimized volume and chose appropriate localization of bulking material (mid and proximal urethra). The goal of bulking is not to "coapt" the urethral mucosa but to obtain static increase in resistance in urethral outlet. Although not absolutely obstructive, the effect of bulking is presumed to be an augmentation effect which lends an element of resistance to a poorly functional urethral sphincter. The authors present their vision of their mutual approaches to bulking in a thorough and complete way and the interested pelvic reconstructionist is urged to consider this as a part of his/her armamentarium.

Roger R. Dmochowski, MD
Mickey Karram, MD

REFERENCES

1. Nygaard I, Thom D, Calhoun E. Urinary incontinence in women. In: Litwin M, Saigal C, editors. Urologic disease in America. Washington, DC: US Government Publishing Office; 2004. p. 71–103.
2. Kong WG, Vasavada SP. Is injection therapy for stress urinary incontinence dead? Yes. Urology 2009;73(1):9–10.
3. Cespedes RD, Serkin FB. Is injection therapy for stress urinary incontinence dead? No. Urology 2009;73(1):11–3.
4. Urogynecologic surgical mesh: update on the safety and effectiveness of transvaginal placement for pelvic organ prolapse. 2011. Available at: http://www.fda.gov/downloads/MedicalDevices/Safety/AlertsandNotices/UCM262760.pdf. Accessed October 15, 2011.
5. Starkman JS, Scarpero H, Dmochowski RR. Emerging periurethral bulking agents for female stress urinary incontinence: is new necessarily better? Curr Urol Rep 2006;7(5):405–13.
6. Chapple CR, Haab F, Cervigni M, et al. An open, multicentre study of NASHA/Dx Gel (Zuidex) for the treatment of stress urinary incontinence. Eur Urol 2005;48(3):488–94.
7. Isom-Batz G, Zimmern PE. Collagen injection for female urinary incontinence after urethral or periurethral surgery. J Urol 2009;181(2):701–4.
8. Chapple CR, Wein AJ, Brubaker L, et al. Stress incontinence injection therapy: what is best for our patients? Eur Urol 2005;48(4):552–65.
9. Koski ME, Enemchukwu EA, Padmanabhan P, et al. Safety and efficacy of sling for persistent stress urinary incontinence after bulking injection. Urology 2011;77(5):1076–80.
10. Kerr L. Bulking agents in the treatment of stress urinary incontinence: history, outcomes, patient populations, and reimbursement profile. Rev Urol 1997; 7:S1–11.
11. Monga AK, Stanton SL. Urodynamics: prediction, outcome and analysis of mechanism for cure of stress incontinence by periurethral collagen. Br J Obstet Gynaecol 1997;104(2):158–62.
12. Appell R. Bulking agents for female stress urinary incontinence. AUA Update Series 2009;28:166–75.
13. Neal DE Jr, Lahaye ME, Lowe DC. Improved needle placement technique in periurethral collagen injection. Urology 1995;45(5):865–6.
14. Rackley R, Elazab A. Bulking agents. In: Davila G, Ghoniem G, Wexner S, editors. Pelvic floor dysfunction. New York: Springer-Verlag; 2005. p. 121–6.
15. Schulz JA, Nager CW, Stanton SL, et al. Bulking agents for stress urinary incontinence: short-term results and complications in a randomized comparison of periurethral and transurethral injections. Int Urogynecol J Pelvic Floor Dysfunct 2004;15(4):261–5.
16. Keegan PE, Atiemo K, Cody J, et al. Periurethral injection therapy for urinary incontinence in women. Cochrane Database Syst Rev 2007;3: CD003881.
17. Faerber GJ, Belville WD, Ohl DA, et al. Comparison of transurethral versus periurethral collagen injection in women with intrinsic sphincter deficiency. Tech Urol 1998;4(3):124–7.
18. Klutke CG, Nadler RB, Andriole GL. Surgeon's workshop: antegrade collagen injection: new technique for postprostatectomy stress incontinence. J Endourol 1995;9(6):513–5.
19. Poon CI, Zimmern PE. Is there a role for periurethral collagen injection in the management of urodynamically proven mixed urinary incontinence? Urology 2006;67(4):725–9 [discussion: 729–30].
20. Strasser H, Marksteiner R, Margreiter E, et al. Transurethral ultrasonography-guided injection of adult autologous stem cells versus transurethral endoscopic injection of collagen in treatment of urinary incontinence. World J Urol 2007;25(4):385–92.
21. Henalla SM, Hall V, Duckett JR, et al. A multicentre evaluation of a new surgical technique for urethral bulking in the treatment of genuine stress incontinence. BJOG 2000;107(8):1035–9.
22. van Kerrebroeck P, ter Meulen F, Larsson G, et al. Efficacy and safety of a novel system (NASHA/Dx copolymer using the Implacer device) for treatment of stress urinary incontinence. Urology 2004;64(2): 276–81.
23. Dmochowski R, Appell RA. Advancements in minimally invasive treatments for female stress urinary incontinence: radiofrequency and bulking agents. Curr Urol Rep 2003;4(5):350–5.
24. Itano N, Sweat S, Lightner D. The use of bulking agents for stress incontinence. AUA Update Series 2002;21:34–9.
25. Murless B. The injection treatment of stress incontinence. J Obstet Gynaecol Br Emp 1938;(45): 521–4.
26. Quackles R. Deux incontinences après adenomectomie gueries par injection de paraffine dans le perinee. Acta Urol Belg 1955;23:259–62 [in French].
27. Sachse H. Treatment of urinary incontinence with sclerosing solutions. Indications, results, complications. Urol Int 1963;15:225–44 [in German].
28. Politano VA, Small MP, Harper JM, et al. Periurethral Teflon injection for urinary incontinence. J Urol 1974; 111(2):180–3.
29. Malizia AA Jr, Reiman HM, Myers RP, et al. Migration and granulomatous reaction after periurethral injection of polytef (Teflon). JAMA 1984;251(24):3277–81.
30. Haab F, Zimmern PE, Leach GE. Urinary stress incontinence due to intrinsic sphincteric deficiency: experience with fat and collagen periurethral injections. J Urol 1997;157(4):1283–6.

31. Lee PE, Kung RC, Drutz HP. Periurethral autologous fat injection as treatment for female stress urinary incontinence: a randomized double-blind controlled trial. J Urol 2001;165(1):153–8.

32. Currie I, Drutz HP, Deck J, et al. Adipose tissue and lipid droplet embolism following periurethral injection of autologous fat: case report and review of the literature. Int Urogynecol J Pelvic Floor Dysfunct 1997;8(6):377–80.

33. Dmochowski RR. Tegress™ urethral implant phase III clinical experience and product uniqueness. Rev Urol 2005;7(Suppl 1):S22–6.

34. Kuhn A, Stadlmayr W, Sohail A, et al. Long-term results and patients' satisfaction after transurethral ethylene vinyl alcohol (Tegress) injections: a two-centre study. Int Urogynecol J Pelvic Floor Dysfunct 2008;19(4):503–7.

35. Hurtado E, McCrery R, Appell R. The safety and efficacy of ethylene vinyl alcohol copolymer as an intra-urethral bulking agent in women with intrinsic urethral deficiency. Int Urogynecol J Pelvic Floor Dysfunct 2007;18(8):869–73.

36. Dyer L, Franco I, Firlit CF, et al. Endoscopic injection of bulking agents in children with incontinence: dextranomer/hyaluronic acid copolymer versus polytetrafluoroethylene. J Urol 2007;178(4 Pt 2):1628–31.

37. Lightner D, Rovner E, Corcos J, et al. Randomized controlled multisite trial of injected bulking agents for women with intrinsic sphincter deficiency: mid-urethral injection of Zuidex via the Implacer versus proximal urethral injection of Contigen cystoscopically. Urology 2009;74(4):771–5.

38. Lightner DJ, Fox J, Klingele C. Cystoscopic injections of dextranomer hyaluronic acid into proximal urethra for urethral incompetence: efficacy and adverse outcomes. Urology 2010;75(6):1310–4.

39. Allergan I. Form 10-K: Annual report for fiscal year 2008. 2009. Available at: http://agn.client.share holder.com/financials.cfm. Accessed May 22, 2012.

40. Radley SC, Chapple CR, Lee JA. Transurethral implantation of silicone polymer for stress incontinence: evaluation of a porcine model and mechanism of action in vivo. BJU Int 2000;85(6):646–50.

41. Ghoniem G, Corcos J, Comiter C, et al. Cross-linked polydimethylsiloxane injection for female stress urinary incontinence: results of a multicenter, randomized, controlled, single-blind study. J Urol 2009;181(1):204–10.

42. Tamanini JT, D'Ancona CA, Netto NR. Macroplastique implantation system for female stress urinary incontinence: long-term follow-up. J Endourol 2006;20(12):1082–6.

43. Zullo MA, Plotti F, Bellati F, et al. Transurethral polydimethylsiloxane implantation: a valid option for the treatment of stress urinary incontinence due to intrinsic sphincter deficiency without urethral hypermobility. J Urol 2005;173(3):898–902.

44. ter Meulen PH, Berghmans LC, van Kerrebroeck PE. Systematic review: efficacy of silicone microimplants (Macroplastique) therapy for stress urinary incontinence in adult women. Eur Urol 2003;44(5):573–82.

45. Tamanini JT, D'Ancona CA, Tadini V, et al. Macroplastique implantation system for the treatment of female stress urinary incontinence. J Urol 2003;169(6):2229–33.

46. Lightner D, Calvosa C, Andersen R, et al. A new injectable bulking agent for treatment of stress urinary incontinence: results of a multicenter, randomized, controlled, double-blind study of Durasphere. Urology 2001;58(1):12–5.

47. Pannek J, Brands FH, Senge T. Particle migration after transurethral injection of carbon coated beads for stress urinary incontinence. J Urol 2001;166(4):1350–3.

48. Madjar S, Sharma AK, Waltzer WC, et al. Periurethral mass formations following bulking agent injection for the treatment of urinary incontinence. J Urol 2006;175(4):1408–10.

49. Chrouser KL, Fick F, Goel A, et al. Carbon coated zirconium beads in beta-glucan gel and bovine glutaraldehyde cross-linked collagen injections for intrinsic sphincter deficiency: continence and satisfaction after extended followup. J Urol 2004;171(3):1152–5.

50. Ghoniem GM, Khater U. Urethral prolapse after Durasphere injection. Int Urogynecol J Pelvic Floor Dysfunct 2006;17(3):297–8.

51. Dmochowski RR, Appell RA. Injectable agents in the treatment of stress urinary incontinence in women: where are we now? Urology 2000;56(6 Suppl 1):32–40.

52. Mayer R, Lightfoot M, Jung I. Preliminary evaluation of calcium hydroxylapatite as a transurethral bulking agent for stress urinary incontinence. Urology 2001;57(3):434–8.

53. Mayer RD, Dmochowski RR, Appell RA, et al. Multicenter prospective randomized 52-week trial of calcium hydroxylapatite versus bovine dermal collagen for treatment of stress urinary incontinence. Urology 2007;69(5):876–80.

54. Lai HH, Hurtado EA, Appell RA. Large urethral prolapse formation after calcium hydroxylapatite (Coaptite) injection. Int Urogynecol J Pelvic Floor Dysfunct 2008;19(9):1315–7.

55. Palma PC, Riccetto CL, Martins MH, et al. Massive prolapse of the urethral mucosa following periurethral injection of calcium hydroxylapatite for stress urinary incontinence. Int Urogynecol J Pelvic Floor Dysfunct 2006;17(6):670–1.

56. von Buelow S, Pallua N. Efficacy and safety of polyacrylamide hydrogel for facial soft-tissue augmentation

in a 2-year follow-up: a prospective multicenter study for evaluation of safety and aesthetic results in 101 patients. Plast Reconstr Surg 2006;118(Suppl 3): 85S–91S.

57. Lose G, Mouritsen L, Nielsen JB. A new bulking agent (polyacrylamide hydrogel) for treating stress urinary incontinence in women. BJU Int 2006;98(1): 100–4.

58. Klarskov N, Lose G. Urethral injection therapy: what is the mechanism of action? Neurourol Urodyn 2008; 27(8):789–92.

59. Lose G, Sorensen HC, Axelsen SM, et al. An open multicenter study of polyacrylamide hydrogel (Bulkamid(R)) for female stress and mixed urinary incontinence. Int Urogynecol J Pelvic Floor Dysfunct 2010;21(12):1471–7.

Midurethral Slings for Stress Urinary Incontinence
A Urogynecology Perspective

Beri Ridgeway, MD, Matthew D. Barber, MD, MHS*

KEYWORDS

- Stress urinary incontinence • Midurethral sling • Tension-free vaginal tape • Pelvic organ prolapse

KEY POINTS

- Retropubic and transobturator midurethral sling procedures are safe and effective treatments for stress urinary incontinence but have different complication profiles.
- History, examination, and additional testing may assist in choosing the correct sling type.
- Appropriate counseling and managing patient expectation are necessary to optimize patient satisfaction.
- Women undergoing surgery for pelvic organ prolapse, both continent and incontinent, may benefit from concurrent midurethral sling placement.

STRESS URINARY INCONTINENCE

Stress urinary incontinence (SUI), the involuntary leakage of urine associated with an increase in intraabdominal pressure (coughing, laughing, and sneezing), affects 12.8% to 46.0% of women.[1] SUI is the most common type of urinary incontinence in women younger than 60 years and accounts for at least half of incontinence in all women. Surgery for SUI represents one of the most common indications for surgery in women with more than 210,000 women undergoing surgery for SUI each year in the United States.[2]

THE MIDURETHRAL SLING

The tension-free vaginal tape (TVT) procedure was first introduced by Ulmsten and colleagues[3] in 1996 and over the subsequent decade, gained worldwide popularity. This operation introduced 2 new concepts to the mechanism of cure for slings: placement at the midurethra and placement

without tension or tension-free. The primary advantage of TVT over other surgical treatments for SUI available at the time, however, is that it could be performed in an outpatient. Often patients can void on the day of surgery and be discharged home without a catheter. Several randomized trials and numerous cohort studies suggest that the TVT procedure has similar cure rates to the Burch colposuspension with a quicker return to normal voiding and fewer postoperative complications.[4–6] The success of the TVT has prompted the development of several similar minimally invasive midurethral slings with varying differences in sling material and surgical approach.

An innovation in the surgical management of SUI is the transobturator tape (TOT) (**Table 1**), which was first described by Delorme[7] in 2001. Similar to TVT, TOT is a minimally invasive midurethral sling that uses a synthetic tape; however, it is placed using a transobturator approach rather than a retropubic one (**Fig. 1**). The impetus for the development of this technique was to reduce

Financial disclosures: None.
Center for Urogynecology and Pelvic Reconstructive Surgery, Obstetrics, Gynecology and Women's Health Institute, Cleveland Clinic, 9500 Euclid Avenue, Desk A81, Cleveland, OH, USA
* Corresponding author.
E-mail address: barberm2@ccf.org

Urol Clin N Am 39 (2012) 289–297
http://dx.doi.org/10.1016/j.ucl.2012.06.002
0094-0143/12/$ – see front matter © 2012 Elsevier Inc. All rights reserved.

Table 1
Transobturator tape versus tension–free vaginal tape.

Special Case	Surgery	Rationale
Mixed urinary incontinence	TOT	TOT improves or does not exacerbate mixed urinary symptoms to the extent TVT may
ISD	TVT	Some but not all data indicate TVT is more effective for ISD
Non-mobile bladder neck	TVT	All sling procedures have lowered effectiveness when the bladder neck is immobile, consider periurethral bulking
With prolapse	TVT or TOT	Limited data support similar effectiveness for either approach
Occult SUI–leaks when prolapse reduced	TVT or TOT or staged	TOT has lower chance of creating new voiding symptoms; staging approach allows treatment of SUI if it develops
Recurrent SUI with history of sling complication or does not want mesh	N/A	May consider Burch, fascial sling or periurethral bulking

Data from Walters MD, Weber AM. Which sling for which SUI patient? OBG Management 2012;24:39.

the risk of bladder perforation as well as eliminate the rare but life-threatening complications of bowel perforation and major vascular injury that have been reported with TVT. Published data are limited regarding the long-term efficacy of this new approach. A meta-analysis evaluating 11 randomized controlled trials comparing retropubic and transobturator approaches demonstrates similar effectiveness in overall and subjective outcomes.[8] Objective outcomes were better with the retropubic approach.

Most recently, the single-incision sling procedure for SUI, sometimes called mini-sling, was introduced with the goal of minimizing risk by avoiding the blind trocar passage through the retropubic or transobturator spaces associated with standard midurethral slings (see **Fig. 1C**). As

such, the single-incision sling procedure has the potential for fewer complications, less postoperative pain, and decreased anesthesia requirements compared with standard sling procedures. One such device, the TVT-SECUR (Ethicon Women's Health and Urology, Somerville, NJ, USA), consists of an 8-cm polypropylene mesh with ends coated with an absorbable fleece material to provide fixation. This device can be placed using a retropubic or "U" approach or a transobturator-like "hammock" approach with clinical trials finding similar cure rates between the U and hammock approaches; however, quality of life and treatment satisfaction outcomes favor the U approach.[9] A recent randomized controlled trial compared a single-incision sling (TVT-SECUR) to TVT, with the primary outcome of subjective cure

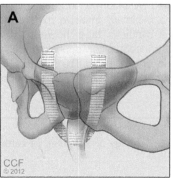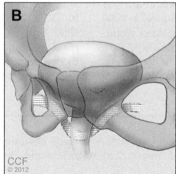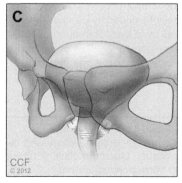

Fig. 1. (*A*) Retropubic midurethral sling. (*B*) Transobturator midurethral sling. (*C*) Single-incision sling. (*Courtesy of* Cleveland Clinic Foundation; with permission.)

of incontinence at 1 year. Results revealed similar subjective cure rates 1 year after surgery but greater postoperative incontinence severity with the single-incision sling compared with TVT.[10] Other available single-incision slings are placed in a transobturatorlike approach using 1 of the fixation devices to anchor the sling into the obturator internus fascia.

Retropubic and transobturator midurethral sling procedures are safe and effective treatments for SUI but have different complication profiles. History, examination, and additional testing, such as urodynamics, can assist a surgeon in choosing the most appropriate sling for an individual patient (**Fig. 2**, **Table 1**).

INDICATIONS FOR SURGERY

Surgery is indicated for the treatment of SUI when conservative treatments have failed to satisfactorily relieve the symptoms, and the patient wishes further treatment in an effort to achieve continence.[11] Although most experts agree that surgery should be delayed until childbearing is complete, the desire for future childbearing should not be considered an absolute contraindication.[11,12] Before surgery, stress incontinence should be objectively documented with direct visualization of urine loss from the urethra with stress. See **Box 1** for the recommended minimum evaluation for women complaining of SUI. Not all patients with urinary incontinence require urodynamic testing before surgery, and emerging data question the utility of urodynamics. However, urodynamics should be considered before surgery if the diagnosis is unclear or the patient is at high-risk for treatment failure or complications (**Box 2**). Traditional teaching requires that urethral hypermobility

be demonstrated with Q-tip testing or some similar method. However, the authors do not consider this an absolute requirement.

Factors that may negatively influence the results of SUI surgery include advancing age, obesity, history of previous incontinence surgery, nonmobile urethra, and preoperative detrusor overactivity (**Box 3**).[13] However, the evidence supporting these negative predictors is generally weak. As such, these factors should not be considered contraindications to continence surgery, but instead be used for patient counseling. Contraindications to SUI surgery include the presence of pure detrusor overactivity and an atonic bladder or a neurogenic bladder (**Box 4**). Also, patients who are otherwise at high risk for postoperative urinary retention who are unable or unwilling to perform self-catheterization may not be good candidates for SUI surgery.

SIMPLE SUI

Simple SUI is a condition in which the patient complains of urinary leakage with coughing, laughing, sneezing, jumping, or exercising. These patients deny symptoms of an overactive bladder and urge urinary incontinence, do not have a history of anti-incontinence procedures, do not have significant pelvic organ prolapse (POP), and demonstrate urethral hypermobility on physical examination. In patients with simple SUI, urodynamics is not likely necessary. The authors evaluate these patients with urinalysis to rule out infection and require that they demonstrate urinary leakage with cough or valsalva. Usually, this evaluation is done during the initial evaluation visit using a cough stress test in the standing position with a full bladder. The authors also check the

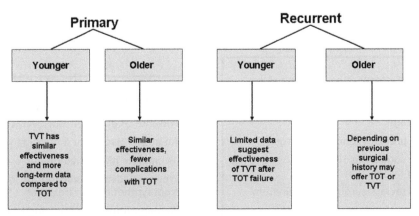

Fig. 2. Primary and recurrent stress incontinence.

Box 1
Preoperative work-up

- Comprehensive history
- Physical examination
- Urinalysis
- Measurement of postvoid residual volume
- Direct visualization of urine loss from the urethra during cough or valsalva
- Urethral hypermobility should be evaluated with Q-tip testing or some similar method

---

Box 3
Risk factors for failure of SUI surgery

- Advancing age
- Obesity
- History of previous incontinence surgery
- Nonmobile urethra
- Preoperative detrusor overactivity

---

residual volume after voiding with a straight catheterization or bladder ultrasound to rule out incomplete bladder emptying. Additional work-up is not usually necessary in patients with simple SUI because it does not add additional information or change the treatment plan. In women with simple SUI, TVT and TOT offer good surgical outcomes and low complication rates. In younger women, the authors typically perform TVT because the data available include long-term follow-up.[14] In addition, emerging data suggest that there may be less sexual pain with TVT compared with TOT.[15] In older women, the authors typically perform TOT because of the excellent subjective outcomes, less postoperative voiding dysfunction, and low complication rates.[16]

MIXED URINARY INCONTINENCE

Approximately one-third of patients with urodynamic stress incontinence have coexisting detrusor overactivity. These patients are said to have mixed urinary incontinence. Obtaining a detailed history in patients with mixed urinary incontinence is critical. The authors attempt to get a clear understanding of what provokes urinary leakage and what type of leakage is most bothersome. Evaluation with urodynamics is indispensable to evaluate

symptoms more thoroughly. Bladder sensation, bladder capacity, and bladder behavior during filling are important factors to consider. In addition, incontinence associated with an increase in intra-abdominal pressure must be demonstrated in the absence of a detrusor contraction because history can be misleading as coughing spells and changes in position can lead to detrusor overactivity. There is some controversy regarding the best management of these patients. Studies have shown that patients with mixed urinary incontinence may have lower cure rates after surgery than those with pure SUI.[17–19] Urge incontinence is resolved in 30% to 60% of women with mixed incontinence after SUI surgery, with 5% to 10% developing worse urge incontinence, and the remainder not changing.[6,20,21] Attempts to use clinical or urodynamic data to predict patients who will improve and who will worsen have been unsuccessful.[22] The authors recommend a trial of medical and behavioral therapy before considering surgery in patients with mixed urinary incontinence because one-third of patients with mixed incontinence can be expected to become dry with conservative therapy alone.[23] In those who have persistent bothersome incontinence after a trial of conservative therapy, surgery can be considered after appropriate patient counseling. Some studies have reported good success in treating mixed urinary incontinence with the retropubic and transobturator slings[24–26] although other studies have reported that the initial benefit for urgency or

---

Box 2
Indications for preoperative urodynamics

- Unclear history
- Advanced age
- History of previous continence surgery
- Symptoms suggestive of detrusor overactivity or voiding dysfunction
- Abnormal sacral neurologic examination
- Increased postvoid residual volume

Box 4
Contraindications to midurethral sling

- Presence of pure detrusor overactivity
- An atonic bladder or a neurogenic bladder
- Incomplete bladder emptying
- Previous adverse reaction or complication from synthetic mesh (relative)
- Planning future child-bearing (relative)

urge incontinence is not sustained over time, compared with the benefit for stress incontinence symptoms.[20,27] In patients with mixed incontinence symptoms, the authors recommend TOT because limited data suggest that the transobturator approach has a lower rate of postoperative urgency and urge incontinence than those of the retropubic approach.[9]

INTRINSIC SPHINCTER DEFICIENCY

Patients with severe urinary incontinence and urodynamic evidence of poor urethral sphincter function are said to have intrinsic sphincter deficiency (ISD), sometimes called type III incontinence or low pressure urethra. Some investigators have suggested that patients with ISD are at risk for poor results after continence surgery. They also suggest that patients who demonstrate a low leak point pressure (<60 cm H_2O) or low maximum urethral closure pressure (<20 cm H_2O) are best served by a procedure, such as a fascial sling, that is more obstructive. These findings are not consistent, however, with some investigators finding no association between the commonly used measures of urethral function and the success of continence surgery.[28–30] In addition, systematic reviews of urethral pressure profilometry and leak point pressure measurement have concluded that these tests are not well standardized and have poor reproducibility.[31,32] Despite this review, many surgeons continue to use the results of urethral function testing in an attempt to provide prognostic information about the success of certain surgical procedures and to triage patients accordingly. TVT may be somewhat more effective for ISD,[33–35] although the data supporting this is not robust and controversy exists on how to make the diagnosis of ISD.[36] Given these issues, the authors do not perform urethral pressure profilometry. In addition the authors do not routinely use leak point pressures to dictate treatment. However, when evaluating a patient with severe SUI symptoms, the authors consider that some studies suggest that patients with ISD have better outcomes with the retropubic approach and usually offer TVT. In addition, the retropubic approach has long-term data to support its effectiveness.

RECURRENT SUI

Evaluation and treatment of women with persistent or recurrent SUI after previous antiincontinence surgery depend on the nature of the original treatment and the presence or absence of associated lower urinary tract symptoms, such as urgency,

frequency, and voiding dysfunction. Although 10% to 20% of women undergoing a midurethral sling procedures have persistent SUI, data to guide appropriate choice of a secondary surgical procedure are limited.[37] In general, women with persistent or recurrent SUI should undergo urodynamics before considering repeat surgical treatment. The operative note from the original surgery is also useful. Cystoscopy is indicated if there is suspicion of urethral or bladder injury. Traditional pubovaginal slings have historically been considered the procedure of choice for the treatment of recurrent SUI although there are no studies currently evaluating their role after failed synthetic midurethral sling procedure. Overall, cure rates for repeat midurethral slings are lower than those for primary surgery.[38] Small uncontrolled case-series suggest that both retropubic and transobturator midurethral slings can be effective salvage procedures, at least in the short-term, with a safety profile similar to that of primary procedures.[37,39,40] One large retrospective series suggests, however, that the retropubic approach has a higher success rate than the transobturator approach for recurrent SUI.[38] Nonetheless, the choice of procedure, in many cases, depends on the procedure that was performed previously. In patients with recurrent SUI after a retropubic colposuspension, some may favor a TOT to minimize the risk of bladder injury associated with retropubic trocar passage. In patients with recurrent SUI after a TOT, the authors recommend a retropubic TVT. Sabadell and colleagues[41] reported good results with the use of retropubic TVT for recurrent SUI after an initial transobturator approach, with overall cure and improvement rates of 86.4% at 12 months and 75% at 36 months, respectively. In patients who have failed a TVT, a repeat TVT or traditional pubovaginal sling are acceptable options. Although data are limited, the authors have also found Burch colposuspension to be effective in this circumstance. In patients who have a fixed urethra, are unsuitable or unwilling to undergo repeat surgery, periurethral bulking can be considered.

POP
POP with Stress Incontinence Symptoms

More than 50% of women presenting with POP also complain of SUI symptoms and an additional 24% have mixed urinary incontinence symptoms.[42] This prevalence of SUI symptoms decreases with advancing POP stage, such that only one-third of women with stage IV POP also present with symptoms of SUI.[42] Existing data indicate that women with POP and SUI undergoing surgery have lower rates of SUI postoperatively if a midurethral sling procedure is performed concurrent with the procedure than if POP surgery is performed alone. Although direct comparisons are uncommon, available data suggest that both TVT and TOT are effective treatments of SUI when performed in conjunction with POP surgery and that the success rates are similar to those receiving SUI surgery alone.[16,26] Hence, in women undergoing POP surgery who also have SUI symptoms and have demonstrated a positive stress test, the authors perform midurethral sling procedure concurrent with the POP surgery. In older patients and patients who also have overactive bladder symptoms or evidence of voiding dysfunction, a transobturator approach is often preferable. In younger patients and patients with recurrent SUI, the authors recommend TVT. There is increasing evidence that transvaginal placement of synthetic mesh to correct anterior vaginal prolapse increases the risk for persistent or worsening SUI postoperatively.[43–46] In one prospective cohort, Fayyad and colleagues[46] noted persistent or worsening SUI in 60% of patients undergoing a transobturator polyproylene mesh kit for anterior POP, when a concomitant midurethral sling procedure was not performed. Although not clear, it is hypothesized that the additional anatomic support provided by the placement of anterior vaginal mesh straightens the bladder neck compromising continence function. So the authors perform TVT routinely in patients undergoing anterior vaginal mesh placement for POP.

POP Surgery in Continent Women

New or de novo SUI occurs after POP surgery in 15% to 25% of women who were continent before surgery.[47,48] Although the precise mechanism by which de novo SUI occurs is not always clear, in many cases, POP surgery unkinks a previously obstructed urethra whose continence mechanism is otherwise compromised.[49] Before POP surgery, many surgeons attempted to predict the patient who is at risk for developing de novo SUI postoperatively by performing urodynamics or a cough stress test with the prolapse reduced. A positive cough stress test after prolapse reduction can be demonstrated in 10% to 80% of continent women with POP.[50–52] This phenomenon has been termed occult, masked, or latent SUI. Although there is some evidence that the presence of occult SUI preoperatively provides some prognostic value about the risk of developing de novo SUI postoperatively, it is by no means a perfect test and no gold standard for prolapse reduction has been established.[53] A recent survey study of 132 women who underwent vaginal prolapse surgery with negative preoperative prolapse reduction testing found that 42% had subjective urinary incontinence after surgery with about a third reporting being moderately or greatly bothered by their symptoms and 5% undergoing additional surgery for these symptoms.[54]

Although surgeons perform a concurrent midurethral sling procedure in continent women with POP who demonstrate occult SUI, there is recent evidence that performing a sling procedure to prevent de novo SUI may also be beneficial for those who have a negative stress test after prolapse reduction preoperatively.[55] The OPUS (Outcomes following vaginal prolapse repair and mid urethral sling) trial randomized 332 continent women with stage 2 to 4 POP undergoing vaginal surgery to receive a prophylactic TVT or sham incisions. Overall, the rate of de novo SUI defined as positive stress test or bothersome symptoms at 3 months was 23.6% in the sling group and 49.4% in the sham group (P<.001), with similar results at 12 months.[55] One-third of patients demonstrated occult incontinence preoperatively. In women with a positive preoperative barrier stress test, 71.9% developed de novo SUI at 3 months in the sham group compared with 29.6% in the TVT group, P value less than.0001 (number need to treat [NNT] = 2.4).[55] In women with negative preoperative barrier stress tests, TVT also resulted in less de novo SUI, albeit less dramatically than those with occult SUI (sham 38.1% vs TVT 20.6%, P = .004; NNT = 5.7).[55] There was no difference in serious adverse events between the groups, but those receiving a prophylactic TVT had higher rates of bladder injury, urinary tract infections, and nonserious bleeding complications. Based on these results, it seems prudent to perform prophylactic midurethral sling procedure in all continent women undergoing surgery for POP who demonstrate occult SUI preoperatively. In women who do not demonstrate occult SUI preoperatively, the authors recommend careful counseling about relative risks and benefits of a prophylactic sling versus a "wait and see" approach in which a sling is placed as a second procedure only in those who develop bothersome SUI postoperatively. Because patients are particularly intolerant of complications from a procedure intended to prevent rather than treat a condition, the authors typically perform a transobturator sling in these patients because of a lower risk of adverse events, particularly bladder injury and postoperative voiding difficulties, relative to TVT. Because of a very low risk of morbidity, this is one area in which the single incision slings may also play a role.

EDITOR'S COMMENTS

Midurethral slings have become the most commonly performed procedures for stress urinary incontinence in North America. These procedures are performed in a variety of ambulatory and in-patient settings and may be performed with or without concomitant prolapse repair. Several types of kits currently exist utilizing mesh and a variety of insertion tools. The authors present their approach to the use of these slings for all types of stress urinary incontinence (pure stress, mixed urinary incontinence, intrinsic sphincter deficiency, complex stress urinary incontinence, the elderly and the obese). Both groups of authors represent experienced senior surgeons who have substantial familiarity with these procedures and who have a tract record of technical expertise and successful outcomes.

In the debate regarding mesh use, and especially in recently released notifications by the Food and Drug Administration, mesh implanted for stress urinary incontinence has been implicated as a potential factor placing women at risk for mesh complications such as erosion and exposure. It is important to note that the American Urologic Association, as well as, the Society of Urodynamics and Female Urology and the American Uro-Gynecologic Society have all presented opinions regarding the appropriateness of mesh for midurethral slings when used in technically competent hands and by surgeons familiar with the presenting symptoms and the perioperative management of the woman undergoing this operation.

Clearly, midurethral slings have become an important component of the overall management of urinary incontinence, however, it is important to realize that no single operation is universally successful for the condition of stress urinary incontinence and so it is advisable to consider secondary options as well as alternative procedures as options for the woman considering surgery for stress urinary incontinence. Midurethral slings, in the appropriate hands, are safe, reproducibly effective and at least equal to results that can be obtained with biologic materials (specifically autologous). However, it is incumbent on the operative surgeon to be familiar with the technique and to obtain appropriate experience with the new variances of these procedures as they emerge (if they are to be adopted by that particular surgeon). The absence of hypermobility may be one risk factor for failure of these types of procedures. Additionally, the vaginal environment (degree of vaginal atrophy) as well as, comorbidities such as diabetes, obesity and other concomitant systemic diseases may also impact wound healing. Management of vaginal erosion can be straightforward and simple although this should be done in an environment where sterility is ensured and adequate instrumentation available.

Midurethral sling will continue to be extensively utilized in the foreseeable future. Surgical choice between retropubic and obturator versions is driven by surgical experience and patient selection.

Roger R. Dmochowski, MD
Mickey Karram, MD

REFERENCES

1. Botlero R, Urquhart DM, Davis SR, et al. Prevalence and incidence of urinary incontinence in women: review of the literature and investigation of methodological issues. Int J Urol 2008;15(3):230–4.
2. Wu JM, Kawasaki A, Hundley AF, et al. Predicting the number of women who will undergo incontinence and prolapse surgery, 2010 to 2050. Am J Obstet Gynecol 2011;205(3):230.e1–5.
3. Ulmsten U, Henriksson L, Johnson P, et al. An ambulatory surgical procedure under local anesthesia for treatment of female urinary incontinence. Int Urogynecol J Pelvic Floor Dysfunct 1996;7:81–5.
4. Ward KL, Hilton P. A prospective multicenter randomized trial of tension-free vaginal tape and colposuspension for primary urodynamic stress incontinence: two-year follow-up. Am J Obstet Gynecol 2004;190(2):324–31.
5. Liapis A, Bakas P, Creatsas G. Burch colposuspension and tension-free vaginal tape in the management of stress urinary incontinence in women. Eur Urol 2002;41(4):469–73.
6. Lapitan MC, Cody DJ, Grant AM. Open retropubic colposuspension for urinary incontinence in women. Cochrane Database Syst Rev 2005;3:CD002912.
7. Delorme E. [Transobturator urethral suspension: mini-invasive procedure in the treatment of stress urinary incontinence in women]. Prog Urol 2001; 11(6):1306–13 [in French].
8. Novara G, Artibani W, Barber MD, et al. Updated systematic review and meta-analysis of the comparative data on colposuspensions, pubovaginal slings, and midurethral tapes in the surgical treatment of female stress urinary incontinence. Eur Urol 2010; 58(2):218–38.
9. Lee KS, Lee YS, Seo JT, et al. A prospective multicenter randomized comparative study between the U- and H-type methods of the TVT SECUR procedure for the treatment of female stress urinary incontinence: 1-year follow-up. Eur Urol 2010;57(6):973–9.
10. Barber MD, Weidner AC, Sokol AI, et al. Single-incision mini-sling compared with tension-free vaginal tape for the treatment of stress urinary incontinence: a randomized controlled trial. Obstet Gynecol 2012; 119(2 Pt 1):328–37.

11. ACOG practice bulletin no. 63. Urinary incontinence in women. Obstet Gynecol 2005;105:1533–45.

12. Brubaker L. Surgical treatment of urinary incontinence in women. Gastroenterology 2004;126(1 Suppl 1): S71–6.

13. Smith ARB, Daneshgari F, Dmochowski R, et al. Surgery for urinary incontinence in women. In: Abrahms P, Cordozo L, Koury S, et al, editors. Incontinence: 3rd International Consultation on Incontinence. Paris: Health Publication Ltd; 2005.

14. Nilsson CG, Palva K, Rezapour M, et al. Eleven years prospective follow-up of the tension-free vaginal tape procedure for treatment of stress urinary incontinence. Int Urogynecol J Pelvic Floor Dysfunct 2008;19(8):1043–7.

15. Petri E, Ashok K. Comparison of late complications of retropubic and transobturator slings in stress urinary incontinence. Int Urogynecol J 2012;23(3): 321–5.

16. Barber MD, Kleeman S, Karram MM, et al. Transobturator tape compared with tension-free vaginal tape for the treatment of stress urinary incontinence: a randomized controlled trial. Obstet Gynecol 2008;111(3):611–21.

17. Colombo M, Zanetta G, Vitobello D, et al. The Burch colposuspension for women with and without detrusor overactivity. Br J Obstet Gynaecol 1996;103(3): 255–60.

18. Scotti RJ, Angell G, Flora R, et al. Antecedent history as a predictor of surgical cure of urgency symptoms in mixed incontinence. Obstet Gynecol 1998;91(1): 51–4.

19. Laurikainen E, Kiilholma P. The tension-free vaginal tape procedure for female urinary incontinence without preoperative urodynamic evaluation. J Am Coll Surg 2003;196(4):579–83.

20. Holmgren C, Nilsson S, Lanner L, et al. Long-term results with tension-free vaginal tape on mixed and stress urinary incontinence. Obstet Gynecol 2005; 106(1):38–43.

21. Segal JL, Vassallo B, Kleeman S, et al. Prevalence of persistent and de novo overactive bladder symptoms after the tension-free vaginal tape. Obstet Gynecol 2004;104(6):1263–9.

22. Brown K, Hilton P. The incidence of detrusor instability before and after colposuspension: a study using conventional and ambulatory urodynamic monitoring. BJU Int 1999;84(9):961–5.

23. Karram MM, Bhatia NN. Management of coexistent stress and urge urinary incontinence. Obstet Gynecol 1989;73(1):4–7.

24. Abdel-fattah M, Mostafa A, Young D, et al. Evaluation of transobturator tension-free vaginal tapes in the management of women with mixed urinary incontinence: one-year outcomes. Am J Obstet Gynecol 2011;205(2):150.e1–6.

25. Palva K, Nilsson CG. Prevalence of urinary urgency symptoms decreases by mid-urethral sling procedures for treatment of stress incontinence. Int Urogynecol J 2011;22(10):1241–7.

26. Richter HE, Albo ME, Zyczynski HM, et al. Retropubic versus transobturator midurethral slings for stress incontinence. N Engl J Med 2010;362(22): 2066–76.

27. Jain P, Jirschele K, Botros SM, et al. Effectiveness of midurethral slings in mixed urinary incontinence: a systematic review and meta-analysis. Int Urogynecol J 2011;22(8):923–32.

28. Bergman A, Koonings PP, Ballard CA. The Ball-Burch procedure for stress incontinence with low urethral pressure. J Reprod Med 1991;36(2): 137–40.

29. Meschia M. Unsuccessful Burch colposuspension: analysis of risk factors. Int Urogynecol J Pelvic Floor Dysfunct 1991;2:19–21.

30. Monga A, Stanton SL. Predicting outcome of colposuspension. A prospective evaluation. Neurourol Urodyn 1997;16:354–5.

31. Weber AM. Leak point pressure measurement and stress urinary incontinence. Curr Womens Health Rep 2001;1(1):45–52.

32. Weber AM. Is urethral pressure profilometry a useful diagnostic test for stress urinary incontinence? Obstet Gynecol Surv 2001;56(11):720–35.

33. Schierlitz L, Dwyer PL, Rosamilia A, et al. Three-year follow-up of tension-free vaginal tape compared with transobturator tape in women with stress urinary incontinence and intrinsic sphincter deficiency. Obstet Gynecol 2012;119(2 Pt 1):321–7.

34. Schierlitz L, Dwyer PL, Rosamilia A, et al. Effectiveness of tension-free vaginal tape compared with transobturator tape in women with stress urinary incontinence and intrinsic sphincter deficiency: a randomized controlled trial. Obstet Gynecol 2008;112(6):1253–61.

35. Rechberger T, Futyma K, Jankiewicz K, et al. The clinical effectiveness of retropubic (IVS-02) and transobturator (IVS-04) midurethral slings: randomized trial. Eur Urol 2009;56(1):24–30.

36. Nager CW, Sirls L, Litman HJ, et al. Baseline urodynamic predictors of treatment failure 1 year after mid urethral sling surgery. J Urol 2011;186(2): 597–603.

37. Walsh CA, Moore KH. Recurrent stress urinary incontinence after synthetic midurethral sling procedure. Obstet Gynecol 2010;115(6):1296–301.

38. Stav K, Dwyer PL, Rosamilia A, et al. Repeat synthetic mid urethral sling procedure for women with recurrent stress urinary incontinence. J Urol 2010;183(1):241–6.

39. Abdel-Fattah M, Familusi A, Fielding S, et al. Primary and repeat surgical treatment for female pelvic

organ prolapse and incontinence in parous women in the UK: a register linkage study. BMJ Open 2011;1(2):e000206.

40. Kuuva N, Nilsson CG. Tension-free vaginal tape procedure: an effective minimally invasive operation for the treatment of recurrent stress urinary incontinence? Gynecol Obstet Invest 2003;56(2):93–8.

41. Sabadell J, Poza JL, Esgueva A, et al. Usefulness of retropubic tape for recurrent stress incontinence after transobturator tape failure. Int Urogynecol J 2011;22(12):1543–7.

42. Slieker-ten Hove MC, Pool-Goudzwaard AL, Eijkemans MJ, et al. The prevalence of pelvic organ prolapse symptoms and signs and their relation with bladder and bowel disorders in a general female population. Int Urogynecol J Pelvic Floor Dysfunct 2009;20(9):1037–45.

43. Sergent F, Sentilhes L, Resch B, et al. [Prosthetic repair of genito-urinary prolapses by the transobturateur infracoccygeal hammock technique: medium-term results]. J Gynecol Obstet Biol Reprod (Paris) 2007;36(5):459–67 [in French].

44. Sergent F, Gay-Crosier G, Bisson V, et al. Ineffectiveness of associating a suburethral tape to a transobturator mesh for cystocele correction on concomitant stress urinary incontinence. Urology 2009;74(4):765–70.

45. Sergent F, Resch B, Al-Khattabi M, et al. Transvaginal mesh repair of pelvic organ prolapse by the transobturator-infracoccygeal hammock technique: long-term anatomical and functional outcomes. Neurourol Urodyn 2010;30(3):384–9.

46. Fayyad AM, North C, Reid FM, et al. Prospective study of anterior transobturator mesh kit (Prolift) for the management of recurrent anterior vaginal wall prolapse. Int Urogynecol J 2011;22(2):157–63.

47. Maher C, Feiner B, Baessler K, et al. Surgical management of pelvic organ prolapse in women. Cochrane Database Syst Rev 2010;4:CD004014.

48. Brubaker L, Cundiff GW, Fine P, et al. Abdominal sacrocolpopexy with Burch colposuspension to reduce urinary stress incontinence. N Engl J Med 2006;354(15):1557–66.

49. Kenton K, Fitzgerald MP, Brubaker L. Striated urethral sphincter activity does not alter urethral pressure during filling cystometry. Am J Obstet Gynecol 2005;192(1):55–9.

50. Haessler AL, Lin LL, Ho MH, et al. Reevaluating occult incontinence. Curr Opin Obstet Gynecol 2005;17(5):535–40.

51. Reena C, Kekre AN, Kekre N. Occult stress incontinence in women with pelvic organ prolapse. Int J Gynaecol Obstet 2007;97(1):31–4.

52. Sinha D, Arunkalaivanan AS. Prevalence of occult stress incontinence in continent women with severe genital prolapse. J Obstet Gynaecol 2007;27(2):174–6.

53. Visco AG, Brubaker L, Nygaard I, et al. The role of preoperative urodynamic testing in stress-continent women undergoing sacrocolpopexy: the Colpopexy and Urinary Reduction Efforts (CARE) randomized surgical trial. Int Urogynecol J Pelvic Floor Dysfunct 2008;19(5):607–14.

54. Al-Mandeel H, Ross S, Robert M, et al. Incidence of stress urinary incontinence following vaginal repair of pelvic organ prolapse in objectively continent women. Neurourol Urodyn 2011;30(3):390–4.

55. Wei JT, Nygaard I, Richter HE, et al. A midurethral sling to reduce incontinence after vaginal prolapse repair. N Engl J Med 2012;366(25):2358–67.

Midurethral Slings for All Stress Incontinence
A Urology Perspective

Eugene Lee, MD, Victor W. Nitti, MD,
Benjamin M. Brucker, MD*

KEYWORDS

- Sling • Midurethral sling • Stress urinary incontinence • Mixed urinary incontinence
- Intrinsic sphincter deficiency • Complex stress urinary incontinence • Elderly • Obese

KEY POINTS

- The midurethral sling (MUS) is the gold standard for stress urinary incontinence (SUI) in the index patient, with equivalent outcomes and minimal adverse events in comparison with traditional SUI procedures.
- With appropriate patient counseling, the MUS can be considered first-line therapy for more complicated situations as well.
- Complicated situations include intrinsic sphincter deficiency, lack of urethral hypermobility, mixed urinary incontinence, prior failed MUS, concomitant pelvic organ prolapse repair, and obese and elderly populations.
- The pubovaginal sling is still preferred for patients in whom synthetic mesh is contraindicated, or in neurogenic SUI whereby obstruction is desired.

Note on the FDA mesh statement

In July 2011, the Food and Drug Administration (FDA) issued a statement directed at transvaginal "surgical mesh implanted to repair pelvic organ prolapse (POP) and/or stress urinary incontinence (SUI)," stating that "serious complications associated with surgical mesh for transvaginal repair of POP are not rare," and its use "has not been shown to improve clinical benefit over traditional non-mesh repair." In particular, the FDA identified vaginal mesh erosion (also called exposure, extrusion or protrusion) and contraction as significant complications, with a higher incidence than that reported in its statement in 2008. On this basis, it recommended consideration of a change in risk classification for transvaginal mesh devices from class II to class III, which could require manufacturers to provide extensive preclinical testing data demonstrating efficacy and safety. The FDA also recommended further clinical studies addressing the risks and benefits of mesh in the treatment of POP and SUI, and expanded postmarket monitoring of mesh-device performance.

The FDA convened a panel to address their statement in September 2011, including presentations from various professional societies including the American Urological Association (AUA), Society for Female Urology and Urodynamics, and American Urogynecologic Society, among others. The AUA and other groups supported the FDA's motion for further clinical studies, rigorous patient consent, appropriate surgeon education and credentialing, and expanded postmarket surveillance of mesh devices. However, the AUA strongly reinforced the need to differentiate between the use of mesh to treat POP versus SUI, citing the existence of extensive data supporting the efficacy of synthetic mesh at the midurethra to treat SUI with minimal morbidity compared with conventional nonmesh procedures. The AUA released a position statement in November 2011 reiterating these points. The FDA is currently considering the panel's recommendations, and a decision is pending.

Department of Urology, New York University, 150 East 32nd Street, Second Floor, New York, NY 10065, USA
* Corresponding author. 150 East 32nd Street, Second Floor, New York, NY 10016.
E-mail address: benjamin.brucker@nyumc.org

Urol Clin N Am 39 (2012) 299–310
http://dx.doi.org/10.1016/j.ucl.2012.05.003
0094-0143/12/$ – see front matter © 2012 Elsevier Inc. All rights reserved.

INTRODUCTION

The midurethral sling (MUS) is now the most commonly performed surgical treatment for stress urinary incontinence (SUI). It is considered the gold standard for patients with genuine SUI. Encouraged by the excellent outcomes and low morbidity in these index patients, clinicians have extended the use of the MUS to treat SUI in more complex situations, such as recurrent SUI, mixed urinary incontinence (MUI), and SUI in the elderly or obese. However, whether an MUS can be recommended for all cases of SUI remains controversial.

This article examines the use of the MUS to treat all forms of SUI, with an emphasis on the nonindex patient. This category includes complex SUI or other circumstances that clinicians commonly encounter. Starting with a brief history of slings, the outcomes of retropubic and transobturator slings in the uncomplicated patient are reviewed. The efficacy and safety of the MUS to treat SUI is then assessed in the following special populations: intrinsic sphincter deficiency (ISD), lack of urethral hypermobility, MUI, recurrent SUI after failed MUS placement, concomitant pelvic organ prolapse (POP) repair, and obese and elderly patients. Based on the available evidence, the discussion herein attempts to identify the populations in whom MUS may not be appropriate in comparison with those who may expect good to excellent outcomes.

HISTORY

In 1997, the AUA Female Stress Incontinence Clinical Guidelines Panel concluded that the retropubic suspensions and pubovaginal sling (PVS) were the most effective treatments for SUI, reflecting the widespread sentiment that these procedures represented the gold standard at that time.[1] Only 2 years earlier, Ulmsten and Petros[2] first described the tension-free vaginal tape (TVT), a retropubic midurethral synthetic sling that was considerably less invasive with high short-term success rates. Because of the relative ease of performance and very good initial results, it quickly became one of the most commonly performed procedures and inspired the development of various other MUSSs.[3] Most notably, in 2001 Delorme[4] introduced the transobturator sling placed through the obturator foramina, which was intended to avoid the retropubic space and its potential major complications.

The first validation of the MUS as a first-line procedure for SUI came from Ward and Hilton,[5] who performed a multicenter randomized controlled trial (RCT) showing no significant differences in efficacy and safety of the TVT compared with the then gold-standard Burch colposuspension. Several RCTs have confirmed their findings, culminating in the most recent meta-analysis by Novara and colleagues,[6] which found that the MUS is more effective than the Burch colposuspension and equally as effective as the PVS in achieving objective cure of SUI. Thus, the MUS has effectively been established as the new gold standard for surgical treatment of SUI.

There are currently even less invasive developments of the MUS, known as minislings or single-incision slings, which are placed through a vaginal incision without any exit incisions. These newer slings are currently under study and have not yet been proved to be equivalent or less morbid than traditional MUS, and as such are not addressed in this review.[7]

ANATOMIC APPROACHES

The Integral theory of Petros and Ulmsten[8] and the Hammock hypothesis of Delancey[9] led to insights on the importance of urethral configuration and its supporting structures in the efficient transmission of closure pressure in maintaining continence, ultimately focusing at the midurethra.[8–10] Based on the Integral theory, the original TVT aimed to reinforce the weakened pubourethral ligaments, restoring compression at the midurethra and resulting in continence.[8] Subsequent ultrasound studies have confirmed this compressive effect at the level of the midurethra, and have also demonstrated a dynamic kinking effect by the MUS based on providing stability at the posterior midurethra.[11,12]

There are 2 main approaches in placing a sling at the level of the midurethra. The retropubic route was used by the original TVT, passing trocars from a midurethral incision through the endopelvic fascia and retropubic space and exiting at the suprapubic area (see **Fig. 1**A for an example of this approach).[2] The transobturator route was subsequently introduced, passing a helical trocar from the groin past the adductor muscle of the leg through the obturator foramen, and exiting the vaginal incision (see **Fig. 1**B for an example of this approach).[4] Numerous technical variations in the direction of trocar passage have been developed for both approaches (**Table 1**).[13]

RESULTS OF MUS IN THE GENERAL POPULATION

There is a vast body of literature reporting on MUS, from which several recent high-quality reviews have provided support for the use of both

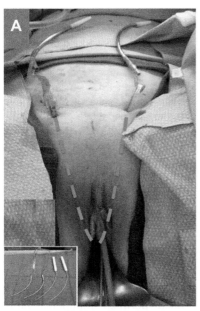 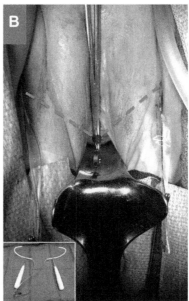

Fig. 1. Examples of the two major approaches to placing a synthetic midurethral sling (MUS). The dashed lines represent the basic path of the sling in each case. (*A*) A retropubic sling has just been placed. The sling will be appropriately adjusted, and the trocars and outer sheath will be removed. The small inset photo shows the components of the device before implantation. (*B*) A transobturator MUS is shown here after both trocars have been passed and then removed. Kelly clamps were placed on each arm of the sling. The small inset photo depicts the device before implantation. The helical nature of the trocar used in the transobturator approach is apparent.

retropubic and transobturator slings to treat SUI.[6,14–17] Most of the early RCTs of MUS, including comparator RCTs to colposuspension and PVS, were performed with a favorable population (the index patient) that excluded conditions such as concomitant prolapse repair, detrusor overactivity (DO), or prior surgery. In brief, in comparing the retropubic and transobturator approaches, the following conclusions can be made based on the Cochrane meta-analysis by Ogah and colleagues[14] regarding the efficacy and complications of MUS in this population:

Table 1
Commonly used midurethral slings

Name	Type	Manufacturer
TVT	Retropubic bottom-top	Ethicon
Advantage	Retropubic bottom-top	Boston Scientific
SPARC	Retropubic top-bottom	AMS
Lynx	Retropubic top-bottom	Boston Scientific
MONARC	Transobturator outside-in	AMS
ObTryx	Transobturator outside-in	Boston Scientific
Aris	Transobturator outside-in	Coloplast
TVT-O	Transobturator inside-out	Ethicon

Adapted from Rapp DE, Kobashi KC. The evolution of midurethral slings. Nat Clin Pract Urol 2008;5:194–201.

Overall summary of Cochrane meta-analysis for retropubic and transobturator slings

Efficacy. For retropubic versus transobturator approach: retropubic slings have a slightly higher objective cure rate (88% vs 84%), but there is no difference in subjective cure rate (83% for both groups in the Cochrane meta-analysis).

Complications. Transobturator slings have a higher incidence of transient groin pain (12%), but retropubic slings have a higher risk of bladder perforation (5.5% vs 0.3%) and postoperative voiding dysfunction (7% vs 4%). The recent review by Novara and colleagues[6] confirmed all of these findings, and also found that retropubic slings have a higher rate of hematoma (odds ratio [OR] 2.62, 95% confidence interval [CI] 1.75–3.57) and vaginal perforation (OR 2.62, 95% CI 1.35–5.08), as well as storage lower urinary tract symptoms (OR 1.35, 95% CI 1.05–1.72).

Based on these data, the literature supports the use of either retropubic or transobturator slings to effectively and safely treat the index patient with SUI, with a slight advantage to the transobturator approach with regard to perioperative and long-term complications. What follows is a discussion of the use of MUS in the treatment of more complex SUI, with the intent of determining whether MUS is appropriate for all forms of SUI.

INTRINSIC SPHINCTER DEFICIENCY AND URETHRAL HYPERMOBILITY

Patients with SUI have traditionally been classified in terms of 2 parameters: defects in the anatomic support of the urethra (urethral hypermobility) versus incompetence of the sphincter itself, commonly referred to as ISD. Current thinking has evolved away from this dichotomy with the understanding that most patients lie on a spectrum with some degree of both hypermobility and ISD.[10] In ISD, the poorly functioning sphincter may be due to aging, previous surgery, radiation therapy, or neurologic insult.

Although there is no standardized definition, ISD has been defined in the literature based on the urodynamic findings of Valsalva leak-point pressure (VLPP) of less than 60 cm H_2O or maximum urethral closure pressure (MUCP) of less than 20 cm H_2O. Women with ISD have been reported to have more severe incontinence with a higher risk of treatment failure, and historically the PVS was recommended in such cases, with cure rates of 80% to 85%.[18,19] Though excluded from most series initially, there are now several studies on both retropubic and transobturator MUS in this population.

Rezapour and colleagues[20] first reported their favorable and durable results using TVT in 49 women with ISD (defined as MUCP <20 cm H_2O, not VLPP) with a cure rate of 74% and significant improvement in 12%, which approaches their success rates in the general population. Of note, only 8 patients did not have urethral hypermobility (as defined by Q-tip test >30°), and of the 7 failures, 5 had fixed urethras. Although the numbers were small, the investigators suggested that lack of hypermobility may be a risk factor for failure.

Subsequently several studies have compared retropubic to transobturator approaches in patients with ISD (defined by VLPP <60 cm H_2O or MUCP <20 cm H_2O). Jeon and colleagues[21] retrospectively compared TVT, transobturator tape (TOT), and the PVS in women with ISD at 2 years' follow-up. Patients with TVT had cure rate of 86.9%, similar to the 87.3% seen with PVS, in

contrast to the TOT group, which had only 34.9% cure (P<.0001). At 31 months, Gungorduk and colleagues[22] found cure rates of 78.3% using TVT versus 52.5% using TOT, and reported that TOT was 5 times more likely to fail than TVT in women with ISD, similar to previously reported short-term results of Miller and colleagues.[23] In the only prospective, randomized study addressing this issue, Schierlitz and colleagues[24] randomized 164 women with ISD to TVT or TOT, with the primary outcome of urodynamic SUI at 6 months. Twenty-one percent of the TVT group had SUI on urodynamics versus 45% in the TOT group (P = .004). Moreover, 13% of women in the TOT group requested a repeat sling, compared with none in the TVT group.

The literature suggests that retropubic slings work well for patients with ISD but obturator slings may not work as well. By contrast, a retrospective study by Rapp and colleagues[25] found no difference between retropubic and transobturator slings in women with ISD with success rates of 76% and 77%, respectively. Costantini and colleagues[26] also reported no difference between TVT and TOT in women with ISD using a subset analysis of their RCT, although it should be emphasized that all of their patients had hypermobility ranging from 43° to 90° by Q-tip test. These investigators found no difference in outcome between 45 TVT patients and 50 TOT patients at 35 months (68% vs 76%, respectively). Although this was a post hoc analysis that was underpowered to detect a difference, the data do suggest that if ISD patients have concurrent hypermobility the results may be different, particularly with the transobturator approach.

A recent study by Haliloglu and colleagues[27] examined the impact of ISD and urethral hypermobility in 65 TOT patients by dividing them into 3 groups: ISD with hypermobility (n = 18), ISD with fixed urethra (n = 16), and hypermobility without ISD (n = 31). At 24 months the 2 groups with hypermobility had similar cure rates, with and without ISD (87.5% and 96.4%, respectively). However, those with no hypermobility had a significantly lower cure rate, at 66.7%. Minaglia and colleagues[28] studied urethral hypermobility independent of ISD in 107 women undergoing TOT, and found that women with urethral mobility of less than 45° were 4 times more likely to have persistent SUI than women with urethral mobility greater than 45° (29.4% vs 6.9%, respectively, P = .005). Hypermobility was also a predictive factor in patients undergoing TVT in a series reported by Fritel and colleagues,[29] with success rates of 92% with Q-tip test greater than 30° versus 70% for Q-tip test less than 30°. ISD defined as MUCP less than 20 cm H_2O had no impact on success rate.

Taken together, retropubic and transobturator MUS procedures appear to be effective in treating patients with ISD and hypermobility. The literature suggests that a less mobile urethra is a risk factor for transobturator sling failure, and in these cases the retropubic approach may be favored.

MIXED URINARY INCONTINENCE

MUI refers to the complaint of involuntary leakage associated with urgency and also with exertion, effort, sneezing, or coughing.[30] Patients with MUI may be difficult to treat, as postoperative incontinence may occur secondary to both recurrent SUI and persistent or de novo urge urinary incontinence (UUI). Moreover, women with MUI who undergo surgery may expect resolution of UUI as well.[31] There are now data and expert consensus to support the use of stress incontinence procedures in patients with MUI and a significant SUI component.[32] Not surprisingly, both retropubic and transobturator MUS has shown to have excellent cure rates for the stress component, reported to range from 85% to 97% in a recent review by Jain and colleagues.[33] Recent research has analyzed the efficacy of MUS in treating the urge component, as well as which factors predict better or worse outcomes.

Duckett and Tamilselvi[34] reported on a series of 46 patients with SUI and DO confirmed on urodynamics. Six months after TVT, 63% reported subjective resolution of urge symptoms, and 47% had objective resolution of DO on postoperative urodynamics. Paick and colleagues[35] reported even higher cure rates in women with MUI undergoing TVT, SPARC, and TOT at 11 months, with resolution of both SUI and UUI in 81.9%, 77.3%, and 78%, respectively. However, they included all patients complaining of UUI with or without DO, and in fact DO was associated with a 3.4-fold risk of treatment failure in this series. Of note, the TOT group had significantly less severe preoperative UUI than both retropubic groups.

In contrast to these promising short-term results, studies with a longer follow-up have demonstrated less encouraging outcomes. Kulseng-Hanssen and colleagues[36] reported on a series of 1113 patients with MUI at 38 months after TVT and found a subjective cure rate of 53.8%. When stratified into patients with predominantly UUI, the subjective cure rate was only 38.4%; however, patients' satisfaction was still 60%. Holmgren and colleagues[37] reported on 112 women with MUI treated with TVT, but with longer follow-up of up to 8 years. In a cross-sectional analysis, 61 women followed for 2 to 3 years had 60% self-reported cure of MUI, but of the 30 women followed for 5 to 8 years only 30% to 40% reported cure. Conversely, Lee and colleagues[38] reported 6-year outcomes in 34 women with MUI, and reported subjective cure rates by validated questionnaire to be similar to those for 107 women with pure SUI (79.4% vs 84.1%).

There are several studies comparing efficacy of retropubic and transobturator slings for the treatment of women with MUI. Gamble and colleagues[39] reported on 305 women with SUI and DO undergoing TOT, TVT, SPARC, or bladder-neck slings. The primary outcome was persistent DO at 3 months. Resolution of DO differed significantly between the groups, with the best results after TOT (47%), followed by retropubic slings (36% after TVT, 37% after SPARC) and bladder-neck slings (14%) ($P<.001$). Subjective cure of UUI was seen in 44% of the whole group, and although cure rates for each sling type were not provided, they reported that sling type predicted persistent UUI. Compared with TOT patients, patients with retropubic and bladder-neck slings were 2 times and 4 times more likely to report persistent UUI, respectively. By contrast, a similar study by Botros and colleagues[40] found no difference in resolution of DO at 3 months in retropubic versus transobturator slings. In a large observational cohort, Lee and colleagues[38] studied 514 women with MUI and 754 women with SUI and urge symptoms (but no UUI) who were treated with retropubic or transobturator slings. At a mean follow-up of 50 months, there was resolution of UUI in 67.7% and urge symptoms in 59.7%. The transobturator approach was a significant predictor for resolution of urgency although it did not affect cure of UUI. Preoperative DO was once again a risk factor for persistent UUI and urgency.

It can be concluded from the available literature that for patients with MUI, MUS effectively treats the SUI and can also cure UUI in at least 50% of the patients in the short term; however, the UUI seems to recur over time. The transobturator approach appears to provide the best control of urgency and DO. However, patients must be counseled extensively because the risk of persistent urge symptoms remains high, particularly in those who have preoperative DO.

RECURRENT SUI

With the widespread use of MUS as primary therapy for SUI and reported failure rates ranging from 5% to 23%, recurrent SUI after failed MUS will likely become an increasingly common condition facing clinicians.[14] The PVS has traditionally been identified as the procedure of choice after failed incontinence surgery based on its superior efficacy over colposuspension, and in this setting reported cure and improvement rates have ranged from 59% to 86%, but data have been lacking on its use in the MUS era.[41–43] Periurethral bulking was recently studied as an option for women with a failed MUS, but cure rate was only 35% at 10 months.[44] There are, however, several recent studies reporting on repeat MUS in this setting, using both retropubic and transobturator approaches.

Liapis and colleagues[45] reported on 31 patients with recurrent SUI after failed MUS who were treated with TVT, and found a 71% self-reported cure rate and 74% objective cure rate by 1-hour pad test. There was a high incidence of ISD defined as MUCP less than 20 cm H_2O (35%), and when this was present with a fixed urethra (Q-tip <30°), the objective cure rate decreased to 40%, versus 63% in patients with concomitant hypermobility. This study did not find an increase in de novo UUI or complications. Abdel-Fattah and colleagues[46] reported on 46 patients with recurrent SUI who were treated with TOT, and found a subjective cure rate by Patient Global Impression of Improvement (PGI-I) of 69.6% and objective cure in 76.5% at 1-year follow-up. On multivariate analysis, MUCP less than 30 cm H_2O was the only risk factor for failure. Biggs and colleagues[47] reported similar acceptable cure rates in their cohort of 27 women, with an 80% success rate based on the PGI-I at mean 27 months' follow-up.

Two retrospective series have compared their outcomes in the primary and repeat setting using both retropubic and transobturator slings. At a mean follow-up of 50 months in 1225 women, Stav and colleagues[48] found a significantly lower subjective cure rate by validated questionnaire in the 77 women undergoing repeat sling compared with those with primary placement (62% vs 86%, respectively, P<.001). There was a significantly higher incidence of ISD in the repeat group (31% vs 13%). Of note, the repeat retropubic sling group had a significantly higher cure rate than the transobturator group (71% vs 48%, respectively), despite their having a higher rate of ISD, although this was not significant (38% vs 21%, respectively). The repeat setting did not have a higher incidence of general postoperative complications, but the rates of de novo urgency (30% vs 14%, P<.001) and de novo UUI (22% vs 5%, P<.001) were significantly higher.

The literature supports the use of MUS for patients with recurrent SUI. Although acceptable cure rates have been reported for both approaches, there are data to suggest that the retropubic approach is preferable; this may be partly due to the high incidence of ISD in this population. It would seem reasonable, then, to consider this plus the circumstances involving a particular patient when deciding on the type of MUS to perform in cases of recurrence.

CONCOMITANT PROLAPSE REPAIR

There continues to be a great deal of controversy regarding the prevention of postoperative SUI in women undergoing POP repair. Forty percent of women with POP also report SUI, and up to 80% who do not report SUI will demonstrate it after prolapse reduction (occult SUI); furthermore, an additional 22% will report de novo SUI after repair.[49–51] These figures are confounded by reports demonstrating that around one-third of patients with either frank or occult SUI do not suffer from incontinence after POP repair.[52,53] Whether a concomitant SUI procedure should be performed in all, some, or no patients undergoing POP repair is under debate, and is beyond the scope of this section. However, the efficacy and safety of using the MUS for patients with SUI also undergoing prolapse repair is reviewed here.

Casiano and colleagues[54] compared their outcomes using a retropubic MUS for documented SUI in 122 women with various types of POP repair versus 159 without POP repair at median 2.7 years' follow-up. At 3 years, there was no difference in self-reported cure of "any" incontinence for concomitant repair versus MUS only (61.6% vs 66.9%, P = .77). However, they did find a higher rate of frequent urination and need for urethrolysis in the concomitant repair group. Meltomaa and colleagues[55] prospectively studied 2 cohorts of women with documented SUI for 3 years. Seventy-five of the women had a TVT alone, and the other cohort of 75 women underwent TVT and concomitant vaginal surgery (including 49 women who underwent a hysterectomy, with or without a vaginal repair, 15 women who had and anterior and/or posterior colporrhaphy, and 11 women who underwent a sacrospinous ligament fixation.) There was no difference in self-reported incontinence cure in the 2 groups (92% vs 87%, respectively, P value not reported). Forty-one percent of the women in each group had urge symptoms, but unlike the series of Casiano and colleagues,[54] there was no difference in postoperative urgency (21% with concomitant vaginal surgery vs 20% with TVT alone). In terms of complications related to the TVT procedure, 5.3% of patients with concomitant vaginal surgery had bladder perforation versus none in the TVT-only group, and a higher rate of transient retention in the POP repair group, but otherwise no differences in TVT-specific complications.

Wang and colleagues[56] prospectively evaluated 140 women randomized to TVT or TOT, of whom 52 underwent concomitant transvaginal POP repair (30 in the TVT group, 22 in the TOT group). Objective cure by cough and pad tests at 1 year were similar for TVT (95% TVT alone vs 90% with POP repair) and also for TOT (93.75% TOT alone vs 86.36% with POP repair) regardless of POP repair. Postoperative complication rates were comparable with those of previous reports of MUS alone. Overall, the results of MUS for symptomatic SUI at the time of prolapse repair also compare favorably with those for bladder-neck suspensions and the PVS performed with prolapse repair, with reported cure rates of 90% to 100% with the traditional procedures.[57,58]

In summary, both retropubic and transobturator slings appear to be effective and safe in the treatment of SUI with concurrent prolapse repair, with no difference in expected cure rate in comparison with patients with isolated SUI.

THE OBESE AND THE ELDERLY

The obese and the elderly share several commonalities that are of special interest when considering the placement of MUS to treat SUI. Not only are both of these populations increasing, but their prevalence of SUI is much higher than in the general population.[59–61] In both cases, there is concern for decreasing therapeutic index, as cure rates may be lower in conjunction with the higher risk of perioperative complications in these at-risk populations.[62,63]

The Obese

A recent meta-analysis of 7 observational studies by Greer and colleagues[64] evaluated the safety and efficacy of TVT in the obese population. Included in the meta-analysis, Rafii and colleagues[65] reported a higher rate of persistent UUI in the obese group (17.9% vs 46%, $P = .02$), and Lovatsis and colleagues[66] found a higher rate of bladder perforations (14% vs 0%, $P = .03$). Skriapas and colleagues[67] did find a significantly higher rate of early postoperative complications in the obese patients (48.4% vs 38.5%, $P = .021$), most of which were minor; however, it should be noted that this also included 2 deep venous thromboses, 1 new-onset arrhythmia, and 1 pneumonia in the obese group versus none in the nonobese group.

In terms of cure rate, all but one study did not find a significant difference at up to 24 months.

The single study showing a difference was by Hellberg and colleagues,[68] who stratified patients into slender (body mass index [BMI] <25), normal (BMI 25–29), obese (BMI 30–34), and very obese (BMI >35) (BMI calculated as weight in kilograms divided by height in meters squared, ie, kg/m^2). At 5.7 years' follow-up, there was a trend toward lower cure rate with increasing BMI, which became significant when comparing the 2 extremes; self-reported cure was 81.2% in slender women, but only 52.1% in the very obese women ($P = .0005$). When these findings were combined with the 6 other studies in the meta-analysis there was a small, but significant difference in cure rates between the obese and nonobese (81% and 85%, respectively $P = .001$).

Recently, data have emerged regarding the use of the transobturator sling in this population. Liu and colleagues[69] retrospectively compared TVT-obturator outcomes in 29 normal, 58 overweight, and 32 obese women as grouped by BMI. At median 24 months' follow-up, they found no difference in objective and subjective cure rate or perioperative complications between the 3 groups. By contrast, Haverkorn and colleagues[70] compared 117 obese women (BMI >30) with 161 normal controls (BMI <30) at minimum 12 months after MONARC transobturator sling. Defining cure using both validated questionnaire and objective cough test, there was a significantly lower cure rate in the obese population (81.2% vs 91.9%, $P<.001$). However, they also reported that the obese women were able to achieve an improvement in quality-of-life indices similar to that of the normal population, suggesting that the difference is not clinically significant.

In summary, the obese population may experience a slightly higher rate of complications, and the very obese may need to be counseled on the possibility of a lower cure rate. However, the literature overall does not support the concerns of a lower therapeutic index for retropubic or transobturator MUS in this population.

The Elderly

In addition to the higher rates of SUI and increased comorbidities seen in the obese population, elderly women must also contend with an increasing prevalence of MUI and ISD, which could potentially lead to a higher risk of adverse outcomes and lower success with MUS for SUI. These concerns have likely contributed to the exclusion of elderly women from most published clinical trials, resulting in limited data in this population.[71] Nevertheless, there are several studies that can help assess whether MUS is an appropriate treatment option for the elderly.

Sevestre and colleagues[72] reported their outcomes after TVT at mean 2-year follow-up in 76 women older than 70 years. Of note, 29% had recurrent SUI after a bladder-neck suspension procedure (Burch, Marschall-Marchetti, or Stamey), 74% had MUCP less than 30 cm H_2O, 31% had MUI, and only 53% had urethral hypermobility. Sixty-seven percent were cured based on validated questionnaire; of the failures, 13.7% had SUI and 18.4% had UUI. There was one bladder perforation but no serious perioperative complications; however, the rate of de novo urgency was 21% and de novo UUI occurred in 5%. The investigators concluded that TVT was a suitable procedure for elderly women, as 82% of the women were satisfied with their procedure; however, cure rate is lower because of the risk of postoperative urgency. In addition to BMI, Hellberg and colleagues[68] also analyzed their TVT series according to age at 5.7 years' mean follow-up. There was a trend toward lower cure rate with increasing age, which became significant when comparing patients older than 75 years with younger women under 60 years old (55.7% vs 79.7%). There was no difference in perioperative complication rate, except that younger women had a slightly higher rate of bladder perforation (2.9% vs 0.9%). Similar to the findings of Sevestre and colleagues,[72] there was a significantly higher rate of de novo urgency in the older women (20.9% vs 13.8%). However, 54% of the elderly women with preoperative urgency had resolution of these symptoms.

There are no current publications that report on transobturator slings for isolated SUI in the elderly population. However, Groutz and colleagues[73] prospectively compared TVT-obturator slings in 97 elderly women older than 70 years with 256 younger women, the majority of whom had concomitant POP repair (90% of the elderly and 70% of the younger cohort). At a mean of 30 months' follow-up, the incidence of persistent SUI was only 5% in both groups, with a similar incidence of overactive bladder in both groups (68% in elderly, 62% in younger). There was also no difference in perioperative complications. There was, however, significantly higher de novo urgency in the elderly (11.9% vs 4.7%) as well as recurrent urinary tract infection (13.7% vs 6.2%).

Taken together, the literature supports the use of MUS to treat SUI in the elderly, provided that patients are counseled appropriately regarding the lower rate of cure as well as the higher risk of de novo urgency.

SPECIAL CONSIDERATIONS

Because of the nature of the MUS as a synthetic sling, there exist a few select clinical situations whereby its use is probably not appropriate, owing to an increased risk of erosion. In the setting of concurrent or prior urethral reconstruction, such as indicated for urethral diverticulectomy, urethrovaginal fistula repair, or urethral injury secondary to prior sling placement or pelvic fracture, the autologous PVS is preferred. Although there are no reports of the MUS being used in this setting, experience with synthetic material in the setting of urethral reconstruction has demonstrated a high rate of erosion.[74] By contrast, excellent outcomes have been reported with the use of PVS in the setting of reconstruction, with an 88% cure rate after diverticulectomy in 16 patients and an 86% cure rate after genitourinary fistula repair in 7 patients, with no reported erosions in either series.[75,76]

The MUS is also not the preferred procedure in the case of the patient with neurogenic incontinence, such as the patient with spina bifida. In this population, already dependent on clean intermittent self-catheterization, a tension-free MUS may not provide the necessary compression to achieve continence between catheterizations. The PVS has been used successfully to provide occlusion at the bladder neck, with a continence rate of 94.44% in this setting.[77,78]

SUMMARY

The MUS has emerged as the new gold standard for the treatment of all SUI. With appropriate counseling, it can be used effectively in complex SUI cases, with minimal morbidity. Introduced over a decade ago as minimally invasive, there are now purportedly even less invasive techniques of placing a sling at the midurethra, and these single-incision slings will now need to be validated against the new gold standard of the MUS. The coming decade may see further improvements in the surgical treatment of both simple and complicated SUI. Situations will undoubtedly still exist whereby a surgeon will elect to perform an alternative intervention for the concomitant surgical correction of SUI when complex reconstruction is performed. These unique situations may include prior synthetic sling extrusion/injury to the urethra, fistula, or cases when obstruction is desirable (such as in a patient already dependent on catheterization). Acknowledging these rare exceptions, the MUS is currently the answer for all SUI.

EDITOR'S COMMENTS

Midurethral slings have become the most commonly performed procedures for stress urinary incontinence in North America. These procedures are performed in a variety of ambulatory and in-patient settings and may be performed with or without concomitant prolapse repair. Several types of kits currently exist utilizing mesh and a variety of insertion tools. The authors present their approach to the use of these slings for all types of stress urinary incontinence (pure stress, mixed urinary incontinence, intrinsic sphincter deficiency, complex stress urinary incontinence, the elderly and the obese). Both groups of authors represent experienced senior surgeons who have substantial familiarity with these procedures and who have a tract record of technical expertise and successful outcomes.

In the debate regarding mesh use, and especially in recently released notifications by the Food and Drug Administration, mesh implanted for stress urinary incontinence has been implicated as a potential factor placing women at risk for mesh complications such as erosion and exposure. It is important to note that the American Urologic Association, as well as, the Society of Urodynamics and Female Urology and the American Uro-Gynecologic Society have all presented opinions regarding the appropriateness of mesh for midurethral slings when used in technically competent hands and by surgeons familiar with the presenting symptoms and the perioperative management of the woman undergoing this operation.

Clearly, midurethral slings have become an important component of the overall management of urinary incontinence, however, it is important to realize that no single operation is universally successful for the condition of stress urinary incontinence and so it is advisable to consider secondary options as well as alternative procedures as options for the woman considering surgery for stress urinary incontinence. Midurethral slings, in the appropriate hands, are safe, reproducibly effective and at least equal to results that can be obtained with biologic materials (specifically autologous). However, it is incumbent on the operative surgeon to be familiar with the technique and to obtain appropriate experience with the new variances of these procedures as they emerge (if they are to be adopted by that particular surgeon). The absence of hypermobility may be one risk factor for failure of these types of procedures. Additionally, the vaginal environment (degree of vaginal atrophy) as well as, comorbidities such as diabetes, obesity and other concomitant systemic diseases may also impact wound healing. Management of vaginal erosion can be straightforward and simple although this should be done in an environment where sterility is ensured and adequate instrumentation available.

Midurethral sling will continue to be extensively utilized in the foreseeable future. Surgical choice between retropubic and obturator versions is driven by surgical experience and patient selection.

Roger R. Dmochowski, MD
Mickey Karram, MD

REFERENCES

1. Leach GE, Dmochowski RR, Appell RA, et al. Female stress urinary incontinence clinical guidelines panel summary report on surgical management of female stress urinary incontinence. J Urol 1997;158:875–80.
2. Ulmsten U, Petros P. Intravaginal slingplasty (IVS): an ambulatory surgical procedure for treatment of female urinary incontinence. Scand J Urol Nephrol 1995;29(1):75–82.
3. Bullock TL, Ghoneim G, Klutke CG, et al. Advances in female stress urinary incontinence: midurethral slings. BJU Int 2006;98(Suppl 1):32–40.
4. Delorme E. Transobturator urethral suspension: mini-invasive procedure in the treatment of stress urinary incontinence in women. Prog Urol 2001; 11(6):1306–13.
5. Ward KL, Hilton P, UK and Ireland TVT Trial Group. A prospective multicenter randomized trial of tension-free vaginal tape and colposuspension for primary urodynamic stress incontinence: 5-year follow up. BJOG 2008;115:226–33.
6. Novara G, Artibani W, Barber MD, et al. Updated systematic review and meta-analysis of the comparative data on colposuspensions, pubovaginal slings, and midurethral tapes in the surgical treatment of female stress urinary incontinence. Eur Urol 2010; 58:218–38.
7. Abdel-Fattah M, Ford JA, Lim CP, et al. Single-incision mini-slings versus standard midurethral slings in surgical management of female stress urinary incontinence: a meta-analysis of effectiveness and complications. Eur Urol 2011;60:468–80.
8. Petros PE, Ulmsten UI. An integral theory of female urinary incontinence. Experimental and clinical considerations. Acta Obstet Gynecol Scand Suppl 1990;153:7–31.
9. Delancey JO. Structural support of the urethra as it relates to stress urinary incontinence: the hammock hypothesis. Am J Obstet Gynecol 1994; 170:1713–23.

10. Plzak L 3rd, Staskin D. Genuine stress incontinence theories of etiology and surgical correction. Urol Clin North Am 2002;29:527–35.

11. Dietz HP, Wilson PD. The "iris effect": how two-dimensional and three-dimensional ultrasound can help us understand anti-incontinence procedures. Ultrasound Obstet Gynecol 2004;23:267–71.

12. Atherton MJ, Stanton SL. A comparison of bladder neck movement and elevation after tension-free vaginal tape and colposuspension. BJOG 2000;107:1366–70.

13. Rapp DE, Kobashi KC. The evolution of midurethral slings. Nat Clin Pract Urol 2008;5:194–201.

14. Ogah J, Cody JD, Rogerson L. Minimally invasive synthetic suburethral sling operations for stress urinary incontinence in women. Cochrane Database Syst Rev 2009;4:CD006375.

15. Sung V, Schleinitz MD, Rardin CR, et al. Comparison of retropubic vs transobturator approach to midurethral slings: a systematic review and meta-analysis. Am J Obstet Gynecol 2007;197:3–11.

16. Latthe PM, Foon R, Toozs-Hobson P. Transobturator and retropubic tape procedures in stress urinary incontinence: a systematic review and meta-analysis of effectiveness and complications. BJOG 2007;114:522–31.

17. Long CY, Hsu CS, Wu MP, et al. Comparison of tension-free vaginal tape and transobturator tape procedure for the treatment of stress urinary incontinence. Curr Opin Obstet Gynecol 2009;21:342–7.

18. McGuire EJ. Urodynamic findings in patients after failure of stress incontinence operation. Prog Clin Biol Res 1981;78:351–3.

19. Maher CF, O'Reilly BA, Dwyer PL, et al. Pubovaginal sling versus transurethral Macroplastique for stress urinary incontinence and intrinsic sphincter deficiency: a prospective randomized controlled trial. BJOG 2005;112:797–801.

20. Rezapour M, Falconer C, Ulmsten U. Tension-free vaginal tape (TVT) in stress incontinent women with intrinsic sphincter deficiency (ISD)—a long-term follow-up. Int Urogynecol J Pelvic Floor Dysfunct 2001;12(Suppl):S12–4.

21. Jeon MJ, Jung HJ, Chung SM, et al. Comparison of the treatment outcome of pubovaginal sling, tension-free vaginal tape, and transobturator tape for stress urinary incontinence with intrinsic sphincter deficiency. Am J Obstet Gynecol 2008;199(1):76 e1–4.

22. Gungorduk K, Celebi I, Ark C, et al. Which type of mid-urethral sling procedure should be chosen for treatment of stress urinary incontinence with intrinsic sphincter deficiency? Tension-free vaginal tape or transobturator tape. Acta Obstet Gynecol Scand 2009;88:920–6.

23. Miller JR, Botros SM, Akl MN, et al. Is transobturator tape as effective as tension-free vaginal tape in patients with borderline maximum urethral closure pressure? Am J Obstet Gynecol 2006;196:1799–804.

24. Schierlitz L, Dwyer PL, Rosamilia A, et al. Effectiveness of tension-free vaginal tape compared with transobturator tape in women with stress urinary incontinence and intrinsic sphincter deficiency: a randomized controlled trial. Obstet Gynecol 2008;112:1253–61.

25. Rapp DE, Govier FE, Kobashi KC. Outcomes following mid-urethral sling placement in patients with intrinsic sphincteric deficiency: comparison of SPARC and MONARC slings. Int Braz J Urol 2009;35(1):68–75.

26. Costantini E, Lazzeri M, Giannantoni A, et al. Preoperative Valsalva leak point pressure may not predict outcome of mid-urethral slings: analysis from a randomized controlled trial of retropubic versus transobturator mid-urethral slings. Int Braz J Urol 2008;34(1):73–81.

27. Haliloglu B, Karateke A, Coksuer H, et al. The role of urethral hypermobility and intrinsic sphincteric deficiency on the outcome of transobturator tape procedure: a prospective study with 2-year follow-up. Int Urogynecol J 2010;21(2):173–8.

28. Minaglia S, Urwitz-Lane R, Wong M, et al. Effectiveness of transobturator tape in women with decreased urethral mobility. J Reprod Med 2009;54(1):15–9.

29. Fritel X, Zabak K, Pigne A, et al. Predictive value of urethral mobility before suburethral tape procedure for urinary stress incontinence in women. J Urol 2002;168:2472–5.

30. Abrams P, Cardozo L, Fall M, et al. The standardization of terminology in lower urinary tract function: report from the standardization sub-committee of the International Continence Society. Neurourol Urodyn 2002;21:167–78.

31. Mallet VT, Brubaker L, Stoddard AM, et al. The expectations of patients who undergo surgery for stress incontinence. Am J Obstet Gynecol 2008;198:308, e1–6.

32. Dmochowski RR, Blaivas JM, Gormley EA, et al. Update of AUA guideline on the surgical management of female stress urinary incontinence. J Urol 2010;183:1906–14.

33. Jain P, Jirschele K, Botros SM, et al. Effectiveness of midurethral slings in mixed urinary incontinence: a systematic review and meta-analysis. Int Urogynecol J 2011;22:923–32.

34. Duckett JR, Tamilselvi A. Effect of tension-free vaginal tape in women with a urodynamic diagnosis of idiopathic detrusor overactivity and stress incontinence. BJOG 2006;113:30–3.

35. Paick JS, Oh SJ, Kim SW, et al. Tension-free vaginal tape, suprapubic arc sling, and transobturator tape in the treatment of mixed urinary incontinence in

women. Int Urogynecol J Pelvic Floor Dysfunct 2008; 19(1):123–9.

36. Kulseng-Hanssen S, Husby H, Shiotz HA. Follow-up of TVT operations in 1,113 women with mixed urinary incontinence at 7 and 38 months. Int Urogynecol J Pelvic Floor Dysfunct 2008;19(3):391–6.

37. Holmgren C, Nilsson S, Lanner L, et al. Long-term results with tension-free vaginal tape on mixed and stress urinary incontinence. Obstet Gynecol 2005; 106:38–43.

38. Lee JH, Cho MC, Oh SJ, et al. Long-term outcome of the tension-free vaginal tape procedure in female urinary incontinence: a 6-year follow-up. Korean J Urol 2010;51:409–15.

39. Gamble T, Botros S, Beaumont J, et al. Predictors of persistent detrusor overactivity after transvaginal sling procedures. Am J Obstet Gynecol 2008;199: 696, e1–7.

40. Botros SM, Miller JJ, Goldberg RP, et al. Detrusor overactivity and urge urinary incontinence following trans obturator versus midurethral slings. Neurourol Urodyn 2007;26(1):42–5.

41. Albo ME, Richter HE, Brubaker L, et al. Burch colposuspension versus fascial sling to reduce urinary stress incontinence. N Engl J Med 2007;356:2143–55.

42. Petrou SP, Frank I. Complications and initial conti- nence rates after a repeat pubovaginal sling proce- dure for recurrent stress urinary incontinence. J Urol 2001;165:1979–81.

43. Groutz A, Blaivas JG, Hyman MJ, et al. Pubovaginal sling surgery for simple stress urinary incontinence: analysis by an outcome score. J Urol 2001;165: 1597–600.

44. Lee HN, Lee YS, Han JY, et al. Transurethral injection of bulking agent for treatment of failed mid-urethral sling procedures. Int Urogynecol J Pelvic Floor Dys- funct 2010;21:1479–83.

45. Liapis A, Bakas P, Creatsas G. Tension-free vaginal tape in the management of recurrent urodynamic stress incontinence after previous failed midurethral tape. Eur Urol 2009;55:1450–8.

46. Abdel-Fattah M, Ramsay I, Pringle S, et al. Evalua- tion of transobturator tension-free vaginal tapes in management of women with recurrent stress urinary incontinence. Urology 2011;77(5):1070–5.

47. Biggs GY, Ballert KN, Rosenblum N, et al. Patient- reported outcomes for tension-free vaginal tape- obturator in women treated with a previous anti-incontinence procedure. Int Urogynecol J Pelvic Floor Dysfunct 2009;20(3):331–5.

48. Stav K, Dwyer PL, Rosamilia A, et al. Long-term outcomes of patients who failed to attend following midurethral sling surgery—a comparative study and analysis of risk factors for nonattendance. Aust N Z J Obstet Gynaecol 2010;50(2):173–8.

49. Long CY, Hsu SC, Wu TP, et al. Urodynamic compar- ison of continent and incontinent women with severe

uterovaginal prolapse. J Reprod Med 2004;49(1): 33–7.

50. Togami JM, Chow D, Winters JC. To sling or not to sling at the time of anterior vaginal compartment repair. Curr Opin Urol 2010;20:269–74.

51. Borstad E, Rud T. The risk of developing urinary stress-incontinence after vaginal repair in continent women. A clinical and urodynamic follow-up study. Acta Obstet Gynecol Scand 1989;68:545–9.

52. Borstad E, Abdelnoor M, Staff AC, et al. Surgical strategies for women with pelvic organ prolapse and urinary stress incontinence. Int Urogynecol J 2010;21:179–86.

53. Reena C, Kekre AN, Kekre N. Occult stress inconti- nence in women with pelvic organ prolapse. Int J Gynaecol Obstet 2007;97:31–4.

54. Casiano ER, Gebhart JB, McGree MM, et al. Does concomitant prolapse repair at the time of midure- thral sling affect recurrent rates of incontinence? Int Urogynecol J 2011;22:819–25.

55. Meltomaa S, Backman T, Haarala M. Concomitant vaginal surgery did not affect outcome of the tension-free vaginal tape operation during a prospec- tive 3-year follow-up study. J Urol 2004;172:222–6.

56. Wang F, Song Y, Huang H. Prospective randomized trial of TVT and TOT as primary treatment for female stress urinary incontinence with or without pelvic organ prolapse in southeast China. Arch Gynecol Obstet 2010;281:279–86.

57. Sze EH, Kohli N, Miklos JR, et al. A retrospective comparison of abdominal sacrocolpopexy with Burch colposuspension versus sacrospinous fixa- tion with transvaginal needle suspension for the management of vaginal vault prolapse and coexist- ing stress incontinence. Int Urogynecol J 1999;10: 390–3.

58. Amundsen CL, Flynn BJ, Webster GD. Anatomical correction of vaginal vault prolapse by uterosacral ligament fixation in women who also require a pubo- vaginal sling. J Urol 2003;169:1770–4.

59. Hunskaar S. A systematic review of overweight and obesity as risk factors and targets for clinical inter- vention for urinary incontinence in women. Neurourol Urodyn 2008;27(8):749–57.

60. Richter HE, Burgio KL, Clements RH, et al. Urinary and anal incontinence in morbidly obese women considering weight loss surgery. Obstet Gynecol 2005;106:1272.

61. Nygaard IE, Lemke JH. Urinary incontinence in rural older women: prevalence, incidence, and readmis- sion. J Am Geriatr Soc 1996;44:1049–54.

62. Sultana CJ, Campbell JW, Pisanelli WS, et al. Morbidity and mortality of incontinence surgery in elderly women: an analysis of Medicare data. Am J Obstet Gynecol 1997;176:344–8.

63. Poirier P, Alpert MA, Fleisher LA, et al. Cardiovas- cular evaluation and management of severely obese

patients undergoing surgery: a science advisory from the American Heart Association. Circulation 2009;120:86.

64. Greer WJ, Richter HE, Bartolucci AA, et al. Obesity and pelvic floor disorders: a systematic review. Obstet Gynecol 2008;112(2 Pt 1):341–9.

65. Rafii A, Darai E, Haab F, et al. Body mass index and outcome of tension-free vaginal tape. Eur Urol 2003; 43(3):288–92.

66. Lovatsis D, Gupta C, Dean E, et al. Tension-free vaginal tape procedure is an ideal treatment for obese patients. Am J Obstet Gynecol 2003;189(6):1601–4.

67. Skriapas K, Poulakis V, Dillenburg W, et al. Tension-free vaginal tape (TVT) in morbidly obese patients with severe urodynamic stress incontinence as last option treatment. Eur Urol 2006;49(3):544–50.

68. Hellberg D, Holmgren C, Lanner L, et al. The very obese woman and the very old woman: tension-free vaginal tape for the treatment of stress urinary incontinence. Int Urogynecol J 2007;18:423–9.

69. Liu PE, Su CH, Lau HH, et al. Outcome of tension-free obturator tape procedures in obese and overweight women. Int Urogynecol J 2011;22(3):259–63.

70. Haverkorn R, Williams B, Kubricht W III, et al. Is obesity a risk factor for failure and complications after surgery for incontinence and prolapse in women? J Urol 2011;185:987–92.

71. Morse AN, Labin LC, Young SB, et al. Exclusion of elderly women from published randomized trials of stress incontinence surgery. Obstet Gynecol 2004; 104:498–503.

72. Sevestre S, Ciofu C, Deval B, et al. Results of the tension-free vaginal tape procedure in the elderly. Eur Urol 2003;44:128–31.

73. Groutz A, Cohen A, Gold R, et al. The safety and efficacy of the "inside-out" trans-obturator TVT in elderly versus younger stress-incontinent women: a prospective study of 353 consecutive patients. Neurourol Urodyn 2011;30:380–3.

74. Morgan JE, Farrow GA, Stewart FE. The Marlex sling operation for the treatment of recurrent stress urinary incontinence: a 16-year review. Am J Obstet Gynecol 1985;151:224–6.

75. Faerber GJ. Urethral diverticulectomy and pubovaginal sling for simultaneous treatment of urethral diverticulum and intrinsic sphincter deficiency. Tech Urol 1998;4:192–7.

76. Carey MP, Goh JT, Fynes MM, et al. Stress urinary incontinence after delayed primary closure of genitourinary fistula: a technique for surgical management. Am J Obstet Gynecol 2002;186:948–53.

77. McGuire EJ, Wang CC, Usitalo H, et al. Modified pubovaginal sling in girls with myelodysplasia. J Urol 1988;139:524.

78. Austin PF, Westney OL, Leng WW, et al. Advantages of rectus fascial slings for urinary incontinence in children with neuropathic bladders. J Urol 2001; 165:2369–71.

Role of Autologous Bladder-Neck Slings
A Urogynecology Perspective

Dani Zoorob, MD[a], Mickey Karram, MD[a,b],*

KEYWORDS

- Stress urinary incontinence • Intrinsic sphincter deficiency • Autologous bladder-neck sling
- Pubovaginal sling

KEY POINTS

- Indications for autologous slings have recently increased.
- Good outcomes have been documented when performed for primary or recurrent SUI.
- Tensioning of autologous slings should be tailored based on the amount of urethral mobility and severity of incontinence.

INTRODUCTION

The concept of using a patient's own tissue as a "sling" to support under the urethra dates to the beginning of the twentieth century; however, it was not until the last quarter of the century that the procedure gained widespread appreciation and evolved into its current identity. Initially the procedure was described as using a strip of mobilized abdominal muscle (either rectus or pyramidalis). One end of the strip was freed from its attachment, passed under the bladder neck, then reaffixed to the abdominal muscle wall, thus forming a U-shaped sling of muscle tissue around the bladder outlet. Subsequently, overlying abdominal fascia was also included in the sling, and eventually replaced the muscle altogether. The final innovation involved using an isolated strip of fascia suspended by free sutures that were then tied to the abdominal wall directly or on top of the abdominal rectus sheath.

Despite its roots as an autologous procedure, many different types of materials have been used as sling substitutions, including various sources of autologous tissue, allograft tissue, xenograft tissue, and synthetic material. Almost all of these attempts at substitution have been made in an effort to limit patient morbidity, as the procedure requires the additional morbidity of a sling tissue harvest site. Nevertheless, in its most popular variety, the pubovaginal sling remains associated with the use of autologous rectus abdominis fascia. Regardless of the material used, the pubovaginal sling is meant to be placed at the junction of the proximal urethra and bladder neck for purposes of supporting the urethra, thus augmenting intraurethral pressure and deficient proximal sphincteric function.

The concept of the autologous pubovaginal sling involves supporting the proximal urethra and bladder neck with a piece of graft material, achieving continence either by providing a direct compressive force on the urethra/bladder outlet or by reestablishing a reinforcing platform or hammock against which the urethra is compressed during transmission of increased abdominal pressure. The sling is suspended with free sutures on each end that are attached either directly to the abdominal wall musculature or, more commonly, tied to each other on the anterior

[a] Department of Obstetrics and Gynecology, Division of Female Pelvic Medicine and Reconstructive Surgery, The Christ Hospital/University of Cincinnati, 231 Albert Sabin Way, Cincinnati, OH 45267, USA; [b] The Christ Hospital, 2123 Auburn Avenue, Suite 307, Cincinnati, OH 45219, USA
* Corresponding author. The Christ Hospital, 2123 Auburn Avenue, Suite 307, Cincinnati, OH 45219.
E-mail address: Mickey.karram@thechristhospital.com

Urol Clin N Am 39 (2012) 311–316
http://dx.doi.org/10.1016/j.ucl.2012.06.009

surface of the abdominal wall. The long-term success of the procedure relies not on the integrity of the suspensory sutures, but rather on the healing and fibrotic process involving the sling, which occurs primarily where the sling passes through the endopelvic fascia.

INDICATIONS

The pubovaginal sling remains an option as a procedure for stress urinary incontinence (SUI). Although pioneered as a surgical option for intrinsic sphincter deficiency (ISD), its indications have been broadened to encompass all types of SUI. Owing to its reliable results and durable outcomes, it is considered to be the one of the main standards of treatment of SUI and has been used extensively as a primary therapy for SUI, both for ISD and urethral hypermobility, as a salvage procedure for recurrent SUI, as an adjunct for urethral and bladder reconstruction, and even as a way to functionally "close" the urethra to abandon urethral access to the bladder altogether. In the authors' opinion, other indications are in patients with SUI who decline to have a synthetic material implanted because of long-term concerns related to synthetic mesh. Moreover, women who have recurrent incontinence after a synthetic sling or have had a complication after a synthetic sling such as a vaginal erosion may be good candidates for the autologous sling. Finally, the authors prefer to use an autologous sling in patients who have been radiated or who have had urethral injuries, and patients who are undergoing either simultaneous or prior urethrovaginal fistula or diverticulum repair.

SLING MATERIALS

Several different types of materials have been tried and investigated for use as a pubovaginal sling. The two most common autologous tissues are rectus abdominis fascia and fascia lata. Both have been extensively studied and have proved to be efficacious and reliable. Of the two, most surgeons prefer rectus fascia as an autologous material because it is easier and quicker to harvest.

Other biological materials that have been used include allogenic (ie, cadaveric) and xenogenic tissues. Cadaveric fascia lata and cadaveric dermis provide reasonable efficacy; however, durability of results remains an issue, as high failure rates have been reported in some studies. Bovine and porcine dermis as well as porcine small intestine submucosa (SIS) have also demonstrated acceptable efficacy for SUI but, again, durability remains a concern.

Synthetic graft materials of various designs and substances have also been used as sling material. As with other types of synthetic graft materials, monofilament, large-pore weave grafts (type 1 mesh) are recommended for implantation in the vagina. Good efficacy can be achieved with synthetic mesh; however, this mesh also poses risks of serious complications, including infection, vaginal extrusion, and genitourinary erosion, and is currently not recommended for use underneath the proximal urethra or bladder neck.

TECHNIQUE FOR HARVEST OF RECTUS FASCIA AND PLACEMENT OF PUBOVAGINAL SLING

1. *Preoperative considerations.* Pubovaginal sling procedures are generally performed under general anesthesia, but spinal or epidural anesthesia is also possible. Full patient paralysis is not warranted, but may facilitate rectus fascia closure after fascial harvest. Perioperative antibiotics are usually administered with appropriate skin and vaginal floral coverage, for example, a cephalosporin or fluoroquinolone. (This has now become a mandated quality-of-care measure in the United States.)

2. *Positioning.* The patient is placed in the low lithotomy position with legs in stirrups, and the abdomen and perineum are sterilely prepared and draped to provide access to the vagina and the lower abdomen. The bladder is drained with a Foley catheter. A weighted vaginal speculum is placed, and either lateral labial retraction sutures are placed or a self-retaining retractor system is used to facilitate vaginal exposure.

3. *Abdominal incision.* An 8- to 10-cm Pfannensteil incision is made (approximately 3–5 cm above the pubic bone) and the dissection is carried down to the level of the rectus fascia with a combination of electrocautery and blunt dissection, sweeping the fat and subcutaneous tissue clear of the rectus tissue.

4. *Fascial harvest.* Harvest of the rectus abdominis fascia can be performed in a transverse or vertical orientation. Typically a fascial segment measuring at least 8 cm in length and 1.5 to 2 cm in width is harvested. The fascial segment to be resected is delineated with a surgical marking pen or electrocautery, then incised sharply with a scalpel, scissors, or electrocautery along the drawn lines. Although virgin fascia is preferred, the presence of fibrotic rectus fascia does not prohibit its use. If resecting the

fascia close and parallel to the symphysis pubis, it is advisable to leave at least 0.5 to 1 cm attached, so as to facilitate closure and approximation to the superior fascial edge. Use of small Army/Navy retractors permits aggressive retraction of skin edges, thus allowing access through a smaller skin incision.

5. *Fascial defect closure.* The fascial defect is closed using a heavy-gauge (#1 or #0) delayed absorbable suture in a running fashion. Mobilization of the rectus abdominis fascial edges may be required to ensure appropriate tension-free approximation. It is important to ensure that adequate anesthesia with muscular relaxation/paralysis are present when the closure is being done.

6. *Preparation of fascia.* To prepare the fascial sling for use, a #1 permanent (eg, polypropylene) suture is affixed to each end using a running stitch to secure the suture to the sling. Defatting of the sling may be done if necessary.

7. *Vaginal dissection.* Vaginal dissection proceeds with a midline or inverted "U" incision. Injectable-grade saline or local analgesic, such as 1% lidocaine, may be used to hydrodissect the subepithelial tissues. Vaginal flaps are created with sufficient mobility so as to ensure tension-free closure over the sling. Dissection is carried laterally and anteriorly until the endopelvic fascia is encountered. The endopelvic fascia is incised and dissected from the posterior surface of the pubis to enter the retropubic space. This dissection can at times be done bluntly but often, especially in recurrent cases, requires sharp dissection with Mayo scissors.

8. *Passing retropubic needles or clamp.* Stamey needles or long clamps are passed through the retropubic space from the open abdominal wound immediately posterior to the pubic bone, approximately 4 cm apart. Distal control of the needles is maintained by finger guidance through the vaginal incision, and the tip of the needle is advanced adjacent to the posterior surface of the pubic bone so as to avoid inadvertent bladder injury. Proper bladder drainage must be assured to minimize injury to the bladder, which may be closely adherent to the pubis, especially if a prior retropubic procedure, as in the case presented, has been previously performed.

9. *Cystoscopy to rule out injury.* Careful cystoscopic examination of the bladder after passing the needles is mandatory to rule out inadvertent bladder injury. As the injuries to the bladder typically occur at the 1 o'clock and 11 o'clock positions, use of the 70° lens is warranted, and the bladder must be completely filled to expand any mucosal redundancy. Wiggling the needles or clamps can help to localize their position relative to the bladder wall.

10. *Deploying the sling.* The free ends of the sutures affixed to the sling are threaded into the ends of the Stamey needles or grasped with the clamp, and each suture is pulled up to the anterior abdominal wall through the retropubic space. Care is taken to maintain the orientation of the sling so that it is centered and flat at the bladder-neck area.

11. Some surgeons prefer to fix the sling in the midline to the underlying periurethral tissue with numerous delayed absorbable sutures. The authors, however, prefer to leave the sling unattached to the underlying urethra and bladder neck.

12. *Tensioning of the sling.* Various techniques for tensioning are applicable. To ensure adequate "looseness," the authors prefer to tie the sutures across the midline while holding a right-angled clamp between the sling material and the posterior urethral surface. Tensioning of the sling may also be accomplished by direct vision of proximal/bladder-neck coaptation with rigid cystoscopy while gently pulling up on the free ends of the sling sutures.

13. The abdominal skin incision is closed with 3-0 and 4-0 absorbable sutures. The vaginal mucosa is closed with 3-0 absorbable sutures. The authors prefer to close the vagina after the tensioning procedure has been completed, whereas some surgeons complete this step before the tensioning.

14. A bladder catheter is left indwelling and a vaginal gauze packing is placed. The catheter and vaginal packing may be removed after 24 hours. If the patient is unable to void, she is taught intermittent self-catheterization or an indwelling Foley is left in place for 1 week.

HARVEST OF AUTOLOGOUS FASCIA LATA

Autologous tissue from the iliotibial fascial band of the lateral thigh (fascia lata) has been used with great success as an alternative to abdominal rectus fascia for a pubovaginal sling. While incurring the morbidity of a secondary incision at a site remote from the abdomen, harvesting fascia lata may be suitable in cases where abdominal fascia may be of poor quality or extensive abdominal procedures have been previously performed, or in patients with significant central obesity or large pannus.

Harvest of fascia lata may require separate positioning, skin preparation, and sterile draping in addition to that for the vaginal procedure. To access the lateral aspect of the distal thigh, the leg is medially rotated and adducted. Two transverse incisions, approximately 5 to 6 cm in length, are made: the distal approximately 4 to 6 cm superior to the lateral femoral condyle and the proximal 8 cm cranially to the first. The incision is carried down through the fatty tissue to the level of the fascia, and the fascia cleared either sharply or bluntly for an appropriate distance to attain a graft 8 × 2 cm in size. The fascial strip is harvested, using both incisions as needed for exposure. Once the graft is removed the fascial defect is not repaired, and the subcutaneous tissue and skin are closed in multiple layers with absorbable suture. A Penrose drain can be secured in place through a separate stab incision and may be removed after 24 hours. Alternatively, a dedicated fascial stripper may be used for graft harvest when a full strip of fascia is desired.

OUTCOMES

The literature shows that pubovaginal slings are highly effective, with success rates between 50% and 75% when followed for up to 10 years.[1] In 2011, a review reported 4-year follow-up with improvement or cure in 100% of patients with uncomplicated stress incontinence and up to 93% in the more complicated cases.[2] The same investigators reported that most failures were due to urge incontinence and happened within the first 6 months postoperatively; 3% of these urge patients were thought to have developed de novo urge incontinence.

Other studies, however, have reported development of de novo urgency and storage symptoms in up to 23% of the patients, with 11% of patients reporting voiding dysfunctions and up to 7.8% requiring long-term self-catheterization.[1] The few randomized controlled trials (RCTs) comparing pubovaginal slings with tension-free vaginal tape (TVT) slings have had flawed methodology, so their outcomes are questionable.[3] Basok and colleagues[4] showed an increased rate of de novo urgency in the pubovaginal sling group compared with the intravaginal slingplasty group, whereas Sharifiaghdas and Mortazavi[5] showed equal efficacy between pubovaginal and TVT retropubic midurethral synthetic slings. The most scientifically valid RCT was by Arunkalaivanan and Barrington[6] in 2003, which showed equal subjective cure rates and complication rates when a biological pubovaginal sling was compared with a TVT sling. In this study, the pubovaginal sling was of porcine origin. When comparing autologous

versus allograft slings, Flynn and Yap[7] showed equal effectiveness in control of stress incontinence over 2 years, with reduced postoperative discomfort in the allograft group. Both groups had recurrent SUI develop in up to 10% of patients. Autologous pubovaginal slings were compared with Burch colposuspension in a multicenter RCT (SISTEr Trial), which showed superiority of fascial slings in controlling incontinence, despite an increased morbidity profile.[8] A meta-analysis in 2010 compared pubovaginal and midurethral synthetic slings, noting equal subjective cure rates as well as equal overall effectiveness.[3]

COMPLICATIONS AND SURGICAL TIPS
Needle Bladder Injuries

Should inadvertent bladder injury occur during retropubic passage of the Stamey needles be recognized on cystoscopy, the needle can simply be withdrawn and repassed through the retropubic space, and the procedure continued as planned. Unrecognized bladder injury can result in serious complications related to foreign-body reactions in the bladder, including suture and sling erosion in the bladder, stone formation, and voiding dysfunction.

Pelvic Visceral Injuries and Blood Loss

Pelvic visceral injuries and pelvic hematomas are rare, and can be avoided or minimized by adequate dissection of the endopelvic fascia and retropubic space, and careful needle passage in close proximity to the posterior surface of the pubic bone with distal needle control by the surgeon's finger. If an inadvertent cystotomy or urethrotomy occurs, the injury should be appropriately repaired. In contrast to synthetic sling placement, which would commonly require aborting the procedure, a biological sling could still be placed after concurrent intraoperative repair of the injury.

Miscellaneous Surgical Complications

Superficial wound infection, subcutaneous seromas, and abdominal fascial hernias are uncommon. In obese patients, the use of a subcutaneous drain may be necessary to prevent fluid loculations. Sling erosions with autologous tissue are exceedingly rare.

Voiding Dysfunction

Transient urinary retention may occur in up to 20% of patients and requires intermittent self-catheterization until resolution (typically 2–4 weeks). Prolonged (persisting longer than 4–6 weeks) postoperative voiding dysfunction, including de novo urgency, urgency incontinence, and/or obstructive symptoms, may occur to some degree in up to 25% of patients. Fewer than 3% of women require subsequent urethrolysis for treatment of prolonged retention/obstructive voiding symptoms. Some surgeons routinely teach patients intermittent self-catheterization in the preoperative period to facilitate its use, if necessary, postoperatively.

Technical Tips

1. Given that substantial bleeding can occur during vaginal dissection, harvesting the autologous fascia and preparing the sling by affixing sutures should be performed first, before vaginal dissection, such that the sling may be inserted and deployed in a timely manner and blood loss can be minimized. Retropubic bleeding occurring during dissection will almost always resolve with sling placement, and time should not be expended with prolonged attempts at hemostasis.

2. When performing an autologous pubovaginal sling procedure in the setting of urethral reconstruction (eg, urethrovaginal fistula or diverticulum resection) or as tissue interposition, harvesting fascia, preparing and deploying the sling with passage of the retropubic sutures, but not tensioning should all be performed before the delicate urethral reconstruction. Once the reconstruction is finished, the sling can be affixed in the appropriate location and tensioned. Damage to the reconstruction can occur through traction or direct injury if the sling is deployed after reconstruction.

3. Surface orientation of the autologous sling material during placement of the graft does not matter; by convention, the body-"side" or underside of the graft is placed on the body-"side" of the patient.

4. Sling tensioning, for most women, can be accomplished with the "2-finger" distance over the fascia. However, in women who have had multiple procedures and have a nonmobile urethra, the sling tension should be more significant, using a 1-fingerbreadth knot with concomitant cystoscopic evidence of an impression ("lip or ledge") being created on the ventrum of the urethra.

SUMMARY

Pubovaginal slings using a biologic sling material (whether autologous, allograft, or xenograft) can be used successfully to manage primary or recurrent stress incontinence.

EDITOR'S COMMENTS

Autologous slings remain a viable alternative for the surgical management of urinary incontinence. Autologous slings can be used both in previously non-operated patients as well as in those who have undergone multiple prior procedures. The technique is well standardized and the editors both make use of smaller sling length (7–8 cm) to reduce the morbidity associated with the harvest site. Autologous slings may be used in circumstances where urethral damage is either encountered or urethral reconstruction is necessary. The American Urological Association's guidelines for female stress urinary incontinence has emphasized the importance of autologous sling use in circumstances of urethral diverticulectomy, concomitant stress incontinence, and urethral reconstruction or in the circumstance of the need for excision of a synthetic sling with associated urethral injury requiring simultaneous management of urinary incontinence.

Autologous slings are not without morbidity and have been shown to have a slightly higher rate of obstructive voiding patterns postoperatively as compared to midurethral slings. They also have morbidity associated with the donor site. A longer time to return to resumption of normal voiding in some patients is experienced and patients should be aware of the potential need for intermediate-term catheterization and dysfunctional voiding until urinary tract normalization occurs postoperatively. As is noted in the two articles on autologous slings, careful attention to detail is important to ensure optimization of this procedure. Sling tensioning is a critical aspect to procedural success and can be varied dependent upon the patient's presentation (degree of hypermobility and associated urethral reconstruction, for instance).

The longest term results available in the medical evidence are related to the sling and demonstrate the robustness of this procedure as an option in the management of urinary incontinence. Clearly, the autologous sling is not indicated for all patients in an era of simpler ambulatory procedures, however, this procedure remains an option in the complicated patient or in the patient who has concerns regarding non-self graft insertion. It is the editors' procedure of choice in complicated reconstructive procedures as well as in those circumstances where urethral patency is suspect.

Roger R. Dmochowski, MD
Mickey Karram, MD

REFERENCES

1. Norton P, Brubaker L. Urinary incontinence in women. Lancet 2006;367:57–67.
2. Blaivas JG, Chaikin DC. Pubovaginal fascial sling for the treatment of all types of stress urinary incontinence: surgical technique and long-term outcome [review]. Urol Clin North Am 2011;38(1):7–15, v.
3. Novara G, Artibani W, Barber MD, et al. Updated systematic review and meta-analysis of the comparative data on colposuspensions, pubovaginal slings, and midurethral tapes in the surgical treatment of female stress urinary incontinence. Eur Urol 2010; 58(2):218–38.
4. Basok EK, Yildirim A, Atsu N, et al. Cadaveric fascia lata versus intravaginal slingplasty for the pubovaginal sling: surgical outcome, overall success and patient satisfaction rates. Urol Int 2008;80:46–51.
5. Sharifiaghdas F, Mortazavi N. Tension-free vaginal tape and autologous rectus fascia pubovaginal sling for the treatment of urinary stress incontinence: a medium-term follow-up. Med Princ Pract 2008;17:209–14.
6. Arunkalaivanan AS, Barrington JW. Randomized trial of porcine dermal sling (Pelvicol implant) vs. tension-free vaginal tape (TVT) in the surgical treatment of stress incontinence: a questionnaire- based study. Int Urogynecol J Pelvic Floor Dysfunct 2003; 14:17–23.
7. Flynn BJ, Yap WT. Pubovaginal sling using allograft fascia lata versus autograft fascia for all types of stress urinary incontinence: 2-year minimum followup. J Urol 2002;167(2 Pt 1):608–12.
8. Albo ME, Richter HE, Brubaker L, et al, Urinary Incontinence Treatment Network. Burch colposuspension versus fascial sling to reduce urinary stress incontinence. N Engl J Med 2007;356:2143–55.

Contemporary Role of Autologous Fascial Bladder Neck Slings: A Urology Perspective

Melissa R. Kaufman, MD, PhD

KEYWORDS

- Pubovaginal sling • Autologous fascia • Urinary incontinence

KEY POINT

- Autologous fascial pubovaginal slings remain a durable therapy for female stress urinary incontinence.
- Fasical slings are particularly indicated for cases of complex intrinsic sphincteric deficiency, concomitant urethral reconstruction, and recurrent incontinence.
- Counseling regarding risks of de novo voiding dysfunction and obstruction is critical to insure outcomes match patient expectations.

INTRODUCTION

Contemporary urologists have witnessed immense advances in the treatment of female stress urinary incontinence (SUI) in the past decade. A plethora of innovative technologies have emerged as a result of increased understanding of the pathophysiology of SUI, with the application of midurethral slings (MUSs) revolutionizing treatment of SUI.[1] Relative ease of the MUS procedure has allowed practitioners not formerly familiar with the intricacies of pubovaginal slings (PVSs) to successfully treat patients with SUI. However, this expansion of technology has been accompanied by increasing incidence of complications related to the use of mesh in women treated for SUI, including vaginal extrusions, erosions into the urinary tract, chronic pain, and sexual dysfunction.[2] Mesh MUSs are not appropriate for every indication, and traditional methods such as the autologous fascial PVS remain the gold standard of treatment based on longevity of results and adaptability of the procedure to a vast array of circumstances. This article reviews the current indications for autologous fascial PVSs and data

regarding sling outcomes, and details the operative technique for fascial harvest and sling placement.

INDICATIONS

The ideal sling would be effective, durable, straightforward to insert, minimally invasive, associated with low morbidity, affordable, and applicable to all types of SUI. Although it is becoming rapidly evident that MUS technologies may possess many of these model sling traits, treatment of all types of SUI is not among the attributes. Numerous criteria should be measured when creating an algorithm for sling placement.[3] Specific clinical scenarios to consider that may be best served by an autologous fascial PVS include women with intrinsic sphincter deficiency and a fixed urethra,[4] simultaneous prolapse repair,[5,6] concomitant urethral surgery such as diverticulectomy or fistula repair,[7,8] and urethral reconstruction secondary to trauma.[9] In all of these high-risk circumstances, use of autologous fascia is preferable over the synthetic MUS tapes. Although significant controversy continues regarding treatment of

Department of Urologic Surgery, Vanderbilt University, A-1302 Medical Center North, Nashville, TN 37232, USA
E-mail address: melissa.kaufman@vanderbilt.edu

Urol Clin N Am 39 (2012) 317–323
doi:10.1016/j.ucl.2012.05.004
0094-0143/12/$ – see front matter © 2012 Elsevier Inc. All rights reserved.

urologic.theclinics.com

MUS failures, the PVS remains a primary option for failed alternative incontinence procedures.[10,11] Autologous slings may also serve as an excellent alternative to bladder neck closure in populations with supravesical diversion, such as suprapubic catheter or bladder augmentation with continent catheterizable channels.[12,13]

Based on panel consensus, the American Urological Association (AUA) guidelines for SUI indicate that synthetic sling surgery is contraindicated in patients with concurrent urethrovaginal fistula, urethral erosion, intraoperative urethral injury, or urethral diverticulum. Although sparse standardized data exist specifically on these special circumstances, panel members recommend preferential use of autologous fascial or other biologic materials in these circumstances.[14]

Although a variety of autologous tissues have been examined through the years, only rectus fascia and fascia lata have substantial evidence to support current consideration. Both autografts by definition have proven noncarcinogenic and nonallergenic, and fascia has been proven a durable medium to potentiate long-term efficacy.[15] Most postoperative complications with autologous fascial harvest are related to abdominal hernia and wound infection.[16]

In addition to autografts, wide arrays of allografts and xenografts have been analyzed for treatment of SUI and pelvic organ prolapse.[16] Although many of these materials have proven to be biocompatible and certainly decrease the morbidity of autologous fascial harvest, long-term efficacy rates may eventually preclude preferential use of these materials, with sparse data available to guide practitioner choice.[14]

OPERATIVE TECHNIQUE

Current AUA guidelines for perioperative antimicrobial treatment include a first- or second-generation cephalosporin or an aminoglycoside with the addition of metronidazole or clindamycin.[17] Deep vein thrombosis prophylaxis should be used per AUA guidelines; however, for most patients, pneumatic compression devices are sufficient.[18] The patient is positioned in the dorsal lithotomy position, with care to not excessively elevate or hyperextend the legs. After appropriate skin preparation, a 16F balloon catheter is inserted into the bladder. Fascial harvest begins with a 6- to 8-cm transverse Pfannenstiel incision approximately 2 cm above the pubic symphysis. Dissection is carried down through subcutaneous tissue until rectus fascia is readily identified. It is important to clear enough adipose and connective

tissue off the rectus fascia so as to allow a clean closure without overdissection and creation of a potential space that may allow seroma formation. Exposure of the fascia by an assistant with Richardson retractors is often sufficient for excellent visualization. Using a surgical marking pen, the fascial sling is marked out as an 8 to 10 cm × 2 cm strip approximately 2 to 3 cm above the pubis (**Fig. 1**). Creating the harvest too close to the pubis will limit the capacity to dissect, and hinder adequate mobility for fascial closure. The fascia is then scored with electrocautery to outline the eventual harvest, because distortion is likely during the harvest (**Fig. 2**). The fascial sling is raised from the rectus muscle and cut with electrocautery. Great care should be taken to not enter the underlying muscle or midline, because often patients have undergone prior operations and have substantial scar tissue in this area (**Fig. 3**). Once the fascia is harvested, it is placed in normal saline on the back table and #1 polydioxanone sutures are secured on each end of the strip in a horizontal mattress fashion at right angles to the fiber direction. These sutures remain long for passage through the retropubic space (**Fig. 4**). Fascial edges are raised with Allis clamps and undermined circumferentially with electrocautery to allow sufficient mobility for a tension-free closure (**Fig. 5**). Fascia may then be approximated in a running fashion with #1 polydioxanone sutures. The wound is packed with saline or antibiotic-soaked sponges and attention is turned to the vaginal portion of the procedure.

For the vaginal dissection, exposure is first obtained with placement of a weighted vaginal speculum. Labial retraction may be required in some instances and achieved with either silk retraction sutures or a ring retractor. A semilunar inverted U incision is marked out on the anterior vaginal wall from the bladder neck, identified with gentle traction of the catheter to identify the

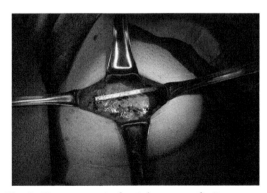

Fig. 1. Measurement of autologous graft site.

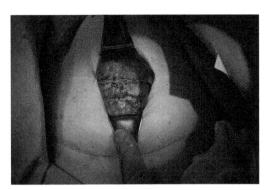

Fig. 2. Scoring of fascial graft.

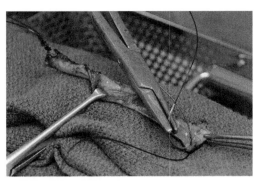

Fig. 4. Suture passage in fascial graft.

balloon, to the mid urethra. The vesicovaginal space is hydrodistended with sterile saline to facilitate the dissection. The initial incision is created with a scalpel, and the avascular plane superficial to the pubocervical fascia is carefully dissected with Metzenbaum scissors with traction from an Allis clamp on the vaginal epithelium (**Fig. 6**). Palpation of the depth of dissection is a critical aspect of the procedure, because a dissection too deep into detrusor fibers will result in not only bleeding but also potential entry into the urethral or bladder lumen. The proper plane on the vaginal wall has a characteristic shiny white appearance.

Dissection is then accomplished laterally toward the ipsilateral shoulder under the vaginal mucosa until the ischiopubic ramus is palpated (**Fig. 7**). The concavity of the scissors should be maintained laterally to avoid damage to the urethra or bladder. Sufficient space is required to pass the sling, which can be approximated by a finger-breadth. Once the pubis is palpated, the scissors are maintained in the superolateral direction toward the ipsilateral shoulder and the endopelvic fascia is pierced directly under the bone. Once the endopelvic fascia is opened, the retropubic space is entered bluntly with finger dissection and a

sweeping motion cranially is used to free the bladder neck and urethral attachments behind the pubis. In complex cases with significant retropubic scarring, it may be preferable to leave the fascial incision open to directly palpate the tract from the abdominal incision and direct guidance with the vaginally placed finger for passage of the suture ligature needle. In reoperative cases, brisk bleeding is not uncommon once the endopelvic fascia is perforated, and is often best managed with direct pressure and expeditious passage of the sling. Ligature passing instruments, such as Stamey needles or Tonsil clamps, are used to pass from the suprapubic incision into the vaginal incision on either side of the bladder neck with direct finger guidance (**Fig. 8**). After ensuring the bladder is empty, a finger is placed into the vaginal incision behind the pubis and the ligature passing instrument is inserted in a stab incision through the rectus fascia approximately 2 cm laterally from midline directly on the pubic bone. The ligature passing instrument is walked along the bone cranially and enters the retropubic space adjacent to bone. Once behind bone, the passer is angled toward the vagina and should be directly

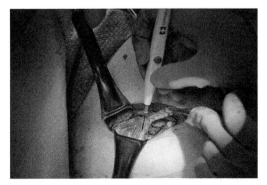

Fig. 3. Raising graft above rectus.

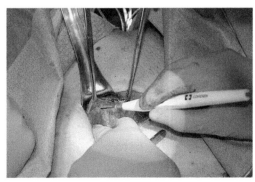

Fig. 5. Mobilization of rectus fascial edges for tension-free closure.

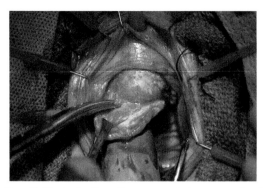

Fig. 6. Vaginal dissection around large urethral diverticulum.

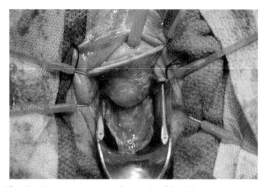

Fig. 8. Ligature passers in vaginal incision.

palpated and guided into the vaginal wound on the fingertip. Once the passer is visible in the vaginal wound, the procedure is repeated on the contralateral side.

A critical component of the procedure is cystoscopy after needle passage. After catheter removal, rigid cystoscopy with both 30° and 70° lenses is undertaken to ensure no injury to the bladder or urethra during dissection or needle passage. Some surgeons additionally administer indigo carmine or methylene blue at this juncture to demonstrate efflux from both ureteral orifices, because the ureters are also at risk with the dissection, particularly in reoperative cases. During cystoscopy, attention should be focused on the dome, anterior wall of the bladder, and bladder neck to assess for the ligature passer within the lumen. If the passer is identified, it should be removed and the bladder drained, and passage may be reattempted with a more lateral entry through the rectus fascia. Patients who have had bladder injury after such trocar passage would likely benefit from several extra days of catheter placement to allow adequate healing.

Once the ligature passers have safely traversed into the vaginal incision, the sutures placed on the ends of the fascial harvest are looped through the passer eyelets (**Fig. 9**). The sling is then brought into position through extraction of the ligature passers back through the suprapubic incision. The ends of the suture are secured with a hemostat and not tied until after the vaginal incision is closed. The sling may be tacked to the periurethral fascia with several interrupted 3-0 absorbable sutures, such as polyglactin, to prevent migration. After irrigation of the vagina, the semilunar incision is closed in a running fashion with 2-0 absorbable sutures.

The sutures attached to the ends of the fascial graft are then extracted into the suprapubic incision and tied to one another over the rectus fascia. Because it is critical that the sling is not placed under excessive tension during this portion, several techniques may be used to ensure appropriate level of traction. First, two fingers may be placed underneath the suture above the rectus fascia to disallow tight approximation during typing. Some authors advocate performing the suture tying with a cystoscope in the bladder, placing downward pressure to depress the vesical

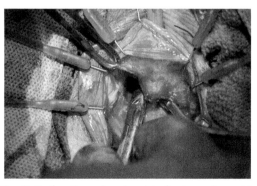

Fig. 7. Perforation of endopelvic fascia under pubic ramus.

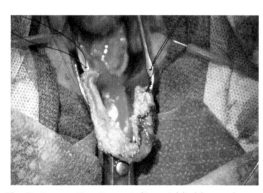

Fig. 9. Preparation to seat sling at bladder neck.

neck and putting the sling on stretch. Whichever maneuver is used, the important point is to secure the sling without tension to decrease postoperative voiding dysfunction. The suprapubic incision is then closed in several layers of absorbable suture. If a large amount of mobilization was required for fascial harvest or closure, or if the patient has significant pannus, the author prefers to use a Penrose drain overnight to prevent seroma formation, which may predispose to wound infection. A vaginal packing moistened with estrogen cream is placed and the bladder remains with catheter drainage for the immediate postoperative period.

POSTOPERATIVE MANAGEMENT

Gauze vaginal packing remains overnight. On postoperative day one, the patient may be given a voiding trial or may be discharged from the hospital with an indwelling catheter, depending on concomitant surgical procedures or comorbidities. Patients who are unable to void after catheter removal should first be instructed on self-intermittent catheterization. Because many transient causes of postoperative urinary retention are possible, such as local pain, edema, retropubic hematoma, and the effects of general anesthesia and narcotics on bladder function, several days of catheterization after pubovaginal sling placement is often required for the patient to regain normal micturition.[19] Most patients regain spontaneous voiding within 1 week. However, for refractory retention, the sling may be loosened or incised in the office or operating room.

Bladder outlet obstruction (BOO) is likely underestimated at approximately 2% after incontinence interventions. Even so, iatrogenic obstruction secondary to surgery for SUI is likely one of the most common causative factors for female BOO.[20] Obscuring analysis of the postoperative patient is the fact that persistent SUI, de novo bladder dysfunction, or even urinary tract infection can produce lower urinary tract symptoms (LUTS) and apparently obstructive symptoms in this population. Meta-analysis reveals the incidence of postoperative obstruction is specific for the type of incontinence procedure performed.[21] For autologous slings, the incidence of postoperative obstruction has been reported to range from 1% to 30%, depending on the individual author's definition of BOO. Overall, the described incidence of retention for more than 1 month after sling placement is 8%, with the risk of these obstructive symptoms persisting long term reported to be less than 5%.

In addition to obstructive voiding symptoms, up to 75% of patients may identify new-onset storage symptoms after SUI surgery.[22] Thus, before secondary surgical interventions to alleviate presumed BOO after SUI surgery, it is doubtless prudent to perform a complete evaluation, including physical examination, cystoscopy, and videourodynamics, although data do not suggest that any single urodynamic parameter will predict which patient will respond positively to urethrolysis.[23] If the patient has demonstrated BOO secondary to placement of an autologous fascial sling, attempts at loosening the sling with application of a traction dilator to the urethra may be successful in the very early postoperative period. This traction approach is not likely to yield encouraging results with midurethral synthetic tapes and should not be attempted with these implants.

The customary approach for treatment of documented long-term BOO after sling procedure for SUI is transvaginal or retropubic urethrolysis, or a combination of the two. The degree of urethral mobilization is surgeon-dependent and ranges from sling incision to substantial explant, but in general these procedures are able to ameliorate obstructive voiding in 70% to 80% of patients, although resolution of further LUTS in this population remains a troublesome entity.[24]

In addition to retention, postoperative concerns after PVS insertion include storage-predominant voiding dysfunction symptoms, vaginal extrusion, nerve injury, sexual dysfunction, fistula development, and de novo prolapse.[19]

OUTCOMES

Although used for more than 100 years, until recently the literature on fascial sling outcomes was consistently devoid of standardized procedures or reporting of outcome measures that surgeons could use to formulate clinical decisions. Fortunately, a landmark multicenter, randomized, controlled trial comparing the Burch colposuspension with the autologous rectus fascial sling conducted by the Urinary Incontinence Treatment Network provided a wealth of well-standardized outcomes to assess efficacy and complications of the PVS.[25] Analysis of a meticulously described group of 326 women randomized to PVS showed a stress incontinence–specific success rate of 66% at 24-month follow-up. Stringent criteria were applied to define success, including no self-reported symptoms of SUI, less than 15-g pad weight in 24 hours, no incontinence documented in a 3-day voiding diary, a negative urinary stress test on physical examination, and no retreatment for urinary incontinence. Although highly effective for SUI, the PVS was accompanied by higher rates of urinary tract infection, urge incontinence, voiding dysfunction, and need for surgical revision to improve voiding when compared with traditional colposuspension. Rates of voiding dysfunction for the autologous sling were 14%, with 24% displaying persistent urge incontinence. However, the 3% rate of de novo urge incontinence was identical to that of colposuspension.

A meta-analysis conducted by the AUA guidelines panel on SUI showed that patients not undergoing concurrent prolapse treatment had estimated cure/dry rates for autologous fascial PVS of 90% at 12 to 23 months and 82% at 48 months or longer.[14] Estimated rates of postsurgical urge incontinence were 33% in patients with preexisting urge incontinence symptoms, with a 9% rate of de novo urge incontinence. Retention rates were estimated at 8%. Complications included urinary tract infection (11%), bladder injury (4%), and wound complications (8%).

In addition to use in complex reconstruction, the autologous fascial PVS may also be considered as first-line therapy. Even in the era of MUS technology, primary use of PVS remains an appropriate option, particularly in situations of intrinsic sphincteric deficiency as defined by severity of Valsalva leak point pressure.[26] Increasing concerns regarding use of mesh for female reconstruction may also lead to patient preference for autologous or biologic materials.

SUMMARY

Fascial slings remain a successful and durable option for treatment of female SUI. With limited risk of disease transmission, extrusion, or complications associated with mesh, use of autologous fascia is an attractive option, particularly for complex reconstructive cases. With generally robust outcomes, the PVS also continues to be a viable option for treatment of primary SUI after appropriate patient counseling regarding risks of BOO and de novo urgency symptoms.

ACKNOWLEDGMENTS

The author wishes to express sincere appreciation for the intraoperative photographs and insightful discussions on female reconstructive surgery provided by Vanderbilt visiting scholar Juan Gabriel De Los Rios Posada.

EDITOR'S COMMENTS

Autologous slings remain a viable alternative for the surgical management of urinary incontinence. Autologous slings can be used both in previously non-operated patients as well as in those who have undergone multiple prior procedures. The technique is well standardized and the editors both make use of smaller sling length (7–8 cm) to reduce the morbidity associated with the harvest site. Autologous slings may be used in circumstances where urethral damage is either encountered or urethral reconstruction is necessary. The American Urological Association's guidelines for female stress urinary incontinence has emphasized the importance of autologous sling use in circumstances of urethral diverticulectomy, concomitant stress incontinence, and urethral reconstruction or in the circumstance of the need for excision of a synthetic sling with associated urethral injury requiring simultaneous management of urinary incontinence.

Autologous slings are not without morbidity and have been shown to have a slightly higher rate of obstructive voiding patterns postoperatively as compared to midurethral slings. They also have morbidity associated with the donor site. A longer time to return to resumption of normal voiding in some patients is experienced and patients should be aware of the potential need for intermediate-term catheterization and dysfunctional voiding until urinary tract normalization occurs postoperatively. As is noted in the two articles on autologous slings, careful attention to detail is important to ensure optimization of this procedure. Sling tensioning is a critical aspect to procedural success and can be varied dependent upon the patient's presentation (degree of hypermobility and associated urethral reconstruction, for instance).

The longest term results available in the medical evidence are related to the sling and demonstrate the robustness of this procedure as an option in the management of urinary incontinence. Clearly, the autologous sling is not indicated for all patients in an era of simpler ambulatory procedures, however, this procedure remains an option in the complicated patient or in the patient who has concerns regarding non-self graft insertion. It is the editors' procedure of choice in complicated reconstructive procedures as well as in those circumstances where urethral patency is suspect.

Roger R. Dmochowski, MD
Mickey Karram, MD

REFERENCES

1. Petros PE, Ulmsten UI. An integral theory of female urinary incontinence. Experimental and clinical considerations. Acta Obstet Gynecol Scand Suppl 1990;153:7–31.
2. Dmochowski RR, Padmanabhan PP, Scarpero HS. Slings: autologous, biologic, synthetic, and midurethral. In: Wein AJ, Kavoussi LR, Novick AC, et al, editors. Campbell's Urology. 10th edition. Philadelphia: Saunders; 2011. p. 2115–67.
3. Wilson WJ, Winters JC. Is there still a place for the pubovaginal sling at the bladder neck in the era of the midurethral sling? Curr Urol Rep 2005;6(5):335–9.
4. Blaivas JG, Chaikin DC. Pubovaginal fascial sling for the treatment of all types of stress urinary incontinence: surgical technique and long-term outcome. Urol Clin North Am 2011;38(1):7–15.
5. Cross CA, Cespedes RD, McGuire EJ. Treatment results using pubovaginal slings in patients with large cystoceles and stress incontinence. J Urol 1997;158(2):431–4.
6. Cross CA, Cespedes RD, McGuire EJ. Our experience with pubovaginal slings in patients with stress urinary incontinence. J Urol 1998;159(4):1195–8.
7. Faerber GJ. Urethral diverticulectomy and pubovaginal sling for simultaneous treatment of urethral diverticulum and intrinsic sphincter deficiency. Tech Urol 1998;4(4):192–7.
8. Leng WW, McGuire EJ. Management of female urethral diverticula: a new classification. J Urol 1998;160(4):1297–300.
9. Blaivas JG, Purohit RS. Post-traumatic female urethral reconstruction. Curr Urol Rep 2008;9(5):397–404.
10. Petrou SP, Frank I. Complications and initial continence rates after a repeat pubovaginal sling procedure for recurrent stress urinary incontinence. J Urol 2001;165(6 Pt 1):1979–81.
11. Giarenis I, Cardozo L. Management of stress urinary incontinence following a failed midurethral tape. Curr Bladder Dysfunct Rep 2011;6:67–9.
12. Gormley EA, Bloom DA, McGuire EJ, et al. Pubovaginal slings for the management of urinary incontinence in female adolescents. J Urol 1994;152(2 Pt 2):822–5 [discussion: 826–7].
13. Austin PF, Westney OL, Leng WW, et al. Advantages of rectus fascial slings for urinary incontinence in children with neuropathic bladders. J Urol 2001;165(6 Pt 2):2369–71 [discussion: 2371–2].
14. Dmochowski RR, Blaivas JM, Gormley EA, et al. Update of AUA guideline on the surgical management of female stress urinary incontinence. J Urol 2010;183(5):1906–14.
15. Woodruff AJ, Cole EE, Dmochowski RR, et al. Histologic comparison of pubovaginal sling graft materials: a comparative study. Urology 2008;72(1):85–9.
16. Gomelsky A, Dmochowski RR. Autograft, allograft, and xenograft slings: how are they different? Contemp Urol 2005;17(5):51–68.
17. Wolf JS Jr, Bennett CJ, Dmochowski RR, et al. Best practice policy statement on urologic surgery antimicrobial prophylaxis. J Urol 2008;179(4):1379–90.
18. Forrest JB, Clemens JQ, Finamore P, et al. AUA Best Practice Statement for the prevention of deep vein thrombosis in patients undergoing urologic surgery. J Urol 2009;181(3):1170–7.
19. Rovner ES. Complications of female incontinence surgery. In: Taneja SS, editor. Complications of urologic surgery. Philadelphia: Saunders Elselvie; 2010. p. 579–92.
20. Gomelsky A, Scarpero HM, Dmochowski RR. Sling surgery for stress urinary incontinence in the female: what surgery, which material? AUA Update Series 2003;22(34):266–76.
21. Leach GE, Dmochowski RR, Appell RA, et al. Female Stress Urinary Incontinence Clinical Guidelines Panel summary report on surgical management of female stress urinary incontinence. The American Urological Association. J Urol 1997;158(3 Pt 1):875–80.
22. McCrery R, Appell R. Transvaginal urethrolysis for obstruction after antiincontinence surgery. Int Urogynecol J Pelvic Floor Dysfunct 2007;18(6):627–33.
23. Lemack GE. Urodynamic assessment of bladder-outlet obstruction in women. Nat Clin Pract Urol 2006;3(1):38–44.
24. Starkman JS, Duffy JW 3rd, Wolter CE, et al. Refractory overactive bladder after urethrolysis for bladder outlet obstruction: management with sacral neuromodulation. Int Urogynecol J Pelvic Floor Dysfunct 2008;19(2):277–82.
25. Albo ME, Richter HE, Brubaker L, et al. Burch colposuspension versus fascial sling to reduce urinary stress incontinence. N Engl J Med 2007;356(21):2143–55.
26. Athanasopoulos A, Gyftopoulos K, McGuire EJ. Efficacy and preoperative prognostic factors of autologous fascia rectus sling for treatment of female stress urinary incontinence. Urology 2011;78(5):1034–8.

Vaginal Prolapse Repair
Suture Repair Versus Mesh Augmentation: A Urogynecology Perspective

Vincent Lucente, MD*, Miles Murphy, MD, MSPH,
Cristina Saiz, MD

KEYWORDS

- Vaginal prolapse repair • Urogynecology • Mesh augmentation • Pelvic organ prolapse
- Transvaginal mesh

KEY POINTS

- There is a growing body of evidence supporting the fact that in order to achieve long term durability in anatomical repair of anterior/apical defects the use of synthetic mesh augmentation is necessary.
- Although the ideal mesh is yet to be developed, current materials pose minimal risk to patients when properly implanted via a transvaginal route.
- Developing and propagating surgeon's expertise to perform transvaginal mesh surgery is no doubt our greatest challenge.

INTRODUCTION

Never before has there been more attention, if not intense debate, surrounding the various approaches to reconstructive pelvic surgery. The recent public health announcement (PHA) release from the Food and Drug Administration (FDA) regarding the use of transvaginal mesh no doubt rekindled the suture repair versus mesh augmentation discussion. Some of this activity is fueled by the age of information where there is almost instantaneous and widespread dissemination of each and every opinion. Further confounding factors are not only the blogging by patients but also the heightened legal climate scrutinizing both the pharmaceutical and medical device industry. All of this occurs within the backdrop of the expanding challenges facing effective surgical training and medical education beyond residency or fellowship to keep pace with the advances in surgical innovation and related technologies. This article highlights the evolving clinical-based experiences of the authors that are primarily grounded in reality-based medicine with consideration and incorporation of evidence-based medicine.[1]

Demographic factors are influencing the expectations and subsequent needs that female patients have regarding their overall pelvic health. Women are not only living longer than ever before but are also adopting more active and robust lifestyles in their senior years. Pelvic organ prolapse (POP) is the hidden epidemic. Demographic studies have shown that women aged more than 80 years are the fastest growing population segment in the United States and Canada. Over the next 30 years, the rate of women who will seek treatment of POP will double.[2] As a result, the sustained biomechanical and physical challenges to the pelvic support structures continue to exceed that experienced by women decades ago. More and more women continue to enter (and remain) in the workforce of physically demanding occupations.

St Luke's Hospital & Health Network, Department of OB/GYN, The Institute for Female Pelvic Medicine & Reconstructive Surgery, Hamilton Court Professional Center, 3050 Hamilton Boulevard, Suite 200, Allentown, PA 18103, USA
* Corresponding author.
E-mail address: vlucente@fpminstitute.com

Urol Clin N Am 39 (2012) 325–333
http://dx.doi.org/10.1016/j.ucl.2012.06.003

Further amplifying risk factors are the epidemic of obesity, history of tobacco exposure, and general reluctance to change delivery practices to mitigate obstetric trauma. Furthermore, basic science research has demonstrated that patients with POP have structurally altered collagen, elastin, laminin, and smooth muscle.[3–7] All of these demographic, genetic, or environmental factors have challenged the durability of traditional suture-based native tissue repair and created the impetus for pelvic reconstructive surgeons to seek the advantages of mesh-augmented repair.

How have we been doing with our suture repair procedures?

- There is an 11.2% lifetime risk of surgical intervention.[8]
- Twenty-nine percent to 40% of reconstructive procedures require surgical reintervention for failure within 3 years.[9]
- Sixty percent of recurrences are at the same site, most being the anterior compartment.[10]
- A total of 32.5% occur at a different site because of an unmasking of an occult support defect.
- Reoperation remains the beginning of a larger issue because women often settle with being *not as bad as before*, not wanting to go through surgery again.

THE RATIONALE BEHIND THE USE OF MESH-AUGMENTED REPAIR

The use of mesh materials in the repair of abdominal wall hernias has been proven to be substantially superior to suture-based repairs, with an associated significant decrease in the recurrence rate when mesh materials are used.[11] Obviously, the female pelvis is substantially different in many aspects when compared with the abdominal wall. Nonetheless, one needs to only consider the basic biophysical model of a human abdominal pelvic cavity to realize the challenge facing any nonmesh repair of the pelvic floor. As a result of our upright biped posture, the abdominal-pelvic cavity in humans is basically a mostly vertical-orientated, cylindrical-shaped body cavity filled with fluid and semisolid or gelatinous structures in which outward and downward vector forces are transmitted as a result of upright posture, diaphragmatic excursions, and gravity. Defects of the nondependent ventral surface of this cylinder, which is composed of dense, regular, connective tissue, carries a high recurrence rate with suture-based repair when compared with mesh repair, thus clearly establishing the medical necessity for the use of mesh. Therefore, it seems highly

implausible that in the most dependent aspect of this vertical cylindrical abdominal-pelvic cavity (the pelvic floor), in which there is mostly loose, irregular, connective tissue, suture-based repair will be able to provide durable anatomic success. This challenge is compounded by the loss of spinal curvature with the aging process, which had served to promote deflection of these downward force vectors, as well as age-related weakening of the levator ani muscle group, which had provided a dynamic trampoline under the connective tissue structures supporting the pelvic organs.

Contributing factors to surgical failure:

- Anatomic
  ○ Denervation, widening of levator hiatus, connective tissue damage
- Tissue Factors (collagen content and structure)
  ○ Genetics, race, age, concomitant disease (connective tissue, diabetes mellitus and so forth)
- Environmental Factors
  ○ Chronic straining, cough, smoking, nutrition, obesity, medications
- Surgical Factors
  ○ Poor choice/execution of procedure, failure to address all defects, suture failure, inadequate convalescence.

We must also recognize that after surgical repair, connective tissue healing or scarring does not replace or add tensile strength back to the original prefailure or nonprolapsed state. Thus, over time, suture repair will only eventually fail to restore and maintain normal anatomic position and function in many patients. In the anterior compartment, this high failure rate with suture repair has been well documented in several well-designed surgical trials.[12]

As mentioned, the vagina does have unique differences when compared with the abdominal wall. Some of these differences challenge both the material scientist bioengineers and the implanting surgeon.

Unique considerations to the vagina in the use of mesh-augmented repair

- Surgical site cannot be sterilized
- Relatively thin tissue overlay with no real fascial layer
- Attachment sites are difficult to surgically access
- Complex 3-dimensional architecture and vector forces
- Subjected to great forces with little or no bony reinforcement (and often poor pelvic floor muscle support)

- Must remain pliable for
  - Surrounding pelvic organ filling/emptying
  - Sexual function.

THE CONSTRUCT OF THE MESH IMPLANT

In addition to the knowledge of pelvic anatomy, it is also important to understand the properties of the individual mesh materials being used.

Characteristics of the ideal prosthetic implant[13]

- Biocompatible and chemically inert
- Does not induce an inflammatory response
- Not physically modified by tissue fluids
- Nonallergenic
- Noncarcinogenic
- Resistant to mechanical stress and infection
- Can be manufactured in the required shape for patients and can be sterilized
- Can prevent adhesion formation over the surfaces in direct contact with viscera
- Better in vivo response than autologous tissue
- No detrimental effect on pelvic function.

Synthetic mesh properties to consider include the following: the core material of the filaments used to construct the mesh, mesh structure (mono vs multi-filament; knitted vs woven), pore size, rigidity, elasticity, tensile strength or burst strength, thickness, and total mesh content per unit area.[14]

Of these parameters, pore size is essential when considering bacterial infection; generally, a pore size of more than 75 mm is desirable to allow the passage of leukocytes that are 9 to 15 μm in size and macrophages that are 16 to 20 μm in size. The problem with weaves and smaller pore sizes is that bacteria (on the order of <1 μm in size) can pass into the material but the hosts defense mechanisms (leukocytes and macrophages) cannot. The classification system by Amid and colleagues[15] is commonly used as the standard for porosity. Currently, most materials used in transvaginal placement are type I (macroporous and monofilamentous). Microporous materials can increase the rate of infection (often thought to be subclinical and perhaps related to exposure development) and can lead to graft encapsulation rather than graft integration.

Additional considerations for type I materials

- Weight (gram/square centimeter)
- Flexural rigidity (milligram/centimeter)
- Elasticity (percentage)
- Inflammatory response
- Degree of contraction (percentage)
- Porosity (total percentage)
- Softness (in vitro/vivo).

Most recently, the importance of changes in the biomechanical stimulus of the host tissue as a response to an implant has been recognized. This alteration in normal mechanical stimuli needed for surrounding host cell viability has been well described in the orthopedic literature as stress shielding. It has now been identified as a potential contributing factor in the outcome of mesh-augmented repairs.[16] This phenomenon occurs when surrounding host cells, such as myocytes and fibroblasts, are overprotected from normal physiologic vector forces that would stimulate cell growth and proliferation. As a result, when these cells are shielded from a desired biomechanical stimulus, they experience degeneration and eventual cell death. This finding sheds light on potential sources of certain complications, such as delayed exposures associated with mesh use. It also adds insight on further material science development in the biochemical properties of materials that may help avoid stress shielding (**Figs. 1** and **2**).

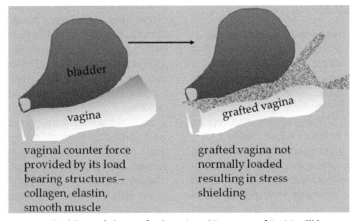

Fig. 1. Mesh results in stress shielding of the grafted vagina. (*Courtesy of* Dr Moalli.)

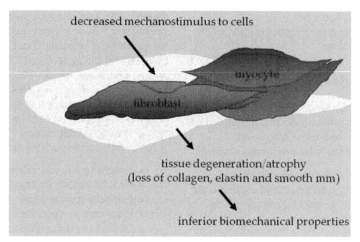

decreased mechanostimulus to cells

myocyte

fibroblast

tissue degeneration/atrophy
(loss of collagen, elastin and smooth mm)

inferior biomechanical properties

Fig. 2. Tissue function declines in grafted vagina. (*Courtesy of* Dr Moalli.)

It is well known that dyspareunia is a potential adverse event following any and all reconstructive pelvic surgery. Unfortunately, in some patients, it can be challenging to completely resolve. In an effort to decrease the rate of de novo dyspareunia that can be associated with transvaginal mesh placement, as well as to improve vaginal elasticity following pelvic reconstruction with mesh augmentation, some manufactures have developed products that contain a combination of both permanent and absorbable or biologic materials. Even though weight itself is not the only factor that dictates the stiffness of the mesh and its burden on the vagina, lighter and partially absorbable materials have been shown to induce less inflammatory reaction, possibly decreasing the mesh contraction/shrinkage effect.[17] Although newer, lighter-weight, and even hybrid synthetic polypropylene implants with sufficient mechanical strength and improved elasticity seem to be promising, a prosthesis that meets all of the criteria of the ideal implant does not currently exist.

THE EVOLVING EVIDENCE: SUTURE VERSUS MESH-AUGMENTED REPAIR

In 2008, a Cochrane review of the surgical management of pelvic organ prolapse in women found that the use of mesh or graft inlays at the time of anterior vaginal wall repair reduces the risk of recurrent prolapse.[18] Since 2008, several studies have been published that continue to support the anatomic superiority of mesh-augmented repairs over suture plication of native tissue (**Table 1**).

As these studies and others substantiated the anatomic superiority of mesh-augmented repairs in comparison with suture-based plication, there was still continued concern that perhaps the anatomic benefit was not worth the reported complications of mesh exposure or dyspareunia.

THE COMPLICATIONS OF EXPOSURE OR DYSPAREUNIA

The most common complication surrounding mesh-augmented repair is that of exposure of the mesh into the vaginal lumen. Obviously, exposure is not a potential complication of suture-only based repairs but it is a well-described and accepted low-rate complication of an abdominal sacrocolpopexy (ASC). In fact, in the often-cited colpopexy and urinary reduction efforts (CARE) trial, the exposure rate was 6.4%.[25] Surgical technique seems to play a significant role in the rate of mesh exposure after transvaginal mesh procedures because these rates vary greatly between studies (anywhere from 0%–29.7%). In fact, in one multicenter randomized control trial, the rate of erosion between sites ranged from 0% to 100%.[23] Because the same mesh and delivery system were used throughout the study, one can conclude that this variation is not a function of the mesh or the delivery system per se but a difference in surgical technique among the in-planting surgeons. In this same study, the investigators demonstrated that in more than half of the mesh exposures, the women were asymptomatic and only one-third required minor outpatient operative intervention. When looking at a large multicenter trial with more than 400 patients conducted by surgeons who perform the index surgery on a regular basis, the risk of exposure requiring a procedure to correct it was 3.2%.[24]

Several studies have reported the rate after transvaginal mesh placement to be higher than that reported in ASC. This finding is no doubt directly related to the technical challenge of achieving placement of the mesh material deep or behind all of the histologic layers composing the vaginal wall when dissecting through the vaginal wall. When the mesh enters the pelvis transabdominally, it

Table 1
Mesh versus no mesh outcomes

	Year	Mesh Type	Number of Patients	Length of Follow-up (mo)	Successful Outcome (%)
Sivaslioglu[19]	2007	Self-cut	45 mesh 45 no mesh	12	Mesh 91 No mesh 72
Nieminen[20]	2008	Self-cut	105 mesh 97 no mesh	24	Mesh 89 No mesh 59
Nguyen[21]	2008	Kit	38 mesh 37 no mesh	12	Mesh 87 No mesh 55
Carey[22]	2009	Self-cut	69 mesh 70 no mesh	12	Mesh 81 No mesh 67
Withagen[23]	2011	Kit	93 mesh 97 no mesh	12	Mesh 90 No mesh 55
Altman[24]	2011	Kit	200 mesh 189 no mesh	12	Mesh 61 No mesh 34

automatically resides behind the full thickness of the vaginal wall. If the surgeon uses a splitting dissection technique (dividing the vaginal wall between the epithelium and muscularis) instead of achieving a full-thickness vaginal wall dissection with entry into the true vesicovaginal space, the exposure rate will be undoubtedly higher than that seen after sacrocolpopexy procedures. Several investigators even recognized this suboptimal dissection during the timeframe of surgical trials, noticing that exposure rates decrease over time (despite the use of the same material), implying that the learning curve of the surgeon is a key factor. This real learning curve was documented in one multicenter trial of 22 surgeons at 13 sites noting a vast difference among exposure rates between the various surgeons despite the investigators being experienced pelvic surgeons.[23]

The adoption of the routine use of precise hydrodissection into the true vesicovaginal space was critical in the authors' development of proper full-thickness surgical dissection of the vaginal wall. The authors have found that the use of a Tuohy needle, commonly used for the placement of epidural anesthesia, is helpful in the consistent and accurate placement of the dissection fluid in the correct anatomic space. The unique periscope shape of the needle tip provides tactile feedback as the needle enters the space; in addition, the 1.0 cm silver/black hash marks provide visual reference to avoid inadvertent advancement of the needle while administering pressure on the syringe to infuse the hydrodissection fluid (**Figs. 3** and **4**). This tool has been most helpful in training surgeons on how to achieve optimal full-thickness dissection. The subsequent surgical steps of sharp and blunt dissection follow the space created by hydrodissection, therefore, it remains the *key* step for optimal dissection to minimize exposure.

Unfortunately, even with optimal full-thickness vaginal dissection during transvaginal mesh procedures or with ASC performed at the time of hysterectomy when the vaginal wall is surgically incised, the potential for exposure exists (**Fig. 5**). At the authors' center they have, over time, lowered the exposure rate to 2.9%, which compares favorably with the reported exposure rate in most ASC studies.[26] In terms of clinical impact to patients, fortunately vaginal exposures are commonly asymptomatic and fairly easily resolved with medical or minimal surgical intervention, often within the office setting.[25] The size and the location of the exposure as well as the quality of the surrounding vaginal tissue and symptom severity

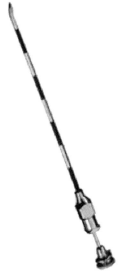

Fig. 3. Tuohy needle.

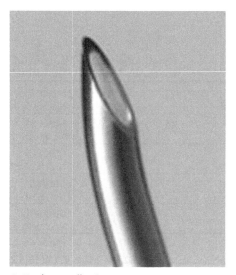

Fig. 4. Tuohy needle tip.

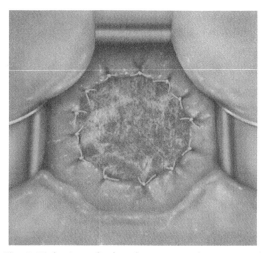

Fig. 6. Biologic graft placed over area where exposed mesh was removed. Note graft is placed below the plane of the surrounding vaginal epithelium.

should be considered when formulating a treatment plan. Small asymptomatic exposures that are below the plane of the epithelium can be managed expectantly with serial observation only or with topical estrogen. Large exposures, or those that protrude through the epithelium, are better managed surgically. For those exposures that are greater than 1 cm in width, a biologic graft may facilitate more-rapid healing (**Figs. 6** and **7**); attempts to undermine the vagina and close over wider exposures are often unsuccessful.

Optimal surgical execution of transvaginal mesh surgery, including correct anatomic dissection, proper sizing of the mesh to the dimensions of the patients, delivery/placement of the material, and adequate setting/adjustment of the graft, does result in a low complication rate. However,

for sexually active patients that develop new-onset dyspareunia, the low rate is irrelevant and the impact on their individual quality of life is significant.

A recent study looking at the incidence of dyspareunia following vaginal prolapse repair with graft materials showed that, in general, the rate of complications was inversely related to the surgeon's case volume.[27] In another study, the dyspareunia score was significantly worse in the nonmesh group at 2 years out. The authors recently reported on a trial performed at their center using synthetic graft placed transvaginally in which the quality-of-life and sexual-health measures significantly improved in women who underwent transvaginal mesh placement for prolapse.[28]

Only a small percentage of patients who develop dyspareunia will require a surgical

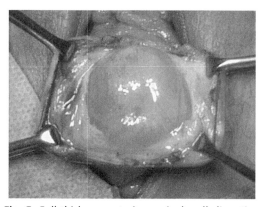

Fig. 5. Full-thickness anterior vaginal wall dissection and exposure of the true vesicovaginal space. Note the yellow color beneath the fluid bleb representing the fat of the areolar tissue within this avascular pelvic space.

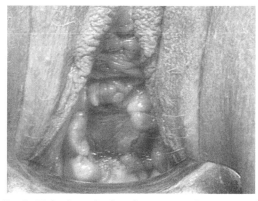

Fig. 7. Biologic graft placed over area where exposed mesh was removed. Note graft is placed below the plane of the surrounding vaginal epithelium.

intervention to remove/revise the graft. Most patients will significantly improve with vaginal estrogen supplementation; pelvic floor muscle therapy; the use of muscle relaxants, such as transvaginal valium suppositories; and trigger point injection of steroid/anesthetic solutions to areas of isolated point tenderness.

2011 FDA NOTIFICATION

On July 13, 2011, the FDA issued an update regarding complications associated with the use of graft materials in the repair of POP. It should be emphasized that the report does not pertain to mesh products used for the surgical management of stress urinary incontinence or for surgical procedures performed via an abdominal approach. However, it seems conflicting that if we use the same graft for repair of POP regardless of surgical route to enter the pelvis, it is acceptable to deliver this material via an abdominal approach with the well-known risks, yet doing it through a transvaginal route (despite favorable or similar risks) is controversial. Honest and experienced implanting surgeon experts agree that it is more often the surgical process in the placement of the material (influenced by the surgeon skill set and case volume) rather than the material itself that contributes to potential complications.

The authors realize that many complications of transvaginal mesh go unreported to the Manufacturer and User Facility Device Experience (MAUDE) database and that the risk of complication with transvaginal mesh procedures is higher than 0.67% (an estimate derived from the number of reported complications by the number of kits consumed during the same time frame). However, the 2011 FDA update implies that this risk of complication is higher than with native tissue repairs. Surgeons who perform native tissue repairs know that the risk of complications is certainly not less than 1%. In fact, when one of the gold standard native tissue repair techniques (the uterosacral ligament suspension) was first described, the risk of ureteral injury alone was 11%. Fortunately, the uterosacral ligament procedure was not banished but rather the technique

was improved on by the shared learning of surgeons. Tragically, as a result of multiple barriers invoked by hospital administrative policies, it is now becoming more and more difficult to effectively learn new surgical techniques or skills from each other in the operating room.

These comments are not intended, in any fashion, to minimize the importance of any surgical complication regardless of its precise prevalence; as surgeons caring for women each day, the authors are keenly aware of the gravity of adverse outcomes to all patients. The authors wish to highlight a fundamental reality within their daily surgical practices that they think is not reflected or acknowledged in the current FDA verbiage: in the surgical management of advanced prolapse, all treatment options involve significant risks. The authors are deeply concerned that the FDA update portrays transvaginal mesh repairs as uniquely hazardous, providing no broader perspective regarding the significant risks or higher recurrence rates associated with its alternatives, such as suture repair.

SUMMARY

We can all agree that, based on evidence within our literature, mesh is clearly needed for long-term success for repair of anterior/apical defects. There is a clear role for transvaginal mesh use in selected patients. In the reality-based medicine that we live in, it is obvious that proper surgical technique is critical. Surgeons must be effectively trained to perform these procedures and must maintain a significant case volume to sustain their proficiency. Clear credentialing and clinical privilege criteria policies are long overdue. Current data, although not robust, is rapidly growing, with several level I studies completed that demonstrate that when transvaginal mesh-augmented repair is used in appropriately selected patients for repair of pelvic organ prolapse, and performed by surgeon experts in this particular technique, the procedure has a favorable risk/benefit ratio when compared with suture repair. New, lighter, more-elastic, hybrid monofilament meshes may offer even better postoperative function in the future.

EDITOR'S COMMENTS

The most controversial aspect regarding prolapse at this time is the use of mesh for surgical augmentation. There is no question that monofilament, macroporous mesh respresents the optimal type of synthetic surgical material for prolapse correction. Other types of mesh are unsuitable for this indication due to the complexities of the vaginal environment and associated wound healing.

The coupling of monofilament mesh with insertion tools to expedite and standardize surgical technique has been proposed over the last decade. Rapid adoption of these "kit" techniques has occurred over the last 5–7 years. Early signals of concern resulted in two separate FDA notifications regarding the use of these kits and mesh in pelvic prolapse correction. The first notification (2008) was informational and intended to increase awareness of mesh related complications. The second notification (2011) was broader in purpose, inclusive of explicit requirements for subsequent clinical trials of mesh and stipulations regarding informed consent and patient education regarding the implantation of mesh. The most recent notification referenced mesh use for prolapse and also for stress incontinence indications. Reports of mesh complications inclusive of exposure, erosion, pain, and sexual dysfunction have increased over this time period as well.

So what does all this mean for the surgical management of prolapse? Surgical experience and understanding of anatomy is critical to successful intervention outcome. Therefore, the kits cannot be expected to decrease the need for experience and surgical knowledge. A clear message arising from this experience is the disconnection between anatomy and function when considering vaginal prolapse. Although the kits have demonstrated successful resolution of anatomic defects in the majority of patients undergoing these procedures, persistent or de novo functional disorders have resulted in patient dissatisfaction and need for secondary interventions. This experience underscores the importance of patient selection and informed consent inclusive of impact on pelvic organ function related to the presenting prolapse and any proposed corrective intervention. Functional symptoms (bowel, bladder, sexual, pain, and prolapse related) may be positively or adversely impacted by any prolapse intervention (mesh related or not) even with objective normalization of anatomy. A woman should be educated to this phenomenon, and the FDA was absolutely correct in urging this as a critical aspect of surgical decision making. The risks of erosion, exposure, dyspareunia or pain induced by mesh implantation have added another layer onto the existing functional impacts of prolapse and also must be factored into the decision to use mesh.

So what is best management of prolapse? Clearly, surgical experience, technical awareness, thorough informed consent, and systematized perioperative care and postoperative management all contribute to patient satisfaction and optimize outcomes. Goal setting for the patient is critical, and that may mean the possibility of persistence of functional symptoms, incomplete resolution of prolapse, and the development of new symptoms even in the most experienced hands. The mere presence of prolapse (absent symptoms) is not an indication for surgery, as the decision for surgery should provide at least the hope for some improvement of bothersome functional symptoms.

How to manage prolapse once the decision has been made for surgery? Plication and interposition procedures are both reasonable options, and interposition can be accomplished with biologic or synthetic materials, based upon surgeon experience, patient preference and presenting anatomic and functional disorders.

Roger R. Dmochowski, MD
Mickey Karram, MD

REFERENCES

1. Vintzileos AM. Evidence-based compared with reality-based medicine in obstetrics. Obstet Gynecol 2009 Jun;113(6):1335–40.
2. Drutz HP, Alarab M. Pelvic organ prolapse: demographics and future growth prospects. Int Urogynecol J Pelvic Floor Dysfunct 2006;17(Suppl 1):S6–9.
3. Ulmsten U, Ekman G, Giertz G, et al. Different biochemical composition of connective tissue in continent and stress incontinent women. Acta Obstet Gynecol Scand 1987;66:455–7.
4. Gilpin SA, Gosling JA, Smith AR, et al. The pathogenesis of genitourinary prolapse and stress incontinence of urine. A histological and histochemical study. Br J Obstet Gynaecol 1989;96:15–23.
5. Norton PA, Boyd C, Deak S. Abnormal collagen ratios in women with genitourinary prolapse. Neurourol Urodyn 1992;11:2–4.
6. Boreham M, Wai CY, Miller RT, et al. Morphometric analysis of smooth muscle in the anterior vaginal wall of women with pelvic organ prolapse. Am J Obstet Gynecol 2002 Jul;187(1):56–63.
7. Chen BH, Wen Y, Zhao Y, et al. Does relaxin contribute to stress urinary incontinence by altering TGF-β expression? Int Urogynecol J 2006;17(Suppl 3):S409.
8. Olson AL, Smith VJ, Bergstrom JO, et al. Epidemiology of surgically managed pelvic organ prolapse and urinary incontinence. Obstet Gynecol 1997;89:501–6.
9. Marchionni M, Bracco GL, Checcucci V, et al. True incidence of vaginal vault prolapse. Thirteen years of experience. J Reprod Med 1999;44:679–84.
10. Clark AL, Gregory T, Smith VJ, et al. Epidemiologic evaluation of reoperation for surgically treated pelvic organ prolapse and urinary incontinence. Am J Obstet Gynecol 2003;189:1261–7.
11. Burger JW, Luijendijk RW, Hop WC, et al. Long-term follow-up of a randomized controlled trial of suture versus mesh repair of incisional hernia. Ann Surg 2004;240:578–83.

12. Nieminen K, Hiltunen R, Takala T, et al. Outcomes after anterior vaginal wall repair with mesh: a randomized, controlled trial with a 3 year follow-up. Am J Obstet Gynecol 2010;203(3):235.e1–8.

13. Cosson M, Debodinance P, Boukerrou M, et al. Mechanical properties of synthetic implants used in the repair of prolapse and urinary incontinence in women: which is the ideal material? Int Urogynecol J Pelvic Floor Dysfunct 2003;14:169–78.

14. Griffis K, Hale D. Grafts in pelvic reconstructive surgery. Clin Obstet Gynecol 2005;48:713–23.

15. Amid PK, Shulman AG, Lichtenstein IL, et al. Biomaterials for abdominal wall hernia surgery and principles of their applications. Langenbecks Arch Chir 1994;379:168–71.

16. Feola A, Abramowitch SD, Stein S, et al. Stress-shielding: the impact of mesh stiffness on vaginal function. AUGS 32nd Annual Meeting paper presentation. Providence (RI), September 14-17, 2011.

17. Ozog Y, Konstantinovic M, Werbrouck E, et al. Shrinkage and biomechanical evaluation of lightweight synthetics in a rabbit model for primary fascial repair. Int Urogynecol J 2011;22:1099–108.

18. Maher C, Baessler K, Glazener CM, et al. Surgical management of pelvic organ prolapse in women: a short version Cochrane review. Neurourol Urodyn 2008;27:3–12.

19. Sivaslioglu AA, Unlubilgin E, Dolen I. A randomized comparison of polypropylene mesh surgery with site-specific surgery in the treatment of cystocoele. Int Urogynecol J Pelvic Floor Dysfunct 2008;19(4):467–71.

20. Nieminen K, Hiltunen R, Heiskanen E, et al. Symptom resolution and sexual function after anterior vaginal wall repair with or without polypropylene mesh. Int Urogynecol J Pelvic Floor Dysfunct 2008;19(12):1611–6.

21. Nguyen JN, Burchette RJ. Outcome after anterior vaginal prolapse repair: a randomized controlled trial. Obstet Gynecol 2008;111(4):891–8.

22. Carey M, Higgs P, Goh J, et al. Vaginal repair with mesh versus colporrhaphy for prolapse: a randomised controlled trial. BJOG 2009;116(10):1380–6.

23. Withagen MI, Milani AL, den Boon J, et al. Trocar-guided mesh compared with conventional vaginal repair in recurrent prolapse: a randomized controlled trial. Obstet Gynecol 2011;117(2 Pt 1):242–50.

24. Altman D, Väyrynen T, Engh ME, et al, Nordic Transvaginal Mesh Group. Anterior colporrhaphy versus transvaginal mesh for pelvic-organ prolapse. N Engl J Med 2011;364(19):1826–36.

25. Brubaker L, Cundiff GW, Fine P, et al, Pelvic Floor Disorders Network. Abdominal sacrocolpopexy with Burch colposuspension to reduce urinary stress incontinence. N Engl J Med 2006;354(15):1557–66.

26. Visco AG, Weidner AC, Barber MD, et al. Vaginal mesh erosion after abdominal sacral colpopexy. Am J Obstet Gynecol 2001;184(3):297–302.

27. Abed H, Rahn DD, Lowenstein L, et al. Incidence and management of graft erosion, wound granulation, and dyspareunia following vaginal prolapse repair with graft materials: a systematic review. Int Urogynecol J 2011;22:789–98.

28. Bhatia N, Murphy M, Lucente VR, et al. A comparison of short term sexual function outcomes for patients undergoing the transvaginal mesh procedure using the standard polypropylene mesh vs a hybrid polypropylene/poliglecaprone mesh. Oral poster presentation SGS Annual Meeting. Tucson (AZ), April 12-14, 2010.

Vaginal Prolapse Repair
Suture Repair Versus Mesh Augmentation: A Urology Perspective

Alex Gomelsky, MD

KEYWORDS

• Vaginal prolapse • Repair • Urine • Incontinence

KEY POINTS

• Pelvic organ prolapse is a prevalent, costly, and bothersome condition.
• Traditional (plication-type) prolapse repairs may be associated with high degrees of anatomic recurrence, but quality of life and symptoms may improve.
• Prolapse repairs augmented with synthetic mesh provide a higher anatomic cure rate, but may be associated with extrusion and erosion.

INTRODUCTION AND EPIDEMIOLOGY OF PELVIC PROLAPSE

An analysis of women who participated in the 2005 to 2006 National Health and Nutrition Examination Survey revealed the weighted overall prevalence of pelvic organ prolapse (POP) to be 2.9%, with the prevalence increasing with age, from 1.6% in women 20 to 39 years of age to 4.1% in women aged 80 years or older.[1] The lifetime risk of undergoing a single operation for prolapse or incontinence by age 80 years has been estimated to be as high as 11.1%, with risk factors being older age, postmenopausal status, multiparity, and obesity.[2] Some US Census Bureau projections estimate that as many as 9.2 million women in the United States will have prolapse by the year 2050, and, as may be expected, the demand for services to care for pelvic floor disorders is also estimated to increase by 45% by the year 2030.[3,4]

The cost of treating POP is also significant, because the direct costs of prolapse surgery were estimated to be $1012 million (in 1997).[5] Furthermore, women with POP have an impaired quality of life (QoL), are more likely to be self-conscious and less likely to feel physically and sexually attractive than normal controls.[6] Taking these factors into account, it is easy to see that the demand for durable and safe surgical options will continue to increase. The main controversy in the realm of POP repair is the role of traditional (plication-type) repairs and augmented repairs, especially with the addition of synthetic mesh. The recent warnings by the US Food and Drug Administration (FDA) regarding the complications of transvaginal mesh implantation for POP repair have raised valid concerns regarding these procedures for pelvic floor reconstruction. Some questions may remain unanswered; however, several conclusions may be drawn regarding the role of different types of POP repair in 2012. Because the role of synthetic mesh in the repair of vaginal vault prolapse with abdominal sacrocolpopexy is beyond the scope of this article, only anterior and posterior compartment POP repairs are discussed.

BRIEF ANATOMY OF PELVIC PROLAPSE
Normal Anatomy

A 3-level system is useful when considering normal vaginal support cephalad to caudad, with

Department of Urology, Louisiana State University Health Sciences Center – Shreveport, 1501 Kings Highway, Shreveport, LA 71130, USA
E-mail address: agomel@lsuhsc.edu

Urol Clin N Am 39 (2012) 335–342
http://dx.doi.org/10.1016/j.ucl.2012.05.005
0094-0143/12/$ – see front matter © 2012 Elsevier Inc. All rights reserved.

levels I and II providing the key support in POP, and level III support responsible for urethral hypermobility and perineal defects, in the anterior and posterior compartments, respectively.[7] The cardinal ligaments anchor the upper vagina and cervix to the pelvic sidewall (level I) and, in the midvagina, the vesicopelvic ligament/pubocervical fascia support the bladder base and the anterior vaginal wall through its attachment to the arcus tendineus fasciae pelvis (ATFP) laterally (level II).

In the posterior compartment, level II support is provided by the direct attachment of the posterior vaginal wall laterally to the levator ani fascia. The vagina is separated from the rectum by the rectovaginal fascia, which is attached laterally to the ATFP in the proximal two-thirds of the vagina and fused proximally with the uterosacral ligaments laterally and the pericervical ring centrally.[7,8]

Anatomic Variations

Weakness in the pubocervical fascia in the setting of an intact lateral attachment of the vesicopelvic ligament to the ATFP produces a central cystocele, whereas a lateral cystocele results from an intact pubocervical fascia and disrupted attachment of the vesicopelvic ligament to the ATFP.[9] Central defects are often associated with loss of level I support at the cardinal ligaments and patients often have a concomitant enterocele. Traditional repair of a central cystocele involves the plication of the pubocervical fascia in the midline (anterior colporrhaphy), whereas a lateral cystocele is repaired with reattachment of the vesicopelvic ligament to the pelvic sidewall (paravaginal repair). Attachment of a mesh graft to the ATFP or obturator internus fascia has the potential to address central and lateral defects simultaneously.

A rectocele may be central, lateral, or combined, and may be addressed with plication of the rectovaginal septum (posterior colporrhaphy). A site-specific rectocele repair involves the repair of discrete rents in the rectovaginal fascia instead of a midline plication.[10] A mesh graft that spans sidewall to sidewall may address all variations of rectoceles.

INTERPOSITION GRAFTING FOR PELVIC PROLAPSE
Background and Anatomy

As pelvic surgeons have gradually noticed similarities between POP and hernias of the abdominal wall, interposition grafting has become an increasingly attractive method to replace or augment standard POP repairs. Advantages of graft augmentation

are that both central and lateral compartment defects can be repaired simultaneously and a graft may be anchored to an apical landmark, or placed suburethrally, to provide concomitant level I and level III support, respectively. Cadaver allografts, xenografts, and synthetic meshes, both absorbable and nonabsorbable, have been used for interposition grafting in both the anterior and posterior compartments.[11]

Owing to the unpredictable long-term outcomes with biologic grafts, permanent synthetic meshes have largely supplanted other materials for interposition grafting. Julian[12] first sutured a polypropylene (Marlex) graft to the obturator/levator fascia to address an anterior compartment defect and reported no anatomic recurrence at 2 years of follow-up. Because synthetic meshes may differ significantly by weave, fiber type, pore size, weight, and stiffness, outcomes may differ substantially with each material. As with midurethral slings (MUS), macroporous, monofilament, polypropylene mesh has the most favorable biocompatibility profile of all the current synthetics. The absence of interstitial pores allows native collagen ingrowth and the large pores allow entry to macrophages and other immune mediators.

Transvaginal Mesh Kits

Owing to the popularity and success of the all-inclusive MUS kits, interest in POP kits has peaked in the last decade. These kits combine mesh for repair of an anterior or posterior compartment defect, trocars for tunneling mesh arms subcutaneously, and suture capturing or anchoring devices to provide simultaneous apical support. The concept behind the kits is to provide a route for a minimally invasive, mesh-augmented, transvaginal POP repair using easily identified landmarks.

The first kit, the posterior intravaginal slingplasty (PIVS; US Surgical, Tyco Healthcare Group, Norwalk, CT, USA), achieved level I support by tunneling a nylon tape through the ischiorectal fossa into an incision in the posterior vaginal fornix.[13] The tunnelers exited through the iliococcygeus muscle near the ischial spines and the deployed tape was sutured to the vaginal vault. Several other commercially manufactured POP kits have been introduced and, although a detailed discussion of specific kit properties is beyond the scope of this article, a comparison of mesh kits is available elsewhere.[11] All of the currently available kits are constructed from type I, macroporous, monofilament polypropylene.

For anterior compartment repair, 2 sets of trocars are typically advanced percutaneously through each obturator foramen into a vaginal incision. The superior trocars exit near the bladder neck, whereas the inferior trocars exit near the ischial spine. Mesh arms are advanced through the skin with the trocars until the body of the mesh is seated under the bladder base in a tension-free position. For posterior compartment repair, 1 set of trocars is passed through bilateral perianal incisions to exit near the ischial spine and the proximal part of the mesh is positioned as described earlier. In the second generation of kit procedures, surgical dissection is performed solely through the vagina under direct vision and there is no percutaneous mesh advancement. In addition, suture passers or specialized trocars attach mesh arms to the sacrospinous ligament for repair of a concomitant apical defect.

OUTCOMES OF PELVIC PROLAPSE REPAIR

The debate over the optimal method to repair POP exists mainly because traditional repairs are perceived to lack durability. In an analysis of the Kaiser Permanente Northwest database, Olson and colleagues[2] found that 29.2% of nearly 400 women underwent reoperation for incontinence or POP and the time intervals between procedures decreased with each subsequent repair. Clark and colleagues[14] determined that the risk of reoperation increased from 12% to 17% in those women who had already failed a previous procedure for SUI or POP. Although 60% underwent reoperation at the same anatomic site, 32.5% of the women developed an occult support defect and underwent reoperation at a different site.

Standard POP Repairs

The reports of success after standard anterior colporrhaphy have been inconsistent. Although some reports cite ~5% long-term recurrence,[15] most studies quote anterior compartment recurrence rates that approach 50%.[16–18] Although no long-term prospective trials are available, anatomic cure rates after isolated rectocele repair are high and typically exceed 85%.[10,19–21] Published outcomes are often difficult to compare because of variations in patient population, surgical technique, definitions of success, and indications for repair. Furthermore, outcomes of POP repair may be confounded by concomitant repairs in other compartments and, as such, should be interpreted cautiously.

Interposition Grafts and Kit Repairs

Despite variations in technique and definitions of success, short-term anatomic cure rates after

interposition grafting with most materials have approached 90%.[11] However, the cure rates with biologic grafts seem to decline with longer periods of follow-up, mirroring the surgical experience after biologic slings.[22] The anatomic outcomes after transvaginal kit repairs have likewise been promising in the short term. A recent meta-analysis encompassing 30 studies with 2653 patients calculated the objective success rates to be 87% to 95% for several different commercial POP kits.[23]

COMPARATIVE STUDIES
Standard Versus Augmented POP Repairs

Studies comparing standard transvaginal POP repairs and those using synthetic or xenograft-derived interposition grafts are summarized in **Table 1**. Several meta-analyses and systematic reviews have evaluated these outcomes. In a 2010 Cochrane Database review, anterior colporrhaphy was associated with more recurrent cystoceles than standard repairs augmented with polyglactin mesh or porcine dermis inlay, polypropylene mesh as an overlay, or armed transobturator mesh.[43] The review also emphasized that, although some data were limited, there were no differences in subjective outcomes, QoL data, de novo dyspareunia, SUI, and reoperation rates for prolapse or incontinence between the augmented and standard procedures.[43] Furthermore, because there are fewer evidence-based outcomes comparing the outcomes after standard posterior colporrhaphy and graft-augmented repair, the review found little evidence supporting interposition grafting in the posterior compartment. An additional meta-analysis encompassing 49 studies and more than 4500 women determined that nonabsorbable synthetic mesh had a significantly lower objective anterior compartment recurrence rate (8.8%) than absorbable synthetic mesh (23.1%) and biologic graft (17.9%).[44]

Augmented Versus Augmented POP Repairs

Data comparing one augmented repair with another is only now emerging. Natale and colleagues[45] performed a randomized controlled trial (RCT) comparing 24-month outcomes of women undergoing anterior colporrhaphy augmented with porcine dermis (Pelvicol) and a polypropylene mesh (Gynemesh PS). The objective recurrence rate was lower in the mesh group (44% vs 28%), whereas the symptomatic improvement was similar. Extrusion was only seen in the mesh group (6.3%) and the dyspareunia rate was slightly higher in the porcine dermis group (12.8% vs 10.4%). Long and colleagues[46]

Table 1
Comparisons of standard and graft-augmented POP repair

Author	Location (N)	Graft (N)	F/U (mo)	Objective Recurrence (%)	Symptomatic Recurrence (%)	Postoperative Complications (%)	
						Extrusion (Graft)	Dyspareunia
Standard Anterior/Posterior Colporrhaphy vs Absorbable Synthetic Mesh-Augmented Repair							
Weber[24] (RCT)	Anterior (35)	Vicryl (35)	23 median	70/58	0/9	N/A	N/A
Sand[25] (RCT)	A&P (70)	Vicryl (73)	12	10/9	N/A	N/A	N/A
Standard Anterior/Posterior Colporrhaphy vs Nonabsorbable Synthetic Mesh-Augmented Repair (Including Kits)							
Hiltunen[26] Niemenen[27] (RCT)	Anterior (97)	PP (104)	12	39/7	18/5	17.3	Dyspareunia score lower in PP group
Sivaslioglu[28] (RCT)	Anterior (45)	PP (45)	12 mean	28/9	P-QoL similar	6.9	0/4.6
Nguyen[29] (RCT)	Anterior (38)	PP + AC (37)	12	45/13	PFDI/PFIQ similar	5	16/9
Carey[30] (RCT)	A&P (70)	PP + A&P (69)	12	34/19	PSI-QoL similar	5.6	15.2/16.7
Niemenen[31] (RCT)	Anterior (97)	PP (105)	36	41/13	65/69	19	8.2/3.8
Altman[32] (RCT)	Anterior (189)	Prolift (200)	12	66/39	38/25	3.2	2/7.3
Sokol[33] (RCT)	AC + VVS (33)	Prolift (32)	12	70/63	9/4	15.6	18.8/6.7
Standard Anterior/Posterior Colporrhaphy vs Xenograft-Augmented Repair							
Gandhi[34] (RCT)	Anterior (78)	Tutoplast + AC (76)	13 median	29/21	31/22	N/A	N/A
Paraiso[35] (RCT)	Posterior (33) SSPC (37)	Bovine pericardium (29)	17.5 mean	14/22/46	16/12/21	N/A	20/14/6
Meschia[36] (RCT)	Anterior (103)	Pelvicol (98)	12	19/7	13/9	1	N/A
Botros[37]	Anterior (89)	Cadaver dermis (102)	>15 mean	23/10	N/A	0	19/14
Guerette[38] (RCT)	Anterior (26)	Bovine pericardium (33)	24	37/24	N/A	N/A	20/15
Hviid[39] (RCT)	Anterior (31)	Pelvicol (30)	12	15/7	3/3	3.3	N/A
Dahlgren[40] (RCT)	Anterior/posterior (60)	Pelvicol (65)	36	57/62 (A) 40/17 (P)	15/16	4.4	N/A
Handel[41]	Anterior (18)	PD (56) PP (25)	13.5 mean	6/36/4	N/A	-/21/4	N/A
Menefee[42] (RCT)	Anterior (32)	PD (31) PP (36)	12/24	58/46/18	13/12/4 (composite)	-/4/14	9/6/6

Abbreviations: AC, anterior colporrhaphy; A&P, anterior and posterior colporrhaphy; F/U (mo), follow up in months; N/A, not available; PD, porcine dermis; PFDI, pelvic floor distress inventory; PFIQ, pelvic floor/incontinence questionnaire; PP, polypropylene; P-QoL, prolapse quality of life questionnaire; RCT, randomized controlled trial; SSPC, site-specific posterior colporrhaphy; Tutoplast, solvent-dehydrated cadaver fascia lata; VVS, vaginal vault suspension.

compared women undergoing 2 POP kit procedures (Perigee and/or Apogee [AMS]; Prolift anterior and/or posterior [Gynecare]) in a nonrandomized trial. Despite significantly longer follow-up periods in the Perigee group (20 vs 12 months), the success rates were not significantly different. The prevalence of detrusor overactivity and urinary symptoms decreased significantly in both groups after surgery. Mesh-related morbidities were also comparable.

COMPLICATIONS OF POP REPAIRS

All POP repairs are associated with varying, but mostly minimal, degrees of significant intraoperative bleeding and inadvertent pelvic organ injury. The incorporation of synthetic grafts, and the use of trocar-guided kits in particular, may be associated with additional and unique complications. A recent meta-analysis of more than 70 studies and case reports assessed the rates of adverse events associated with graft use.[47] These adverse events included bleeding (0%–3%), visceral injury (1%–4%), urinary tract infection (0%–19%), graft extrusion (0%–30%), and fistula formation (1%). The data were insufficient regarding sexual, voiding, or defecatory dysfunction.

Another recent systematic review identified 110 MEDLINE studies that reported on graft erosion, wound granulation, and/or dyspareunia after prolapse repair using graft materials.[48] The rate of graft extrusion was 10.3% (range 0%–29.7%; synthetic 10.3%, biologic 10.1%) and the rate of wound granulation was 7.8% (range 0%–19.1%; synthetic 6.8%, biologic 9.1%), whereas dyspareunia was described in 70 studies for a rate of 9.1% (range 0%–66.7%; synthetic 8.9%, biologic 9.6%). It must also be mentioned that pelvic pain and dyspareunia in women with POP may be multifactorial and may persist or worsen regardless of the type of repair performed.[49] Furthermore, RCTs confirm that the rate of de novo or persistent dyspareunia after standard repairs often exceeds that of augmented POP repairs (see **Table 1**).

CONCERNS OVER TRANSVAGINAL MESH IMPLANTATION

Because synthetic mesh implantation for transvaginal POP repair has increased significantly, the reporting of associated surgical complications has been closely scrutinized. In the last several years, the French Health Authority, the Society of Gynecologic Surgeons Systematic Review Group, and the FDA have all issued warnings

regarding the unique complications associated with mesh use in the pelvis.[11] The FDA recommended that surgeons (1) obtain specialized training for each mesh placement technique; (2) inform patients that surgical mesh implantation is permanent, and that some mesh complications may require additional surgery; and (3) provide patients with a written copy of the patient labeling from the surgical mesh manufacturer, if available.

More recently, on July 13, 2011, the FDA released a second Safety Communication in response to the reporting of more complications associated with transvaginal mesh placement (http://www.fda. gov/MedicalDevices/Safety/AlertsandNotices/ ucm262435.htm). The FDA update stated that adverse events for POP mesh repair are not rare, as was previously reported, and brought into question the relative effectiveness of meshed versus unmeshed repairs. The FDA once again encouraged physicians to seek specialized training, consider risks, advise patients appropriately, and diligently diagnose and report complications.

On September 8, 2011, the FDA convened the Obstetrics and Gynecology Devices Panel of the Medical Devices Advisory Committee, to which the Mesh Device Manufacturers' Working Group comprising industry representatives and selected pelvic surgeons presented their case to the FDA for the safety, efficacy, and continued classification of mesh as a class II device for POP. On January 3, 2012, the FDA mandated that postmarket surveillance studies will be required of all previously approved and currently available vaginal mesh devices for POP. No devices were recalled and they remain in use, and the FDA continues to assess whether to reclassify future transvaginal mesh devices for POP to class III. The FDA set a deadline of February 1, 2012, for submissions of 522 studies by manufacturers regarding clinical study plans and protocols to satisfy postmarket requirements for transvaginal mesh. Companies will be charged with providing safety and efficacy data compared with native tissue POP repair.

SUMMARY

The ideal procedure for POP repair would be associated with a low chance of long-term anatomic recurrence in the corrected compartment and should not predispose the patient to de novo SUI or POP in other compartments. The procedure should also improve the woman's QoL and subjective symptoms of pelvic floor dysfunction. Furthermore, the repair should be safe and not be associated with significant immediate and long-term morbidity. Because there are multiple options for surgical POP correction, the debate over the optimal repair persists.

A consensus may be close on several fronts. First, standard anterior colporrhaphy has a high rate of anatomic recurrence but the improvement in subjective indices and QoL is similar to that after augmented repairs. Second, nonabsorbable synthetic mesh is associated with significantly lower anatomic recurrence rates than other grafts. Third, there is currently insufficient information to support interposition grafting of any type in the posterior compartment. Fourth, mesh use is associated with vaginal extrusion; however, the rate of persistent or de novo dyspareunia may be similar to standard repairs in the short term.

In conclusion, each procedure for POP repair has strong advantages and potential detractors. It is here that the surgeon's experience should dictate the decision-making process and a detailed informed consent discussion should take place. Judicious patient selection, adequate surgeon training, comfort with variations in pelvic anatomy, and the ability to address postoperative complications are vital to the success of any POP surgery.

EDITOR'S COMMENTS

The most controversial aspect regarding prolapse at this time is the use of mesh for surgical augmentation. There is no question that monofilament, macroporous mesh respresents the optimal type of synthetic surgical material for prolapse correction. Other types of mesh are unsuitable for this indication due to the complexities of the vaginal environment and associated wound healing.

The coupling of monofilament mesh with insertion tools to expedite and standardize surgical technique has been proposed over the last decade. Rapid adoption of these "kit" techniques has occurred over the last 5–7 years. Early signals of concern resulted in two separate FDA notifications regarding the use of these kits and mesh in pelvic prolapse correction. The first notification (2008) was informational and intended to increase awareness of mesh related complications. The second notification (2011) was broader in purpose, inclusive of explicit requirements for subsequent clinical trials of mesh and stipulations regarding informed consent and patient education regarding the implantation of mesh. The most recent notification referenced mesh use for prolapse and also for stress incontinence indications. Reports of mesh complications inclusive of exposure, erosion, pain, and sexual dysfunction have increased over this time period as well.

So what does all this mean for the surgical management of prolapse? Surgical experience and understanding of anatomy is critical to successful intervention outcome. Therefore, the kits cannot be expected to decrease the need for experience and surgical knowledge. A clear message arising from this experience is the disconnection between anatomy and function when considering vaginal prolapse. Although the kits have demonstrated successful resolution of anatomic defects in the majority of patients undergoing these procedures, persistent or de novo functional disorders have resulted in patient dissatisfaction and need for secondary interventions. This experience underscores the importance of patient selection and informed consent inclusive of impact on pelvic organ function related to the presenting prolapse and any proposed corrective intervention. Functional symptoms (bowel, bladder, sexual, pain, and prolapse related) may be positively or adversely impacted by any prolapse intervention (mesh related or not) even with objective normalization of anatomy. A woman should be educated to this phenomenon, and the FDA was absolutely correct in urging this as a critical aspect of surgical decision making. The risks of erosion, exposure, dyspareunia or pain induced by mesh implantation have added another layer onto the existing functional impacts of prolapse and also must be factored into the decision to use mesh.

So what is best management of prolapse? Clearly, surgical experience, technical awareness, thorough informed consent, and systematized perioperative care and postoperative management all contribute to patient satisfaction and optimize outcomes. Goal setting for the patient is critical, and that may mean the possibility of persistence of functional symptoms, incomplete resolution of prolapse, and the development of new symptoms even in the most experienced hands. The mere presence of prolapse (absent symptoms) is not an indication for surgery, as the decision for surgery should provide at least the hope for some improvement of bothersome functional symptoms.

How to manage prolapse once the decision has been made for surgery? Plication and interposition procedures are both reasonable options, and interposition can be accomplished with biologic or synthetic materials, based upon surgeon experience, patient preference and presenting anatomic and functional disorders.

Roger R. Dmochowski, MD
Mickey Karram, MD

REFERENCES

1. Nygaard I, Barber MD, Burgio KL, et al, Pelvic Floor Disorders Network. Prevalence of symptomatic pelvic floor disorders in US women. JAMA 2008; 300:1311–6.
2. Olsen AL, Smith VJ, Bergstrom JO, et al. Epidemiology of surgically managed pelvic organ prolapse and urinary incontinence. Obstet Gynecol 1997;89:501–6.
3. Wu JM, Hundley AF, Fulton RG, et al. Forecasting the prevalence of pelvic floor disorders in U.S. women: 2010 to 2050. Obstet Gynecol 2009;114: 1278–83.
4. Luber KM, Boero S, Choe JY. The demographics of pelvic floor disorders: current observations and future projections. Am J Obstet Gynecol 2001;184: 1496–501.
5. Subak LL, Waetjen LE, van den Eeden S, et al. Cost of pelvic organ prolapse surgery in the United States. Obstet Gynecol 2001;98:646–51.
6. Jelovsek JE, Barber MD. Women seeking treatment for advanced pelvic organ prolapse have decreased body image and quality of life. Am J Obstet Gynecol 2006;194:1455–61.
7. Delancey JO. Anatomic aspects of vaginal eversion after hysterectomy. Am J Obstet Gynecol 1992;166: 1717–24.
8. Leffler KS, Thompson JR, Cundiff GW, et al. Attachment of the rectovaginal septum to the pelvic sidewall. Am J Obstet Gynecol 2001;185:41–3.
9. Dmochowski RR, Gomelsky A. Cystocele and anterior vaginal prolapse. In: Graham SD, Glenn JF, Keane TE, editors. Glenn's urologic surgery. 6th edition. Philadelphia: Lippincott Williams & Wilkins; 2004. p. 339–48.
10. Cundiff GW, Weidner AC, Visco AG, et al. An anatomic and functional assessment of the discrete defect rectocele repair. Am J Obstet Gynecol 1998; 179:1451–6.
11. Gomelsky A, Penson DF, Dmochowski RR. Pelvic organ prolapse (POP) surgery: the evidence for the repairs. BJU Int 2011;107:1704–19.
12. Julian TM. Efficacy of Marlex mesh in the repair of severe, recurrent vaginal prolapse of the anterior midvaginal wall. Am J Obstet Gynecol 1996;175:1472–5.
13. Petros PE. Vault prolapse II: restoration of dynamic vaginal supports by infracoccygeal sacropexy, an axial day-case vaginal procedure. Int Urogynecol J Pelvic Floor Dysfunct 2001;12:296–303.
14. Clark AL, Gregory T, Smith VJ, et al. Epidemiologic evaluation of reoperation for surgically treated pelvic organ prolapse and urinary incontinence. Am J Obstet Gynecol 2003;189:1261–7.
15. Beck RP, McCormick S, Nordstrum L. A 25 year experience with 519 anterior colporrhaphy procedures. Obstet Gynecol 1991;78:1011–4.
16. Shull BL, Capen CV, Riggs MW, et al. Preoperative and postoperative analysis of site-specific pelvic support defects in 81 women treated with sacrospinous ligament suspension and pelvic reconstruction. Am J Obstet Gynecol 1992;166:1764–71.
17. Paraiso MF, Ballard LA, Walters MD, et al. Pelvic support defects and visceral and sexual function in women treated with sacrospinous ligament suspension and pelvic reconstruction. Am J Obstet Gynecol 1996;175:1423–31.
18. Maher C, Baessler K. Surgical management of anterior vaginal wall prolapse: an evidence based literature review. Int Urogynecol J Pelvic Floor Dysfunct 2006;17:195–201.
19. Kenton K, Shott S, Brubaker L. Outcome after rectovaginal fascia reattachment for rectocele repair. Am J Obstet Gynecol 1999;181:1360–3.
20. Singh K, Cortes E, Reid WM. Evaluation of the fascial technique for surgical repair of the isolated posterior vaginal wall prolapse. Obstet Gynecol 2003;101:320–4.
21. Maher CF, Qatawneh A, Baessler K, et al. Midline rectovaginal fascial plication for repair of rectocele and obstructed defecation. Obstet Gynecol 2004; 104:685–9.
22. Gomelsky A, Scarpero HM, Dmochowski RR. Sling surgery for stress urinary incontinence in the female: what surgery, which material? AUA Update Series 2004;21. Lesson 34.
23. Feiner B, Jelovsek JE, Maher C. Efficacy and safety of transvaginal mesh kits in the treatment of prolapse of the vaginal apex: a systematic review. BJOG 2009;116:15–24.
24. Weber AM, Walters MD, Piedmonte MR, et al. Anterior colporrhaphy: a randomized trial of three surgical techniques. Am J Obstet Gynecol 2001;185:1299–304.
25. Sand PK, Koduri S, Lobel RW, et al. Prospective randomized trial of polyglactin 910 mesh to prevent recurrence of cystoceles and rectoceles. Am J Obstet Gynecol 2001;184:1357–62.
26. Hiltunen R, Nieminen K, Takala T, et al. Low-weight polypropylene mesh for anterior vaginal wall prolapse: a randomized controlled trial. Obstet Gynecol 2007;110:455–62.
27. Niemenen K, Hiltunen R, Heiskanen E, et al. Symptom resolution and sexual function after anterior vaginal wall repair with or without polypropylene mesh. Int Urogynecol J Pelvic Floor Dysfunct 2008; 19:1611–6.
28. Sivaslioglu AA, Unlubilgin E, Dolen I. A randomized comparison of polypropylene mesh surgery with site-specific surgery in the treatment of cystocoele. Int Urogynecol J Pelvic Floor Dysfunct 2008;19:467–71.
29. Nguyen JN, Burchette RJ. Outcome after anterior vaginal prolapse repair: a randomized controlled trial. Obstet Gynecol 2008;111:891–8.
30. Carey M, Higgs P, Goh J, et al. Vaginal repair with mesh versus colporrhaphy for prolapse: a randomized controlled trial. BJOG 2009;116:1380–6.

31. Nieminen K, Hiltunen R, Takala T, et al. Outcomes after anterior vaginal wall repair with mesh: a randomized, controlled trial with a 3 year follow-up. Am J Obstet Gynecol 2010;203:235.e1–8.

32. Altman D, Väyrynen T, Engh ME, et al. Anterior colporrhaphy versus transvaginal mesh for pelvic-organ prolapse. N Engl J Med 2011;364:1826–36.

33. Sokol AI, Iglesia CB, Kudish BI, et al. One-year objective and functional outcomes of a randomized clinical trial of vaginal mesh for prolapse. Am J Obstet Gynecol 2012;206:86.e1–9.

34. Gandhi S, Goldberg RP, Kwon C, et al. A prospective randomized trial using solvent dehydrated fascia lata for the prevention of recurrent anterior vaginal wall prolapse. Am J Obstet Gynecol 2005;192:1649–54.

35. Paraiso MF, Barber MD, Muir TW, et al. Rectocele repair: a randomized trial of three surgical techniques including graft augmentation. Am J Obstet Gynecol 2006;195:1762–71.

36. Meschia M, Pifarotti P, Bernasconi F, et al. Porcine skin collagen implants to prevent anterior vaginal wall prolapse recurrence: a multicenter, randomized study. J Urol 2007;177:192–5.

37. Botros SM, Sand PK, Beaumont JL, et al. Arcus-anchored acellular dermal graft compared to anterior colporrhaphy for stage II cystoceles and beyond. Int Urogynecol J Pelvic Floor Dysfunct 2009;20:1265–71.

38. Guerette NL, Peterson TV, Aguirre OA, et al. Anterior repair with or without collagen matrix reinforcement: a randomized controlled trial. Obstet Gynecol 2009;114:59–65.

39. Hviid U, Hviid TV, Rudnicki M. Porcine skin collagen implants for anterior vaginal wall prolapse: a randomised prospective controlled study. Int Urogynecol J 2010;21:529–34.

40. Dahlgren E, Kjolhede P. Long-term outcome of porcine skin graft in surgical treatment of recurrent pelvic organ prolapse. An open randomized controlled multicenter study. Acta Obstet Gynecol Scand 2011;90:1393–401.

41. Handel LN, Frenkl TL, Kim YH. Results of cystocele repair: a comparison of traditional anterior colporrhaphy, polypropylene mesh and porcine dermis. J Urol 2007;178:153–6.

42. Menefee SA, Dyer KY, Lukacz ES, et al. Colporrhaphy compared with mesh or graft-reinforced vaginal paravaginal repair for anterior vaginal wall prolapse. Obstet Gynecol 2011;118:1337–44.

43. Maher C, Feiner B, Baessler K, et al. Surgical management of pelvic organ prolapse in women. Cochrane Database Syst Rev 2010;(4). CD004014.

44. Jia X, Glazener C, Mowatt G, et al. Efficacy and safety of using mesh or grafts in surgery for anterior and/or posterior vaginal wall prolapse: systematic review and meta-analysis. BJOG 2008;115:1350–61.

45. Natale F, La Penna C, Padoa A, et al. A prospective, randomized, controlled study comparing Gynemesh®, a synthetic mesh, and Pelvicol®, a biologic graft, in the surgical treatment of recurrent cystocele. Int Urogynecol J Pelvic Floor Dysfunct 2009; 20:75–81.

46. Long CY, Hsu CS, Jang MY, et al. Comparison of clinical outcome and urodynamic findings using "Perigee and/or Apogee" versus "Prolift anterior and/or posterior" system devices for the treatment of pelvic organ prolapse. Int Urogynecol J 2011; 22:233–9.

47. Sung VW, Rogers RG, Schaffer JI, et al, Society of Gynecologic Surgeons Systematic Review Group. Graft use in transvaginal pelvic organ prolapse repair: a systematic review. Obstet Gynecol 2008; 112:1131–42.

48. Abed H, Rahn DD, Lowenstein L, et al, Systematic Review Group of the Society of Gynecologic Surgeons. Incidence and management of graft erosion, wound granulation, and dyspareunia following vaginal prolapse repair with graft materials: a systematic review. Int Urogynecol J 2011; 22:789–98.

49. Weber AM, Walters MD, Piedmonte MR. Sexual function and vaginal anatomy in women before and after surgery for pelvic organ prolapse and urinary incontinence. Am J Obstet Gynecol 2000; 182:1610–5.

Robotic/Laparoscopic Prolapse Repair
Role of Hysteropexy: A Urogynecology Perspective

Olga Ramm, MD, MS[a,b], Kimberly Kenton, MD, MS[a,b],*

KEYWORDS

- Sacrocolpopexy • Hysteropexy • Pelvic reconstruction • Pelvic organ prolapse
- Female pelvic medicine and reconstructive surgery • Pelvic floor disorders • Laparoscopy
- Minimally invasive gynecology

KEY POINTS

- Uterine preserving surgery for pelvic organ prolapse may be appropriate for select, appropriately counseled women.
- Short and long-term patient related and anatomic outcomes of hysteropexy (with and without mesh) are needed, including possible complications related to uterine and cervical preservation.
- Surgeons should have a thorough understanding of uterine and cervical disease and fertility prior to counseling women regarding uterine preserving prolapse surgery.

INTRODUCTION

Although the uterus is now known to be a passive bystander rather than the cause of pelvic organ prolapse (POP), POP continues to be the leading cause of hysterectomy performed for benign causes in United States women older than 50 years.[1,2] In the late nineteenth and early twentieth century, before the advent of sterile surgical techniques and preoperative antibiotics, gynecologic surgeons attempted to treat prolapse without hysterectomy to avoid the danger of entering the peritoneal cavity. These early efforts at hysteropexy included uterine ventrofixation, uterine interposition, vaginal colpocleisis, and the Manchester-Fothergill operation, among others; however, all of these procedures lack durability.[3,4] As intraperitoneal surgery became increasingly safe in the latter part of the twentieth century,

hysterectomy became a routine part of POP repair, so much so that most currently available surgical outcome data concern women who underwent hysterectomy with pelvic floor repair or had post-hysterectomy prolapse repair.

As women lead longer and more active lives, pelvic reconstructive surgeons increasingly shifted attention to the long-term outcomes and durability of POP repairs. Sacrocolpopexy has emerged as the gold standard for POP repair, with a recent Cochrane review on surgical treatment of pelvic organ prolapse concluding that sacrocolpopexy was associated with better anatomic outcomes, lower rates of recurrent prolapse, longer time to prolapse recurrence, and less postoperative dyspareunia.[5] However, open abdominal sacrocolpopexy was also associated with longer recovery time and hospital stay.[5] Both of these disadvantages may

a Division of Female Pelvic Medicine & Reconstructive Surgery, Department of Obstetrics & Gynecology, Loyola University Chicago, Stritch School of Medicine, 2160 South First Avenue, Maywood, IL 60153, USA; b Department of Urology, Loyola University Chicago, Stritch School of Medicine, 2160 South First Avenue, Maywood, IL 60153, USA
* Corresponding author. Division of Female Pelvic Medicine & Reconstructive Surgery, Department of Obstetrics & Gynecology, Loyola University Chicago, Stritch School of Medicine, 2160 South First Avenue, Maywood, IL 60153.
E-mail address: kkenton@lumc.edu

Urol Clin N Am 39 (2012) 343–348
http://dx.doi.org/10.1016/j.ucl.2012.06.008

be mitigated by laparoscopic/robotic approaches, making sacrocolpopexy a common choice for primary prolapse repair. As physicians and patients turn toward minimally invasive operations, they have raised the question of why the uterus, a normal organ without intrinsic pathology, must be removed at the time of POP repair. Several investigators published articles on the feasibility of laparoscopic/robotic sacrohysteropexy. The long-term outcomes and implications of hysteropexy are not well studied, and the practice of uterine preservation at the time of pelvic floor repair is currently deemed controversial. The aim of this article is to highlight the techniques, outcomes, advantages, and potential problems surrounding minimally invasive hysteropexy.

HISTORICAL PERSPECTIVE

In the late 1800s, Drs Donald and Fothergill described the Manchester operation.[6] The Manchester operation consists of a circumferential vaginal incision, exposing then amputating the distal cervix and suturing the upper cervix or lower uterine segment to the transected cardinal ligaments for support. Shortly thereafter, Dr Thomas Watkins published his description of the Watkins interposition procedure for uterovaginal prolapse.[7] After the bladder was dissected from the uterus through an anterior colpotomy incision, the uterus was severely anteverted until the uterine fundus was pulled through the colpotomy and sutured to the anterior vaginal wall; this method was also applied to the surgical treatment of vesicovaginal fistulas. The only uterine-sparing vaginal operation still currently in use is the sacrospinous hysteropexy, which can be performed with or without mesh augmentation.[8–10]

In 1930, Arthur Giles[11] published on the outcomes following abdominal hysteropexy, which he described as the fixation of the anterior lower uterine segment to the fascia and muscle of the anterior abdominal wall using silk sutures. His case series contained an impressive 1424 women, including 135 who went on to achieve pregnancy and 111 who delivered following the hysteropexy. Uterine position was evaluated following delivery and was noted to be "normal" or "satisfactory" in 97% of cases, prompting Giles to conclude that "pregnancy has no appreciable effect in producing a return of displacement after hysteropexy has been performed." Fixation of the uterine fundus or the round ligaments to the anterior abdominal wall have since fallen out of favor, because of uterine elongation and lack of effectiveness in the treatment of prolapse over time.[3] In 1993, Joshi[12] described a retrospective cohort of 20 women with uterine suspension to the pectineal ligament with mersilene mesh. Five of these women went on to have a full-term vaginal delivery; long-term prolapse outcomes following the pregnancy and delivery are unknown.

MINIMALLY INVASIVE TECHNIQUES

Robotic/laparoscopic hysteropexy can be performed using sutured native tissue as well as mesh. Maher and colleagues[13] described laparoscopic plication of the uterosacral ligaments to obliterate the posterior cul-de-sac and elevate the cervix posteriorly in 43 women. With 12 ± 7 months follow-up, 81% were subjectively cured and 79% objectively cured of prolapse. Outcomes are limited by short-term follow-up and lack of validated outcome measures.

Because of its durability, robotic or laparoscopic sacrocolpopexy is the most commonly performed robotic pelvic reconstructive procedure.[14] Several investigators have published on the feasibility of laparoscopic/robotic sacrohysteropexy with varying techniques.[15–17] Most commonly, a rectangular piece of mesh is attached to the posterior aspect of the lower uterine segment and the cervix, extending to just below the level of the uterosacral ligaments, then pexed to the anterior longitudinal ligament at the sacral promontory. The anterior mesh is often Y-shaped, with the single arm attached to the anterior cervix and lower uterine segment, then split into 2 arms, each of which is passed through a window created within the broad ligament, then secured to the anterior longitudinal ligament. Based on data derived from open sacrocolpopexy, anatomic outcomes are better if a permanent mesh is attached to the anterior and posterior vaginal walls (not just the apex), then to the sacrum with permanent sutures.[18,19] Open techniques that do not place the mesh anteriorly are associated with up to 30% anterior vaginal wall recurrence rates.[18] Similarly, sacral sutures are sometimes replaced by tacking devices during robotic and laparoscopic procedures; however, available comparative studies use sutures on the sacrum, so the outcomes after using sacral tacks are unknown.[18,20]

OUTCOMES

There is no level I evidence regarding the impact of uterine preservation on the effectiveness or longevity of prolapse repair, and all available information is based on individual-center case series. Maher and colleagues[13] published their 1-year outcomes of laparoscopic uterosacral hysteropexy in 43 women, reporting an 80% objective and subjective cure rate. Two women in this series completed term pregnancies and were delivered by elective cesarean without recurrence of prolapse during the short follow-up time. In 2001, Leron and Stanton[21] published their case series of 12 women with second- or third-degree uterine prolapse who were treated with open sacrohysteropexy using anteriorly and posteriorly placed Teflon mesh. Although no objective outcomes are reported, more than 50% of women reported that the operation improved their life, and the investigators concluded that mesh-augmented sacrohysteropexy is both feasible and safe. Long-term outcomes of open sacrohysteropexy are limited to a follow-up time of 3 to 5 years and report a 93% success rate (prolapse<Stage 2).[22,23] A single-site study of 55 women with greater than stage 2 prolapse undergoing open (n = 47) or laparoscopic (n = 8) sacrohysteropexy with mesh placed anteriorly and posteriorly suggests high success rates. Objective cure, defined as cervix at least 6 cm inside the hymen and no prolapse beyond the hymen, was approximately 87% with all recurrences being anterior or posterior.[22] Rosen and colleagues[24] published the only comparative study addressing the impact of laparoscopic uterine preservation on prolapse outcomes in 2008. Sixty-four women with stage 2 to 4 POP scheduled for laparoscopic pelvic floor repair self-selected to undergo hysterectomy versus uterine preservation. At 12 months, 13% of those in the hysterectomy group had recurrent prolapse compared with 21% in the hysteropexy group. This study is limited by lack of standardization of surgical technique, with some patients undergoing "global pelvic floor repair," others having single-compartment repair, and others with additional vaginal procedures, limiting generalizability of these data. Laparoscopic and robotic sacrohysteropexy are increasingly performed despite the limited data on outcomes. Even fewer data are known regarding the pregnancy rates and outcomes after sacrohysteropexy; however, there is a case report of a successful pregnancy carried to term following laparoscopic sacrohysteropexy.[16] The patient's prolapse recurred after 2 years, at which time she was treated with a hysterectomy and sacrocolpopexy.

UNIQUE CONSIDERATIONS
Fertility

As previously outlined, there are several case reports of successful pregnancies achieved following hysteropexy.[11,12,16] For those women wishing to preserve their fertility but substantially bothered by prolapse to warrant surgical intervention, hysteropexy can be discussed as an option.

These discussions must underscore the paucity of data available on the impact of hysteropexy on conception rates, rates of preterm delivery, and complications at the time of delivery. The likelihood of recurrent prolapse following pregnancy and delivery must also be addressed. The best mode of delivery following pelvic floor repair is unknown; the authors recommend an individualized approach, taking into consideration obstetric indications and complications, future fertility plans, and patient preference. These conversations are probably best had in conjunction with the patient's obstetrician to balance obstetric risks and benefits regarding pelvic floor repair. Similarly, if the sacrohysteropexy includes anteriorly placed mesh, the obstetrician should be advised as to the location of the mesh, as it may affect the surgical approach and planning for cesarean delivery. Standard practice at present suggests that women undergo surgical repair of their pelvic floor disorders after they have completed childbearing and use conservative treatments, such as pessary, until that time.

Mesh Complications

When performing a concomitant hysterectomy, the majority of reconstructive surgeons now prefer supracervical hysterectomy to total hysterectomy to decrease the risk of mesh complications.[25–27] A large multicenter cohort of women undergoing open sacrocolpopexy reported a nearly 5-fold increase in vaginal mesh erosion with concomitant total hysterectomy compared with sacrocolpopexy alone for vault prolapse.[25] Similarly, a retrospective case series reported 7-fold higher mesh-erosion rates after sacrocolpopexy with concomitant total hysterectomy (8%) than after sacrocolpopexy with supracervical hysterectomy (0) or vault suspension (0).[26] Recently, a retrospective series of 188 women undergoing minimally invasive sacrocolpopexy (laparoscopic or robotic) reported mesh erosion/exposure rates of 10%.[27] Subgroup analyses comparing 3 groups (concomitant supracervical hysterectomy, concomitant vaginal hysterectomy, and post-hysterectomy) found a 5.7-fold increased odds of mesh erosion in the vaginal hysterectomy group (23%) compared with supracervical hysterectomy (5%) and post-hysterectomy groups (5%). Erosion rates with abdominally placed polypropylene mesh approximate 3%.[28] It stands to reason that avoiding the hysterectomy altogether and performing hysteropexy may decrease mesh-exposure rates even further. Two of 55 patients in the previously discussed series of sacrohysteropexies had vaginal mesh exposures requiring revision.[22]

Cervical Disease

Women who choose pelvic floor repair with uterine preservation must be up to date with routine cervical screening,[29] including a recent normal Papanicolaou (pap) test, and be carefully queried for a history of cervical dysplasia. Those who have a history of cervical dysplasia, especially cervical intraepithelial neoplasia grade II or higher, should be counseled regarding the need for continued surveillance with pap tests and/or colposcopy, in accordance with American Society for Colposcopy and Cervical Pathology guidelines. Persistent or progressive high-grade dysplasia refractory to local excision may necessitate a hysterectomy, which can be complicated by a prior hysteropexy, especially if the procedure was augmented with permanent mesh. Surgeons should educate and provide patients with a copy of the operative report in the event that the patient needs hysterectomy in the future, as vaginal hysterectomy may be challenging.

Uterine Disease

Leaving the uterus in situ at the time of pelvic floor repair also allows for the development of endometrial or myometrial abnormality, especially if the repair is performed in younger women with decades of future life expectancy. Although there are several available medical therapies for leiomyomata, fibroids continue to be the leading cause of benign hysterectomy in the United States.[1] How previous hysteropexy with or without mesh will influence medical management of leiomyomata or affect surgical risk of hysterectomy is unknown. Endometrial carcinoma is the most common gynecologic malignancy, and its treatment requires surgical excision and staging.[30] Prior hysteropexy may affect surgical risks associated with this procedure. Upward of 80% of endometrial cancers are diagnosed in stage I[29] because the disease causes uterine bleeding in

precancerous (endometrial hyperplasia) and early stages. Thus, any woman planning pelvic floor repair should be queried about a recent history of postmenopausal uterine bleeding or irregular uterine bleeding if premenopausal, and those who report abnormal uterine bleeding should be further evaluated with an endometrial biopsy and/or pelvic ultrasonography before any surgical procedure.[31,32] The rate of endometrial cancer in asymptomatic women planning POP repair is low (0.6%), rendering preoperative screening methods ineffective in this population.[30] Women can further be reassured by the low likelihood of developing endometrial cancer following uterine-preserving pelvic floor repair, with a review of 517 women who underwent vaginal hysterectomy as a part of POP repair in the United Kingdom reporting a 0.8% malignancy rate.[33] However, if women choose uterine-sparing surgical treatment of prolapse at increasingly younger ages, their chances of developing a uterine malignancy may increase.

SUMMARY

Uterine-preserving procedures, including sacrohysteropexy, are increasingly performed for pelvic organ prolapse. Limited data are available to guide surgeons and patients regarding long-term pelvic floor outcomes and complications of sacrohysteropexy; however, early data suggest hysteropexy may be an option in carefully selected women. Comparative long-term outcomes studies capturing objective, symptom-based, and quality-of-life outcomes as well as short-term and long-term complications are necessary.

In addition to prolapse outcomes and complications, women choosing sacrohysteropexy should be counseled regarding the importance of appropriate gynecologic surveillance for uterine and cervical pathology as well as the potential impact hysteropexy (especially with permanent mesh) may have on future hysterectomy and fertility in women of reproductive age.

EDITOR'S COMMENTS

Robotics represents the most advanced and most expensive of the current technologies available for pelvic floor surgical indications. Initially used as a minimally invasive replacement for open sacralcolpopexy, robotics is now being essayed for ureteral re-implantation, vesicovaginal fistula repair, and even excision of eroded or problematic mesh. While all of these indications are reasonable and certainly allow more rapid convalescence, risk/benefit ratios and medical economic costs must be factored into the overall calculation of value based care around the use of the robot.

The authors present their robotic approaches to apical prolapse, inclusive of lessons learned and technical tips. Both groups have been among the earliest adopters and now represent some of the most experienced units performing these procedures for vaginal prolapse. The outcomes are commendable and demonstrate the importance of apical fixation for vaginal vault stabilization. The addition of mesh arm extension represents an approach for simultaneous management of associated anterior and posterior defects. Additionally, extended posterior mesh arms may be fashioned to stabilize the perineum and posterior cul-de-sac (sacralcolpoperineopexy).

However, several variables regarding robotic prolapse repair must be addressed. A learning curve for performing sacralcolpopexy exists and this curve is accentuated by the addition of robotics. Both the procedure and the associated robotic technique require separate technical acquisition skills and therefore it is preferable to have some experience with sacralcolpopexy prior to initiating robotic assistance. As surgical and robotic simulation labs improve – many of these skills can now be acquired simultaneously. Robotic peritoneal access skills are critical to successful procedural performance, and these skills may also be acquired initially in the simulation lab experience, followed by structured and mentored live surgical experience. The recognition of thermal and crush injuries is another critical aspect of surgical safety, and therefore familiarity and facility with the robotic surgical instrumentation is essential to successful robotic surgery.

The most important question, however, is not whether robotics *can* be performed for all the noted pelvic floor procedures, but whether this approach *should* be done. Medical economics will enter into this decision in the very near future and may actually lead to restricted use of this technique to high volume centers with experienced teams. Also familiarity with base procedure (ie, sacralcolpopexy) is critical, and the occasional performance of reconstructive procedures just because a surgical robot is available may not provide the best outcomes. Additionally, the presence of an experienced team and structured perioperative process cannot be underestimated, and a commitment to the development of both aspects is critical to a successful robotic surgical program.

Roger R. Dmochowski, MD
Mickey Karram, MD

REFERENCES

1. Wu JM, Hundley AF, Fulton RG, et al. Forecasting the prevalence of pelvic floor disorders in U.S. Women: 2010 to 2050. Obstet Gynecol 2009; 114(6):1278–83.

2. Smith FJ, Holman CD, Moorin RE, et al. Lifetime risk of undergoing surgery for pelvic organ prolapse. Obstet Gynecol 2010;116(5):1096–100.

3. Durfee RB. Suspension operations for treatment of pelvic organ prolapse. Clin Obstet Gynecol 1966; 9(4):1047–61.

4. O'Conor J. A mode for ventrofixation of the uterus for the relief of prolapses. Ann Surg 1915;62(4): 479–80.2.

5. Maher C, Feiner B, Baessler K, et al. Surgical management of pelvic organ prolapse in women. Cochrane Database Syst Rev 2010;4:CD004014.

6. Conger GT, Keettel WC. The Manchester-Fothergill operation, its place in gynecology: a review of 960 cases at University Hospitals, Iowa City, Iowa. Am J Obstet Gynecol 1958;76:634–40.

7. Cashman BZ. The combined Manchester-Watkins interposition operation in the treatment of prolapse of the uterus. Am J Obstet Gynecol 1946;51:706.

8. Maher CF, Cary MP, Slack MC, et al. Uterine preservation or hysterectomy at sacrospinous colpopexy for uterovaginal prolapse? Int Urogynecol J Pelvic Floor Dysfunct 2001;12:381–4.

9. Dietz V, de Jong J, Huisman M, et al. The effectiveness of the sacrospinous hysteropexy for the primary treatment of uterovaginal prolapse. Int Urogynecol J Pelvic Floor Dysfunct 2007;18:1271–6.

10. Gamble TL, Aschkenazi SO, Nguyen A, et al. Bilateral graft-augmented sacrospinous hysteropexy: d1-year anatomic and functional outcomes following surgery for uterine preservation. J Pelvic Med Surg 2008;14:275.

11. Giles AE. The effect of hysteropexy upon a subsequent pregnancy, and of pregnancy upon a previous hysteropexy. Proc R Soc Med 1930;23(8):1170–7.

12. Joshi VM. A new technique of uterine suspension to pectineal ligaments in the management of uterovaginal prolapse. Obstet Gynecol 1993;81:790–3.

13. Maher CF, Carey MP, Murray CJ. Laparoscopic suture hysteropexy for uterine prolapse. Obstet Gynecol 2001;97(6):1010–4.

14. Visco AG, Advincula AP. Robotic gynecologic surgery. Obstet Gynecol 2008;112(6):1369–84.

15. Price N, Stack A, Jackson SR. Laparoscopic hysteropexy: the initial results of a uterine suspension procedure for uterovaginal prolapse. BJOG 2010; 117(1):62–8.

16. Lewis CM, Culligan P. Sacrohysteropexy followed by successful pregnancy and eventual reoperation for prolapse. Int Urogynecol J 2012;23(7):957–9.

17. Faraj R, Broome J. Laparoscopic sacrohysteropexy and myomectomy for uterine prolapse: a case report and review of the literature. J Med Case Rep 2009;3:99.

18. Brubaker L. Sacrocolpolexy and the anterior compartment: support and function. Am J Obstet Gynecol 1995;176(6):1690–6.

19. Geller EJ, Siddique S, Wu J, et al. Comparison of short-term outcomes of robotic sacrocolpopexy versus abdominal sacrocolpopexy. J Pelvic Med Surg 2008;14(4):233–4.

20. Paraiso M, Chen C, Jelovsek JE, et al. Conventional laparoscopic versus robotic-assisted laparoscopic sacral colpopexy: a randomized controlled trial. Female Pelvic Med Reconstr Surg 2010;16(5):S58.

21. Leron E, Stanton SL. Sacrohysteropexy with synthetic mesh for the management of uterovaginal prolapse. BJOG 2001;108:629–33.

22. Costantini E, Lazzeri M, Zucchi A, et al. Five-year outcome of uterus sparing surgery for pelvic organ prolapse repair: a single-center experience. Int Urogynecol J 2011;22(3):287–92.

23. Barranger E, Fritel X, Pigne A. Abdominal sacrohysteropexy in young women with uterovaginal prolapse: long-term follow-up. Am J Obstet Gynecol 2003; 189(5):1245–50.

24. Rosen DM, Shukla A, Cario GM, et al. Is hysterectomy necessary for laparoscopic pelvic floor repair. A prospective study. J Minim Invasive Gynecol 2008;15(6):729–34.

25. Cundiff GW, Varner E, Visco AG, et al. Risk factors for mesh/suture erosion following sacral colpopexy. Obstet Gynecol 2008;199(6):688.e1–5.

26. Bensinger G, Lind L, Guess M, et al. Abdominal sacral suspensions: analysis of complications using permanent mesh. J Pelvic Med Surg 2005;11(2):66.

27. Tan-Kim J, Menefee SA, Luber KM, et al. Prevalence and risk factors for mesh erosion after laparoscopic-assisted sacrocolpopexy. Int Urogynecol J Pelvic Floor Dysfunct 2011;22(2):205–12.

28. Nygaard IE, McCreery R, Brubaker L, et al. Abdominal sacrocolpopexy: a comprehensive review. Obstet Gynecol 2004;104(4):805–23.

29. Available at: http://www.asccp.org/Consensus Guidelines/tabid/7436/Default.aspx. Accessed April, 2012.

30. Ramm O, Gleason JL, Segal S, et al. Utility of preoperative endometrial assessment in asymptomatic women undergoing hysterectomy for pelvic floor dysfunction. Int Urogynecol J 2012;23(7):913–7.

31. American College of Obstetricians and Gynecologists practice bulletin 14: management of anovulatory bleeding. Washington, DC: American College of Obstetricians & Gynecologists; 2009.

32. Renganathan A, Edwards R, Duckett JR. Uterus conserving prolapse surgery—what is the chance of missing a malignancy? Int Urogynecol J 2010; 21(7):819–21.

33. Barrett RJ 2nd, Harlan LC, Wesley MN, et al. Endometrial cancer: stage at diagnosis and associated factors in black and white patients. Am J Obstet Gynecol 1995;173(2):414–22.

Robotic/Laparoscopic Prolapse Repair and the Role of Hysteropexy: A Urology Perspective

Kimberly L. Burgess, MD, Daniel S. Elliott, MD*

KEYWORDS

- Pelvic organ prolapse • Uterine prolapse • Robotics • Surgical procedures • Operative

KEY POINTS

- The abdominal sacrocolpopexy offers high long term success for the management of apical prolapse and can be performed using an open, laparoscopic, or robotic approach.
- The laparoscopic and robotic approaches offer decreased blood loss and decreased length of hospital stay with similar complication rates compared to the open procedure.
- Hysteropexy may be used to treat uterine prolapse in select patients with decreased morbidity compared to pelvic organ prolapse repair performed with concomitant hysterectomy.

INTRODUCTION

Approximately 11% of women will undergo a surgical procedure for the treatment of pelvic organ prolapse (POP) or urinary incontinence by age 80 years.[1] There are varying reports of the incidence of vaginal vault prolapse following hysterectomy, with Marchionni and colleagues[2] reporting the incidence of vaginal vault prolapse at 4.4% following hysterectomy based on examination. When hysterectomy was performed for prolapse, the subsequent incidence of vaginal vault prolapse was 11.6%.[2] It is estimated that 1 in 9 women will undergo a hysterectomy in their lifetime.[3] Following hysterectomy, the median time to vault prolapse is reported at around 15.8 years (range 0.4–48.4 years).[4] There are multiple surgical approaches available to manage apical prolapse, with many studies evaluating for the repair that offers the most effective, safe, and durable treatment, as the reoperation rate for POP may be as high as 30%.[1] Goals of surgical repair for POP include relief of symptoms, restoration of support to pelvic structures, prevention of new defects in pelvic support, prevention of new symptoms, and improvement or maintenance of urinary, bowel, and sexual function.[5] Surgical treatment options include both vaginal and abdominal approaches along with the option of laparoscopic and robotic procedures. Abdominal sacrocolpopexy (ASC) has been found in multiple studies to have high long-term success rates for repair of severe vault prolapse,[6] and the focus of this article is describing laparoscopic sacrocolpopexy (LSC) and robotic sacrocolpopexy (RSC). The role of hysteropexy for the treatment of POP is also discussed.

RELEVANT ANATOMY AND EVALUATION

POP is defined as the descent of one or more of the pelvic organs. It is estimated that 50% of parous women lose pelvic floor support.[1,7] Swift showed in an observational study that 50% of women presenting for an annual pelvic examination had stage II to III POP. The study consisted of 497 women with a mean age of 44 years, and the incidence increased to 74% with age older

The authors have nothing to disclose.
Department of Urology, Mayo Clinic, 200 First Street Southwest, Rochester, MN 55905, USA
* Corresponding author.
E-mail address: elliott.daniel@mayo.edu

Urol Clin N Am 39 (2012) 349–360
http://dx.doi.org/10.1016/j.ucl.2012.05.006
0094-0143/12/$ – see front matter © 2012 Elsevier Inc. All rights reserved.

than 70 years.[8] Parity, increased age, constipation, and obesity are some of the reported risk factors for developing POP,[3,5] with obesity being the primary risk factor for developing post-hysterectomy vaginal vault prolapse in one study.[2] In this report, the incidence of obesity was 45% among those who developed prolapse following hysterectomy, compared with 10.5% in those who did not develop vaginal vault prolapse.[2]

There are multiple structures providing support for the female pelvic organs including bone, muscle, and endopelvic fascia. The pelvic floor consists of the pelvic diaphragm, made up of the levator ani group, coccygeus muscles, and surrounding fascia.[9,10] From these structures, a shelf of muscle is formed that attaches to the pelvic side wall by the arcus tendineus fasciae pelvis that runs between the pubic symphysis and the ischial spine. The upper vagina rests on this shelf, creating its natural axis, which is horizontal. Vaginal prolapse may occur when this axis is altered.[5,9] DeLancey[11] described 3 levels of vaginal support within the pelvis: level I or apical support, level II or lateral support, and level III or distal support. Suspension of the vaginal apex is the result of level I support, and apical or vaginal vault prolapse is the consequence when this level of support is lost.[11] There are ligamentous supports to the female pelvic organs also, with the upper vagina and the uterus having support from the cardinal and uterosacral ligaments.[12] The cardinal ligaments extend between the cervix and pelvic side wall while the uterosacral ligaments run from the sacrum to the cervix and vaginal fornices, and these structures can be damaged by a hysterectomy.[5,10,12] **Fig. 1** illustrates vaginal vault prolapse.

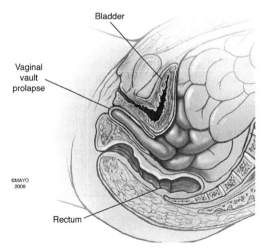

Fig. 1. Vaginal vault prolapse. (*Courtesy of* Mayo Clinic, Rochester, Minnesota.)

Symptoms of POP include pelvic bulge, pelvic pressure, pelvic pain, back pain, voiding complaints, bowel symptoms, dyspareunia, or difficulty walking or sitting.[3,7,13] The most common presenting symptom is pelvic bulge, which is reportedly present in 94% to 100% of patients.[4,14] Obtaining a thorough history and proper counseling of the patient can help reduce postoperative patient dissatisfaction, especially in cases where patients falsely attribute symptoms to their prolapse that, in actuality, are caused by unrelated medical conditions. In such cases patients may have false expectations, compromising the success of the procedure performed. A thorough pelvic examination is vital in the evaluation for POP, and one should distinguish between anterior, apical, and posterior prolapse, which is important in determining the appropriate treatment. Care should also be taken to evaluate for voiding dysfunction such as urinary incontinence, as Mayne and Assassa[15] reported that up to 45% of women older than 40 years have symptoms of voiding dysfunction, and up to 26% of these women will have clinically significant symptoms. Identifying the presence of voiding dysfunction is important, as concomitant procedures may need to be considered at the time of prolapse repair and these coexisting conditions may affect the patient's expectations. Having the patient stand, if they are physically able, during the physical examination is preferred, and the patient should be asked to strain during the examination to assess the maximum degree of prolapse along with the function of the pelvic muscles.[1] If the patient has any evidence of anterior prolapse, the examiner should reduce the prolapse and instruct the patient to Valsalva to evaluate for the presence of urinary incontinence, as there are reports of stress urinary incontinence (SUI) being present concomitantly in up to 38% and urge incontinence in 26% of those with POP.[4,16,17] One should also consider checking a postvoid residual, as there is a risk of preoperative urinary retention, particularly in older women. It is reported that 89% of these women will have resolution of their urinary retention following treatment of their POP.[18] The staging used to grade POP is:

Stage 0: No prolapse present
Stage I: Distal portion of prolapse greater than 1 cm above hymen
Stage II: Distal portion of prolapse within 1 cm of hymen, either above or below
Stage III: Distal portion of prolapse greater than 1 cm below hymen but not complete eversion
Stage IV: Complete vaginal eversion.

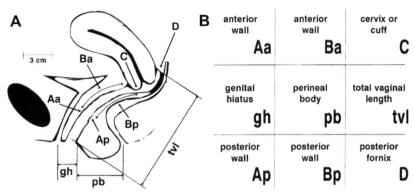

Fig. 2. POP-Q staging system. (*A*) Six sites (points Aa, Ba, C, D, Bp, and Ap), genital hiatus (gh), perineal body (pb), and total vaginal length (tvl) used for pelvic organ support quantitation. (*B*) Grid for recording quantitative description of pelvic organ support. (*Reprinted from* Bump RC, Mattiasson A, Bo K, et al. The standardization of terminology of female pelvic organ prolapse and pelvic floor dysfunction. Am J Obstet Gynecol 1996;175(1):12–3; with permission.)

The pelvic organ prolapse quantification (POPQ) system standardizes the staging of POP (**Fig. 2**) using reference points within the vagina to characterize the level and location of prolapse present. Using this system, point C represents the cervix or vaginal cuff; a negative value is assigned when prolapse is proximal to the hymen, and a positive number assigned when prolapse extends distal to the hymen.[5,19]

TREATMENT OPTIONS AND GOALS OF REPAIR

Treatment consists of obliterative or restorative procedures. Colpocleisis, an obliterative procedure, is an option for patients who no longer desire sexual intercourse or have other medical comorbidities that make more invasive procedures less appealing, while still offering the patient a high success rate reported at 90% to 100%.[18] The goals of a restorative procedure, which can be performed via a transvaginal or transabdominal approach, are restoration of vaginal anatomy with preservation of vaginal axis, length, and function.[20,21] When approaching vaginal vault prolapse transvaginally, treatment consists of fixation of the vaginal apex to the sacrospinous ligaments, uterosacral ligaments, or ileococcygeus muscles. Traditional advantages of a transvaginal approach compared with ASC included decreased operative time, recovery time, and cost, and avoidance of an abdominal incision.[7,22] Not all of these advantages hold true with the introduction of minimally invasive repairs such as LSC and RSC, and a significant disadvantage with a transvaginal repair is the consistently lower long-term success rate in comparison with an abdominal approach.[23]

The mainstay of transabdominal repairs for the management of vaginal vault prolapse is ASC, which provides high success rates and durable results. When success is defined as a lack of apical prolapse, long-term success is obtained in 78% to 100% of patients following ASC.[6] A Cochrane review of the surgical management of POP identified 40 randomized controlled trials comparing vaginal sacrospinous ligament suspension with ASC, and found that there was a decreased incidence of recurrent vaginal vault prolapse and dyspareunia with ASC. Also, in patients with persistent apical prolapse the stage was lower following ASC versus vaginal repair.[7] The ASC consists of fixation of mesh to the anterior and posterior aspects of the vaginal apex that extends to the sacral promontory. Among synthetic grafts, monofilament, large-pore polypropylene mesh (Type 1) grafts have the lowest rate of erosion reported.[5] Advantages of the ASC in managing vaginal vault prolapse are support of the vault to the anterior surface of the sacrum preserving (or restoring) the normal axis of the vagina, preservation of maximal vaginal depth, and strength to weakened native tissue with the use of synthetic suspensory material. Preservation of vaginal depth is important in patients who desire continued sexual activity, particularly in patients with an already foreshortened vagina from previous surgery. **Fig. 3** illustrates the end result following sacrocolpopexy.

LAPAROSCOPIC SACROCOLPOPEXY

With the introduction of less invasive approaches, sacrocolpopexy has become a more attractive option because it provides a highly successful repair

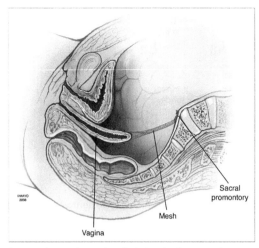

Fig. 3. The end result of abdominal sacrocolpopexy. (*Courtesy of* Mayo Clinic, Rochester, Minnesota.)

along with a better cosmetic result and a shorter recovery time. In recent years there has been a significant amount of data published evaluating LSC and RSC and the outcomes after these procedures. Regarding conventional laparoscopy for the repair of vaginal vault prolapse, published comparative studies evaluating LSC versus ASC show similar success rates along with similar complication rates.[24,25] In a study by Klauschie and colleagues,[25] patients were evaluated for mean improvement in reference point C in the POPQ grading system following LSC and ASC, with no significant difference noted between the 2 groups. High anatomic success along with high patient satisfaction was reported in a review of 11 series of LSC, which included more than 1000 patients, with mean anatomic success rate of 92% (range 75%–100%) and mean patient satisfaction of 94.4% (range 79%–98%).[26] Another benefit of a laparoscopic approach other than better cosmesis is the enhanced view of pelvic anatomy secondary to magnification and the increased field of view.[27,28]

The surgical procedure is described here; however, as with any procedure, there are variations depending on the surgeon's preference and experience. Patients are placed in the lithotomy position and then are put into steep Trendelenburg position to allow a view of the pelvis free of small bowel.[29] First, pneumoperitoneum is obtained and ports are placed. Of note, the associated pneumoperitoneum can facilitate the dissection of an associated enterocele by producing ballooning of the enterocele.[20] One may use any of the multiple port configurations described in the literature. A few of these configurations are

described here, with one possible layout consisting of a 10-mm umbilical port for the camera, two 5-mm ports placed two-thirds of the distance between the umbilicus and anterior superior iliac spine on each side, and either a 5- or 10-mm port halfway between the umbilicus and pubic symphysis.[29,30] Another configuration is placement of a 10-mm camera port at the umbilicus, two 5-mm ports placed 5 cm above and medial to the anterior superior iliac spine on each side, a 5-mm port placed halfway between the lateral and umbilical ports on one side, and a 10-mm port placed in the same position on the contralateral side.[16] In a recent randomized controlled trial comparing LSC with RSC, 4 ports were placed for an LSC: a 5-mm umbilical port for the camera, two 10- or 12-mm ports in the lower quadrants, and one 5-mm port placed lateral to the rectus muscle 9 cm subcostally on one side.[31] Once port placement is complete, the sigmoid is retracted to the left, allowing identification of the sacral promontory. The sacral promontory is identified and the overlying peritoneum is incised, which is then carried inferiorly into the pelvis staying lateral to the rectum and being careful to avoid the right ureter.[29] When working in the area of the sacrum, care should be taken to avoid damaging the presacral veins, as significant hemorrhage may occur.[5,13,20] Attention is then turned to the vaginal apex, and at this point placement of a vaginal retractor aids in identifying the limits of the vaginal vault by deflection of the vagina. **Fig. 4** shows an example of a customized hand-held retractor, although others describe using retractors such as an end-to-end anastomotic sizer or ring forceps.[5,20] The dissection of the anterior and posterior vaginal walls starts with incising the peritoneum over the vaginal apex. Anteriorly, the bladder is dissected off of the vagina for at least a few centimeters, using forceps and scissors with electrocautery, and this should be a relatively bloodless plane. Posteriorly, the rectovaginal space is entered and rectum is dissected away from the posterior vagina.[13] Like the various port-placement configurations that may be used, there are also variations in the graft placed. The authors prefer to use a preformed Y-shaped piece of mesh whereas some use separate strips of mesh for the anterior and posterior vagina.[5] There are also groups that report only placing mesh along the posterior vaginal wall,[28,30] and one series reports attachment of the posterior mesh to the levator ani instead of the posterior vagina.[16] Suture material should be nonabsorbable, and full-thickness sutures are placed in an interrupted fashion to securely attach the mesh graft to the vaginal

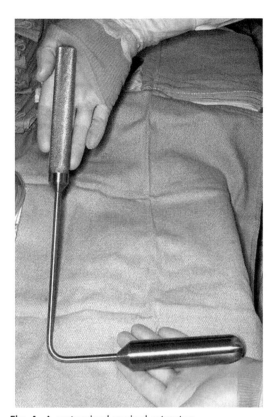

Fig. 4. A customized vaginal retractor.

apex. Interrupted sutures are then placed through the anterior longitudinal ligament and periosteum of the sacrum, avoiding the presacral veins. These sutures are used to secure the long arm of the Y-shaped graft to the sacral promontory while avoiding excessive tension on the vaginal apex. Knots may be tied with either an intracorporeal or extracorporeal technique, depending on the surgeon's preference. The mesh may be secured to the sacral promontory using tacks rather than sutures.[12,28] As one of the reported disadvantages of LSC is knot tying, one may consider using a disposable suturing device, such as the Endo-stitch (US Surgical Corp., Norwalk, CT, USA) to make laparoscopic suturing easier. The last step of the procedure is closing the peritoneum over the graft.

Decreased postoperative pain, blood loss, and length of hospital stay are advantages of LSC compared with the open ASC.[20,24,26,27] A review of LSC including 11 different series found that the overall average rate of recurrent prolapse requiring reoperation was 6.2% at a mean follow-up of 24.6 months.[26] A recent study involving 4 centers in France reported quality-of-life outcomes at 1 year following LSC, with anatomic

success in 94%, a patient satisfaction rate of 98.6%, and significant improvement in quality-of-life scores.[32] As already mentioned, one of the major disadvantages reported with this technique is the difficulty associated with laparoscopic knot tying along with a steep learning curve, resulting in increased operative time in comparison with the open approach.[20,26,27] According to Paraiso and colleagues,[24] for surgeons choosing to adopt a conventional laparoscopic approach the rate-limiting step is the learning curve associated with laparoscopic suturing and knot tying. One reason for advocating use of the surgical robot is that suturing is reportedly easier compared with a conventional laparoscopic approach. A study comparing suturing tasks using standard laparoscopy versus robotic assistance showed that whereas laparoscopic novices performed better with all tasks assessed when using the robot, laparoscopic experts demonstrated improvement only in their economy of movement or path length, with no difference noted in speed or smoothness of the task with the use of the surgical robotic system.[33] It was noted that the early learning curve associated with standard laparoscopy was eliminated in laparoscopic novices with use of the robotic system and, therefore, the decision to use a standard laparoscopic or robotic approach to perform a sacrocolpopexy may depend on the surgeon's baseline laparoscopic skills.[33] An expert laparoscopist may not gain significant benefit with robotic assistance. Another aspect that needs to be taken into account when deciding between surgical approaches is the associated cost, and the increased operative time along with the use of disposable instruments has been reported to result in LSC having an increased cost compared with ASC.[34] Another potential disadvantage of laparoscopy or robotics is the risk of anesthesia-related complications that may occur secondary to the pneumoperitoneum, which is not a risk associated with an open approach.[27] Overall, LSC has been shown to be a safe and effective alternative to ASC, with the benefit of being less invasive.

ROBOTIC SACROCOLPOPEXY

The daVinci surgical robot (Surgical Intuitive, Sunnyvale, CA, USA) was approved by the Federal Drug Administration in 2005 for use in gynecologic surgery.[19] The features offered by the daVinci robotic surgical system compared with standard laparoscopy include 3-dimensional imaging, instruments with 7 degrees of freedom that may offer improved dexterity, and tremor filtration.[19,35–37] These factors provide an ergonomic environment for the surgeon that may simplify the performance of complex laparoscopic tasks particularly with laparoscopic novices, as discussed earlier. Overall the goal of RSC, like other approaches, is to provide the most durable repair while minimizing the morbidity associated with transabdominal procedures.

As for LSC, it is important to understand that variations of the RSC procedure exist and only one approach is presented here. As described for LSC, the patient is placed in the dorsal lithotomy position. A face-shield plate may be used to protect the endotracheal tube and the patient's face from potential trauma from the robotic scope, which is larger than a standard laparoscopic scope. Pneumoperitoneum is attained at the umbilicus. After obtaining pneumoperitoneum, ports are placed, beginning with placement of a 12-mm periumbilical port, which may be placed under direct vision to avoid visceral or vascular injury. The remaining ports, as shown in **Fig. 5**, are placed as follows: one 12-mm port right subcostal lateral to the rectus muscle, one 5-mm port 1 hand-breadth inferior laterally, and two 8-mm robotic ports placed lateral to the rectus muscle 2 finger-breadths superior to the iliac crest. Another option for port configuration, as described by Paraiso and colleagues,[31] consists of a shallow "W" formation with a 12-mm umbilical port for the scope, a 12-mm port placed subcostally at the level of the umbilicus lateral to the rectus muscle on the right, one 8-mm robotic port placed at this same location on the contralateral side, and two 8-mm robotic ports just lateral to the rectus on each

side in the lower quadrants. Whichever port configuration is used, it is important to make sure that there is enough space between the robotic ports so that the robotic arms will not collide. One method to ensure this is to verify that ports are spaced a hand-breadth or 8 to 9 cm apart. The patient is placed into steep Trendelenburg position and the robot is docked with the base positioned at the foot of the bed. Similar to the LSC approach, the sigmoid colon is reflected cephalad and to the left followed by incision of the posterior peritoneum, exposing the sacral promontory. Sometimes it is helpful to place a retracting suture through an appendix epiploica of the sigmoid to help expose the sacral promontory, or the third arm can be used to provide traction. At this point, mobilization of the vagina is performed with the aid of a hand-held vaginal retractor, such as the customized retractor discussed previously and shown in **Fig. 4**. The anterior mobilization involves dissection of the bladder from the anterior vaginal wall using forceps and scissors with electrocautery. This dissection is performed as distal as possible toward the introitus, which will maximize the support given by the mesh graft. Posteriorly, the peritoneal reflection is incised to mobilize the posterior vaginal wall away from the rectum and also carried distally. After adequate vaginal mobilization, attention is turned to the sacral promontory where the dissection should expose the periosteum, which is accomplished with careful attention to avoid presacral veins, as discussed previously, although this dissection can also be performed before the vaginal dissection. Next,

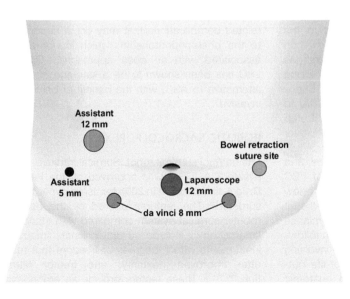

Fig. 5. Example of port placement configuration for robotic sacrocolpopexy. The bowel retraction suture site (*yellow circle*) also represents a potential site for a third robotic-arm port.

the polypropylene Y-graft is brought into the field through the 10-mm port but, as discussed with LSC, there are other graft configurations that may be used. The graft is then sutured with interrupted full-thickness sutures at the vagina using 1.0 Gore-Tex Suture with the 30° lens and vaginal retractor to maximize exposure for placement of the sutures. The long arm of the Y-graft is then sutured to the periosteum of the sacral promontory using approximately 3 interrupted sutures, with careful attention to avoid any undue tension on the vagina. Finally, the posterior peritoneum is closed over the mesh graft with a running absorbable suture.[2,35,37–39]

Improved cosmesis, decreased hospital stay, and decreased blood loss are the main advantages of RSC, just as for LSC. The reported disadvantages of RSC are increased operative time and cost.[19,40] The daVinci robotic system offers features such as articulating instruments, which may decrease the learning curve associated with complex tasks using conventional laparoscopy. As already mentioned, the decrease in the learning curve is most significant with laparoscopic novices.[33] Akl and colleagues[36] reported that operative time decreased by 25.4% after the first 10 RSC cases. An equivalent level of apical support is obtained with RSC as for ASC, and RSC has a comparable rate of complications, making this a safe and effective option for repair of vaginal vault prolapse.[19] RSC also offers a durable repair with 100% anatomic success, defined as apical support, in the authors' series, and with a patient satisfaction rate of 95%.[35]

The main disadvantage of the robotic approach is the increased cost compared with the other abdominal approaches, although there is some conflicting data in this regard. A cost-minimization analysis by Judd and colleagues[40] comparing ASC, LSC, and RSC revealed that the robotic procedure cost $1155 more than the laparoscopic procedure and $2716 more than the open procedure, with the increased cost being related to the expense of using disposable instruments and increased operative time. On the other hand, a recently published base case analysis reported overall cost savings of 10% with RSC versus ASC, and concluded that the robotic approach is equally or less costly than the open approach from a hospital-cost perspective.[41] The most important variables associated with the cost were the number of robotic cases performed at an institution, length of hospital stay, and operative time, and this study found that the decreased cost noted in the model data was also present in the institutional billing.[41]

A question one may ask is which of the 2 minimally invasive procedures, LSC or RSC, is the better approach. The answer to this will be partly individualized to surgeons, based on their laparoscopic experience and skill level with complex laparoscopic tasks along with their access to equipment. Paraiso and colleagues[31] recently published their data from a randomized controlled trial comparing LSC with RSC, which found no difference in complications or vaginal support between the 2 procedures but did find the operative time to be significantly longer in the robotic group, along with an associated increased cost. It should be noted that the surgeons in this study were experienced in laparoscopy.[31]

ROLE OF HYSTEROPEXY

A common treatment option for uterine prolapse has been a hysterectomy, but this does not address the underlying defect in the pelvic support that resulted in the uterine descent,[42,43] and is associated with a 15% to 20% rate of POP recurrence.[2] There is a growing number of women who desire uterine preservation, particularly young patients with symptomatic POP.[44] Reasons for this include preservation of fertility, maintenance of anatomy, and maintenance of positive body image.[42,43] A prospective observational trial of 51 women treated with laparoscopic hysteropexy for uterovaginal prolapse revealed significant improvement in their symptoms of prolapse, sexual well-being, and related quality of life as measured using the International Consultation on Incontinence Questionnaire for vaginal symptoms (ICIQ-VS).[43] Repair of vaginal vault prolapse with uterine preservation allows the restoration of vaginal length without changing the caliber of the vagina.[43] Decreased morbidity, operative time, blood loss, and length of hospital stay are also advantages of this procedure in comparison with repair of POP with concomitant hysterectomy.[42,45] With uterine preservation, women should continue to undergo uterine and cervical cancer surveillance, which is one disadvantage of this procedure.[42] Although women maintain fertility status with uterine preservation, a disadvantage is that it is recommended that these women proceed with a cesarean section if they become pregnant because the mesh from the repair may prevent cervical dilation.[43] It is important that patients are properly counseled regarding the continued need for cancer surveillance and recommendations, and potential risks associated with future pregnancies, before undergoing this procedure. Success rates ranging from 94.7% to 100% have been reported with laparoscopic hysteropexy.[43,46,47] It has also been shown that a robotic approach is a safe and feasible option for performing a hysteropexy.[44]

For a standard laparoscopic approach, patient positioning and port placement are similar to those for LSC previously described. Vitobello and colleagues[44] described their technique for a robotic hysteropexy with the following port placement: 12-mm umbilical camera port, two 8-mm robotic ports each a hand-breadth away from the umbilical port, and one 12-mm subcostal port on the left. After access to the peritoneal cavity and pneumoperitoneum is obtained, the peritoneum overlying the sacral promontory is identified and incised, and dissection is carried down until the periosteum is visualized. The peritoneal incision is then taken down into the pelvis on the right, lateral to the sigmoid colon and medial to the right uterosacral ligament, with avoidance of the right ureter until the posterior vagina is reached.[46] The plane anterior to the cervix between the bladder and anterior vaginal wall may then be developed along with developing the rectovaginal space posterior to the cervix. A uterine manipulator may be used to place the uterus in an anteverted and anteflexed position to aid in access to the posterior vagina.[44,47] There are multiple options available for mesh placement at the level of the cervix and vagina, with some groups reporting placement of mesh to the anterior cervix only, such as described by Price and colleagues,[43] whereas others report placing mesh only posteriorly. This positioning obviously affects which plane (anterior, posterior, or both)

needs to be developed before mesh placement, and as described with sacrocolpopexy, sutures should be of full thickness and nonabsorbable. Some of the descriptions of posterior-only mesh placement include attaching mesh from the posterior vaginal fornix to the uterine isthmus,[44] attachment of mesh to the rectovaginal fascia and distal portion of the uterosacral ligaments at the level of the cervix,[46] or fixation of mesh to the rectovaginal fascia and posterior cervix at the level of the internal cervical os.[48] Zucchi and colleagues[42] describe attaching separate pieces of mesh to both the anterior and posterior vaginal walls. Any mesh that is placed anterior to the uterus is bifurcated, so that arms of the mesh can be passed on each side of the uterus through windows that are created at the cervicouterine junction in the broad ligament to reach the sacrum. An example of this is shown in **Fig. 6**.[42,43,49] Using interrupted sutures or tacks, the mesh is then attached to the sacral promontory without placing excessive tension on the vagina in a similar fashion to that described for LSC and RSC.[42–44,46] The peritoneum is closed over the mesh graft as in the previously described procedures.[42,43,46] There is also a report of a meshless procedure or suture hysteropexy whereby suture is placed in a running fashion from the posterior cervix to the sacrum along the right uterosacral ligament.[47]

COMPLICATIONS

Some of the procedures have unique complications that can be associated with them, such as

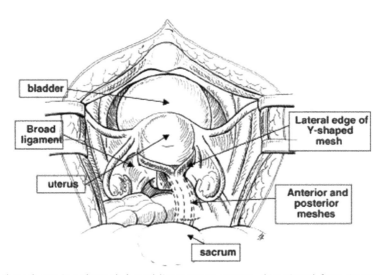

Fig. 6. Bifurcated mesh passing through broad ligament to sacrum. (*Reprinted from* Costantini E, Mearini L, Bini V, et al. Uterus preservation in surgical correction of urogenital prolapse. Eur Urol 2005;48(4):644; with permission.)

the risk of converting a laparoscopic or robotic procedure to an open one, although most of the potential complications are possible with each of the approaches. There are multiple reasons that a case may need to be converted to an open approach, and a review of 11 series of LSC noted that the rate of conversion to an open procedure and operative time both decreased as surgeons' experience increased.[26] Most published studies report a conversion rate of less than 3% and even as low as 0%, although there are data with conversion rates as high as 5%.[16,19,26,35,36,46] Another unique complication with laparoscopic and robotic approaches is the possibility for developing a port-site hernia, although incision hernias can occur with any repair.[25,35] Paraiso and colleagues[31] reported that 9% of the patients in the RSC cohort developed abdominal wall pain that required trigger-point injection. Comparison studies assessing open versus laparoscopic approaches have shown no significant difference between the observed complication rate associated with each approach.[12,19,25]

Complications can be divided into early versus late complications, with intraoperative complications included in the early group. Some potential early complications are injury to pelvic structures, infection, thrombotic events, hemorrhage, and ileus. The bowel, bladder, and ureters are all susceptible to injury during a sacrocolpopexy or hysteropexy, and if the injury is identified intraoperatively a primary repair can often be used to manage the injury. To evaluate for possible bladder injury, cystoscopy can be performed once the case is complete, and during cystoscopy one can also verify efflux of urine from both ureteral orifices. In a systematic review published by Nygaard and colleagues,[6,25,28,30] which included 65 studies of open ASC, the mean incidence of bladder injury was 3.1%.[6] The rate of reported bladder injury ranges from 0.4% to as high as 15.8% in published series evaluating the outcomes of ASC. The randomized controlled trial by Paraiso and colleagues[31] comparing LSC with RSC had equal incidence of cystotomy, 6% with either approach. The systematic review by Nygaard and colleagues[6] found that ureteral injury occurs less often, with mean incidence of 1%, and a robotic series noted the occurrence of ureteral injury in 1 of 80 patients (1.2%).[36] Bowel injury reportedly occurs in up to 2.5% of patients undergoing ASC or hysteropexy for the management of apical POP.[6,16,36,46,47] The mean incidence of bowel injury in the already mentioned systematic review of open ASC was 1.6%,[6] and the LSC versus RSC trial reported an incidence

of 1.5%.[31] Urinary tract infections occur in up to 26% of patients in some series, with a median rate of 11%.[6] In the randomized controlled trial wound infection occurred in 3%, abscess occurred in 3%, and urinary tract infections occurred in 12% of patients.[31] Bleeding or need for transfusion, ileus, and deep vein thrombosis are other possible early complications occurring in 4.6%, 3.6%, and 3.3% of patients, respectively, according to the systematic review on open ASC.[6]

After the immediate postoperative period, complications that may arise include small-bowel obstruction, mesh erosion, and incisional hernia, with an incidence of 1.1%, 3.4%, and 5%, respectively, as published in the systematic review on ASC.[6] The LSC versus RSC randomized controlled trial had a small-bowel obstruction rate of 3% and erosion rate of 3%.[31] Evaluating published series in terms of the mesh erosion rate among all abdominal approaches, the rate varies widely from less than 1% to as high as 12%.[6,16,25,26,31,35,36,42,46,50] The development of de novo SUI, urge incontinence, or other voiding dysfunction not present preoperatively represents another set of potential complications that may occur in women following the repair of POP. A Cochrane review of the surgical management of POP found the incidence of de novo SUI to be 15%, with new overactive bladder symptoms in 12% and new voiding dysfunction in 12% of patients.[7] A series of 80 patients who underwent LSC showed an incidence of postoperative de novo SUI in 6.3% of patients who did not receive any type of concomitant anti-incontinence procedure, which the investigators noted was 16.2% of the patients who had tested negative for SUI preoperatively.[32] Concomitant procedures are frequently performed at the time of apical prolapse, particularly procedures for incontinence, which were performed in 71% of women in the trial by Paraiso and colleagues[31] comparing LSC and RSC. Of note, one series found that SUI present preoperatively resolved in half of the women following LSC although no concomitant continence had been performed.[28] A controversial topic is whether to perform concomitant continence procedures in stress-continent women at the time of POP repair. When assessed using meta-analysis, concomitant continence surgery did not significantly decrease the rate of postoperative SUI.[7] On the other hand, a large randomized study did show that performing a Burch colposuspension in stress-continent women resulted in a decreased incidence of postoperative SUI.[51] Offering concomitant continence procedures such as a midurethral sling at the time of

POP repair to stress-continent women is an option as long as the patient is properly of counseled the possible risks associated with the additional procedure that may be unnecessary. In women with preoperative SUI, even if occult SUI, strong consideration should be given to addressing this aspect at the time of the apical repair to avoid the need for additional procedures in the future.

SUMMARY

Laparoscopic and robotic sacrocolpopexy are both excellent options for managing vaginal vault prolapse, with either of these options providing high rates of anatomic success and patient satisfaction. Each of these have their advantages and disadvantages, and part of the decision to proceed with one option over the other will likely depend on the surgeon's preference, laparoscopic experience with complex tasks, and access to equipment such as the surgical robotic system. A patient's preferences should also play a role in the decision-making process, along with evaluation of concomitant voiding dysfunction and other medical comorbidities. A patient's preference particularly plays a large role in deciding whether uterine preservation would be an option for management of POP. Hysteropexy may play a role in younger women with symptoms of POP who have a desire to maintain their fertility status or avoid the potential complications of a hysterectomy. A minimally invasive treatment option, whether it is standard laparoscopy or a robotic approach, may come at an increased cost but with the added benefits of improved cosmesis, decreased length of stay, and decreased blood loss. Patients should be provided with good preoperative counseling so that they have appropriate expectations, which can help reduce postoperative dissatisfaction. Variations of the current treatment options may continue to be developed, as there are reports of single-port laparoscopic sacrocolpopexy.[52]

EDITOR'S COMMENTS

Robotics represents the most advanced and most expensive of the current technologies available for pelvic floor surgical indications. Initially used as a minimally invasive replacement for open sacralcolpopexy, robotics is now being essayed for ureteral re-implantation, vesicovaginal fistula repair, and even excision of eroded or problematic mesh. While all of these indications are reasonable and certainly allow more rapid convalescence, risk/benefit ratios and medical economic costs must be factored into the overall calculation of value based care around the use of the robot.

The authors present their robotic approaches to apical prolapse, inclusive of lessons learned and technical tips. Both groups have been among the earliest adopters and now represent some of the most experienced units performing these procedures for vaginal prolapse. The outcomes are commendable and demonstrate the importance of apical fixation for vaginal vault stabilization. The addition of mesh arm extension represents an approach for simultaneous management of associated anterior and posterior defects. Additionally, extended posterior mesh arms may be fashioned to stabilize the perineum and posterior cul-de-sac (sacralcolpoperineopexy).

However, several variables regarding robotic prolapse repair must be addressed. A learning curve for performing sacralcolpopexy exists and this curve is accentuated by the addition of robotics. Both the procedure and the associated robotic technique require separate technical acquisition skills and therefore it is preferable to have some experience with sacralcolpopexy prior to initiating robotic assistance. As surgical and robotic simulation labs improve – many of these skills can now be acquired simultaneously. Robotic peritoneal access skills are critical to successful procedural performance, and these skills may also be acquired initially in the simulation lab experience, followed by structured and mentored live surgical experience. The recognition of thermal and crush injuries is another critical aspect of surgical safety, and therefore familiarity and facility with the robotic surgical instrumentation is essential to successful robotic surgery.

The most important question, however, is not whether robotics *can* be performed for all the noted pelvic floor procedures, but whether this approach *should* be done. Medical economics will enter into this decision in the very near future and may actually lead to restricted use of this technique to high volume centers with experienced teams. Also familiarity with base procedure (ie, sacralcolpopexy) is critical, and the occasional performance of reconstructive procedures just because a surgical robot is available may not provide the best outcomes. Additionally, the presence of an experienced team and structured perioperative process cannot be underestimated, and a commitment to the development of both aspects is critical to a successful robotic surgical program.

Roger R. Dmochowski, MD
Mickey Karram, MD

REFERENCES

1. Olsen AL, Smith VJ, Bergstrom JO, et al. Epidemiology of surgically managed pelvic organ prolapse and urinary incontinence. Obstet Gynecol 1997;89:501.
2. Marchionni M, Bracco GL, Checcucci V, et al. True incidence of vaginal vault prolapse. Thirteen years of experience. J Reprod Med 1999;44:679.
3. Elliott DS. Diagnosis and management of apical prolapse. In: Goldman HB, Vasavada SP, editors. Female urology: a practical clinical guide. Totowa (NJ): Humana Press Inc; 2007. p. 297–305. Chapter 21.
4. Webb MJ, Aronson MP, Ferguson LK, et al. Posthysterectomy vaginal vault prolapse: primary repair in 693 patients. Obstet Gynecol 1998;92:281.
5. Herschorn S. Campbell's urology. 9th edition. Philadelphia: Saunders; 2007. p. 2187–233. Chapter 66.
6. Nygaard IE, McCreery R, Brubaker L, et al. Abdominal sacrocolpopexy: a comprehensive review. Obstet Gynecol 2004;104:805.
7. Maher C, Feiner B, Baessler K, et al. Surgical management of pelvic organ prolapse in women. Cochrane Database Syst Rev 2010;4:CD004014.
8. Swift SE. The distribution of pelvic organ support in a population of female subjects seen for routine gynecologic health care. Am J Obstet Gynecol 2000;183:277.
9. Fischer M, Padmanabhan P, Rosenblum N. Anatomy of pelvic support. In: Goldman HB, Vasavada SP, editors. Female urology: a practical clinical guide. Totowa (NJ): Humana Press Inc; 2007. p. 3–18. Chapter 1.
10. Albo M, Dupont MC, Raz S. Transvaginal correction of pelvic prolapse. J Endourol 1996;10:231.
11. DeLancey JO. Anatomic aspects of vaginal eversion after hysterectomy. Am J Obstet Gynecol 1992;166:1717.
12. Miklos JR, Moore RD, Kohli N. Laparoscopic surgery for pelvic support defects. Curr Opin Obstet Gynecol 2002;14:387.
13. Addison WA, Timmons MC. Abdominal approach to vaginal eversion. Clin Obstet Gynecol 1993;36:995.
14. Timmons MC, Addison WA, Addison SB, et al. Abdominal sacral colpopexy in 163 women with posthysterectomy vaginal vault prolapse and enterocele. evolution of operative techniques. J Reprod Med 1992;37:323.
15. Mayne CJ, Assassa RP. Epidemiology of incontinence and prolapse. BJOG 2004;111:2.
16. Rozet F, Mandron E, Arroyo C, et al. Laparoscopic sacral colpopexy approach for genito-urinary prolapse: experience with 363 cases. Eur Urol 2005;47:230.
17. Karram M, Goldwasser S, Kleeman S, et al. High uterosacral vaginal vault suspension with fascial reconstruction for vaginal repair of enterocele and vaginal vault prolapse. Am J Obstet Gynecol 2001;185:1339.
18. Abbasy S, Kenton K. Obliterative procedures for pelvic organ prolapse. Clin Obstet Gynecol 2010;52:86.
19. Geller EJ, Siddiqui NY, Wu JM, et al. Short-term outcomes of robotic sacrocolpopexy compared with abdominal sacrocolpopexy. Obstet Gynecol 2008;112:1201.
20. Scarpero HM, Cespedes RD, Winters JC. Transabdominal approach to repair of vaginal vault prolapse. Tech Urol 2001;7:139.
21. Deval B, Haab F. What's new in prolapse surgery? Curr Opin Urol 2003;13:315.
22. Maher C, Baessler K, Glazener CM, et al. Surgical management of pelvic organ prolapse in women: a short version Cochrane review. Neurourol Urodyn 2008;27(1):3–12.
23. Benson JT, Lucente V, McClellan E. Vaginal versus abdominal reconstructive surgery for the treatment of pelvic support defects: a prospective randomized study with long-term outcome evaluation. Am J Obstet Gynecol 1996;175:1418.
24. Paraiso MF, Walters MD, Rackley RR, et al. Laparoscopic and abdominal sacral colpopexies: a comparative cohort study. Am J Obstet Gynecol 2005;192:1752.
25. Klauschie JL, Suozzi BA, O'Brien MM, et al. A comparison of laparoscopic and abdominal sacral colpopexy: objective outcome and perioperative differences. Int Urogynecol J Pelvic Floor Dysfunct 2009;20:273.
26. Ganatra AM, Rozet F, Sanchez-Salas R, et al. The current status of laparoscopic sacrocolpopexy: a review. Eur Urol 2009;55:1089.
27. Mahran MA, Herath RP, Sayed AT, et al. Laparoscopic management of genital prolapse. Arch Gynecol Obstet 2011;283:1015.
28. North CE, Ali-Ross NS, Smith AR, et al. A prospective study of laparoscopic sacrocolpopexy for the management of pelvic organ prolapse. BJOG 2009;116:1251.
29. Gaston R, Ramsden A. Surgery illustrated-surgical atlas. Laparoscopic sacrocolpopexy. BJU Int 2011;107:500.
30. Price N, Slack A, Jackson SR. Laparoscopic sacrocolpopexy: an observational study of functional and anatomical outcomes. Int Urogynecol J 2011;22:77.
31. Paraiso MF, Jelovsek JE, Frick A, et al. Laparoscopic compared with robotic sacrocolpopexy for vaginal prolapse. Obstet Gynecol 2011;118:1005.
32. Perez T, Crochet P, Descargues G, et al. Laparoscopic sacrocolpopexy for management of pelvic organ prolapse enhances quality of life at one year: a prospective observational study. J Minim Invasive Gynecol 2011;18:747.

33. Chandra V, Nehra D, Parent R, et al. A comparison of laparoscopic and robotic assisted suturing performance by experts and novices. Surgery 2009;147:830.

34. Paraiso MF, Walters MD. Laparoscopic surgery for stress urinary incontinence and pelvic organ prolapse. Clin Obstet Gynecol 2005;48:724.

35. Shimko MS, Umbreit EC, Chow GK, et al. Long-term outcomes of robotic-assisted laparoscopic sacrocolpopexy with a minimum of three years follow-up. J Robotic Surg 2011;5:175.

36. Akl MN, Long JB, Giles DL, et al. Robotic-assisted sacrocolpopexy: technique and learning curve. Surg Endosc 2009;23:2390.

37. Elliott DS, DiMarco DS, Chow GK. Female urologic robotic surgery. In: Faust RA, editor. Robotics in surgery. New York: Nova Science Publishers, Inc; 2007. p. 137–46. Chapter 8.

38. Elliott DS, Krambeck AE, Chow GK. Long-term results of robotic-assisted laparoscopic sacrocolpopexy for the treatment of high grade vaginal vault prolapse. J Urol 2006;176:655.

39. DiMarco DS, Chow GK, Gettman MT, et al. Robotic-assisted laparoscopic sacrocolpopexy for treatment of vaginal vault prolapse. Urology 2003; 63:373.

40. Judd JP, Siddiqui NY, Barnett JC, et al. Cost-minimization analysis of robotic-assisted laparoscopic and abdominal sacrocolpopexy. J Minim Invasive Gynecol 2010;17:493.

41. Elliott CS, Hsieh MH, Sokol ER, et al. Robot-assisted versus open sacrocolpopexy: a cost-minimization analysis. J Urol 2012;187:638.

42. Zucchi A, Lazzeri M, Porena M, et al. Uterus preservation in pelvic organ prolapse surgery. Nat Rev Urol 2010;7:626.

43. Price N, Slack A, Jackson SR. Laparoscopic hysteropexy: the initial results of a uterine suspension procedure for uterovaginal prolapse. BJOG 2010; 117:62.

44. Vitobello D, Siesto G, Bulletti C. Robotic sacral hysteropexy for pelvic organ prolapse. Int J Med Robot 2012;8(1):114–7.

45. Rosen DM, Shukla A, Cario GM, et al. Is hysterectomy necessary for laparoscopic pelvic floor repair? a prospective study. J Minim Invasive Gynecol 2008; 15:729.

46. Rosenblatt PL, Chelmow D, Ferzandi TR. Laparoscopic sacrocervicopexy for the treatment of uterine prolapse: a retrospective case series report. J Minim Invasive Gynecol 2008;15:268.

47. Krause HG, Goh JT, Sloane K. Laparoscopic sacral suture hysteropexy for uterine prolapse. Int Urogynecol J 2006;17:378.

48. Daneshgari F, Paraiso MF, Kaouk J, et al. Robotic and laparoscopic female pelvic floor reconstruction. BJU Int 2006;98:62.

49. Costantini E, Mearini L, Bini V, et al. Uterus preservation in surgical correction of urogenital prolapse. Eur Urol 2005;48:642.

50. Beer M, Kuhn A. Surgical techniques for vault prolapse: a review of the literature. Eur J Obstet Gynecol Reprod Biol 2004;119:144.

51. Brubaker L, Nygaard I, Richter HE, et al. Two-year outcomes after sacrocolpopexy with and without burch to prevent stress urinary incontinence. Obstet Gynecol 2008;112:49.

52. White WM, Goel RK, Swartz MA, et al. Single-port laparoscopic abdominal sacral colpopexy: initial experience and comparative outcomes. J Urol 2009;74:1009.

Posterior Compartment Prolapse: A Urogynecology Perspective

Monica L. Richardson, MD, MPH*,
Christopher S. Elliot, MD, PhD, Eric R. Sokol, MD

KEYWORDS

- Posterior compartment prolapse • Posterior colporrhaphy • Rectocele • Enterocele
- Perineorrhaphy

KEY POINTS

- Symptomatic women of posterior compartment prolapse may present with complaints of vaginal bulge, constipation, tenesmus, splinting, and fecal incontinence.
- A clinical examination is generally sufficient in the workup of posterior compartment prolapse, and imaging studies should be reserved for cases whereby symptoms do not correlate with the physical examination.
- Defecatory dysfunction, quality of life, and sexual function can significantly improve after surgical repair with either traditional or site-specific colporrhaphy.

INTRODUCTION

In 2010 an estimated 166,000 women underwent surgical repair for pelvic organ prolapse.[1] Of these women, an estimated 52% had a rectocele procedure as part of their repair.[2] In women undergoing rectocele repair, the most common presenting symptoms beyond vaginal bulge are those of defecatory dysfunction, including constipation (46%), tenesmus (32%), splinting (39%), and fecal incontinence (13%).[3] In addition, dyspareunia is present in 29%. Although the symptoms of posterior vaginal prolapse do not directly correlate with the degree of the prolapse,[4] repair of a rectocele alleviates the associated symptoms in most patients.[5–7]

WORKUP
Clinical Examination

The pelvic examination is performed in the dorsal lithotomy position. The posterior wall is assessed while supporting the vaginal apex and anterior wall with a separated posterior blade of a bivalve speculum. The authors currently use the Pelvic

Organ Quantification System (POPQ) to objectively measure prolapse during maximal Valsalva effort (**Fig. 1**).[8] The POPQ system has been adopted by the American Urogynecologic Society, Society of Gynecologic Surgeons, International Urogynecological Association, and International Continence Society.[9]

The POPQ measurements Ap and Bp measure the posterior vaginal wall. Point Ap is located in the midline of the posterior vaginal wall, 3 cm proximal to the posterior hymen. The quantitative value of point Ap is anywhere from -3 to $+3$ cm from the hymeneal ring, depending on the extent of posterior wall prolapse. Point Bp is the most distal (ie, most dependent) position of any part of the upper posterior vaginal wall between point Ap and the vaginal cuff or posterior vaginal fornix. This value can range from -3 (no prolapse) to more than $+3$ (up to the total vaginal length) if associated with a vault prolapse beyond the hymeneal ring.

A rectal examination aids in detecting specific defects in the posterior vaginal wall and can help identify an enterocele or sigmoidocele. In addition, one can evaluate for an enterocele by evaluating

Financial disclosures: None.
Division of Urogynecology and Pelvic Reconstructive Surgery, Stanford University School of Medicine, 300 Pasteur Drive, H-333, Palo Alto, CA 94305, USA
* Corresponding author.
E-mail address: monicar@stanford.edu

Urol Clin N Am 39 (2012) 361–369
http://dx.doi.org/10.1016/j.ucl.2012.06.005

urologic.theclinics.com

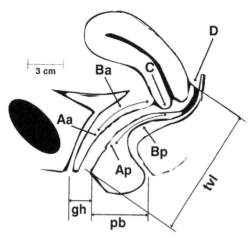

Fig. 1. Six sites (points Aa, Ba, C, D, Bp, and Ap), genital hiatus (gh), perineal body (pb), and total vaginal length (tvl) are used for quantification of pelvic organ support. (*From* Bump RC, Mattiasson A, Bø K, et al. The standardization of terminology of female pelvic organ prolapse and pelvic floor dysfunction. Am J Obstet Gynecol 1996;175(1):10; with permission.)

the patient in a standing position because the small bowel will enter the enterocele sac. It is also important to evaluate for rectal intussusception or rectal prolapse. In addition, a rectal examination can help evaluate the integrity of the perineal body and anal sphincter tone.

Imaging

A thorough clinical examination is an accurate way of evaluating for posterior compartment defects. Imaging studies are occasionally useful if there is a concern for other abnormality, or if there is recurrent posterior compartment prolapse. The use of ancillary studies may also be helpful for patients who complain of fecal incontinence or report defecatory dysfunction and do not have a posterior compartment prolapse on clinical examination.

Defecography

Defecography provides a 2-dimensional view of rectal emptying efficiency and allows for the quantification of rectal measurements. The size of the rectocele is determined by measuring the distance between the anterior border of the anal canal and the maximal point of the bulge of the rectal wall into the posterior vaginal wall. Anything less than 2 cm is considered normal, and a rectocele is considered large if the rectal wall protrudes more than 3.5 cm.[10–12] The clinical utility of defecography is limited, and diagnosis of anterior rectocele correlates with level of experience of the person reading the test.[13] One study of elderly patients

found no association between abnormalities found on defecogram and symptoms.[14] Another suggested only a limited correlation between the radiologic findings and clinical outcomes after surgical repair.[15] The authors do not typically obtain defecography studies unless they are considering a diagnosis of pelvic floor dyssynergia, whereby the puborectalis or external anal sphincter muscle is paradoxically contracted on rectal examination, or identifying a sigmoidocele.

Magnetic Resonance Imaging

Dynamic magnetic resonance imaging (MRI) offers high-quality images of the pelvic soft tissues and viscera, and can be used to evaluate posterior compartment prolapse. However, the lack of standardization in grading posterior prolapse, the high cost of MRI, and its poor correlation with clinical staging makes its routine use problematic.[16,17] MRI does continue to be used in the research setting. Because clinical examination has a high sensitivity for detecting rectoceles, the authors generally do not order MRI for the routine evaluation of posterior compartment prolapse.

Endoanal Ultrasonography

On clinical examination, diminished resting or squeeze tone of the distal anal canal and suspicion of a sphincter disruption may prompt an endoanal ultrasonogram. This modality can aid in the detection of a sphincter defect (either internal or external), and also allows visualization of the puborectalis muscle.[18] The finding of a defect in the sphincter complex in an appropriate patient with complaints of fecal incontinence may prompt consideration of a sphincteroplasty.

TREATMENT

Treatment should be pursued only if the patient's prolapse is symptomatic. She should be counseled regarding potential outcomes with expectant management and pessary use. Pessary fittings have been found to be successful in the treatment of symptomatic pelvic organ prolapse. In one study of 100 consecutive patients with symptomatic pelvic organ prolapse, pessaries were successfully fitted in 73% of patients, with 92% still being satisfied at a 2-month follow-up. Patients successfully fitted with pessaries noted significant decreases in vaginal bulge (90% down to 3%; $P<.001$), pressure (49% down to 3%; $P<.001$), and splinting to defecate (14% down to 0%; $P = .001$).[19] The authors offer virtually all of their patients a pessary trial before discussing the possibilities of surgical treatment.

Posterior Colporrhaphy

The goal of posterior transvaginal repair is to relieve symptoms relevant to the anatomic support defect. Patients often present with complaints of a vaginal bulge or obstructed defecation. In plicating the endopelvic fascia (also known as the Denonvillier fascia), the strength of the posterior vaginal wall is increased, eliminating the vaginal bulge and allowing for better stool emptying.[20] The surgical technique of traditional posterior colporrhaphy has been previously reviewed in this journal.[21] In brief, a small diamond-shaped incision is made from the perineum to the posterior vaginal mucosa beyond the hymen after injection of a hemostatic solution, and the skin is excised. The posterior vaginal mucosa is undermined and a midline incision is made past the apex of the rectocele. The posterior vaginal epithelium is then dissected in a thin plane off of the Denonvillier fascia, with the dissection carried laterally to the levator muscles. Plication of the edges of the Denonvillier fascia over the herniated rectum is performed with interrupted stitches of 2-0 delayed absorbable sutures (the authors use 2-0 Vicryl) from the upper edge of the rectocele to the perineal body. The vaginal epithelium is trimmed if necessary and then closed to the hymen with a running 2-0 delayed absorbable suture. Perineorrhaphy is performed as appropriate, and the reconstructed rectovaginal septum is attached to the reconstructed perineal body. The rest of the vaginal and perineal skin is then closed.

Perineorrhaphy

A perineorrhaphy is often necessary when treating posterior compartment prolapse. The rectovaginal fascia normally attaches to the perineal body, although detachment is often seen in women with posterior compartment defects. Compromise of this attachment can lead to perineal descent and a relaxed perineum. During a perineorrhaphy, the bulbocavernosus and transverse perinei muscles are brought together in the midline of the perineal body with absorbable sutures. The authors typically also attach the reconstructed rectovaginal septum to the reconstructed perineal body. A well-performed perineorrhaphy helps prevent perineal descent with bowel movements, and reduces the need for defecatory splinting. Although vaginal dimensions did not predict dyspareunia in a study of sexually active women undergoing posterior repair,[22] care should be taken to avoid an overaggressive perineorrhaphy, which can constrict the vaginal opening and lead to dyspareunia.[23]

Endorectal Repair

Colorectal surgeons typically approach posterior compartment defects through a transanal approach. The first endorectal rectocele repair was described in 1968 by Sullivan and colleagues.[24] An endorectal repair is done with the patient in the prone jack-knife position. An anal retractor is inserted to expose the anterior rectal wall. Two transverse incisions are made; the first is in the rectal mucosa at or near the dentate line and the second is made cephalad, above the prolapsed defect. One vertical incision is made in the midline. Mucomuscular flaps are developed on each side of the vertical incision. The rectovaginal septum is reapproximated using vertical plication sutures with a 3-0 polyglycolic acid suture. The rectal flaps are trimmed and the incision is closed with a running 5-0 polyglycolic acid suture. (Adapted from Khubchandani and colleagues.[25])

Posterior Colporrhaphy Versus Endorectal Repair

Colorectal and gynecologic surgeons traditionally perform rectocele repairs using different surgical approaches (transanal and transvaginal, respectively). The disadvantages of a transanal approach include the inability to repair prolapse in other vaginal compartments concurrently, limited exposure, the inability to access high rectoceles and enteroceles, and a possible increased risk of rectovaginal fistula formation. An advantage of a transanal approach is the ability to perform concurrent rectal procedures in the same positioning. Early retrospective reviews suggested that the transanal and transvaginal approaches have similar symptomatic outcomes and complication rates.[20] However, more recent evidence suggests that the transanal approach is not durable, with a 50% anatomic recurrence rate at a mean 6 years of follow-up: much higher than in series of transvaginal repairs.[26] In addition, there are concerns of decreased anal sphincter integrity following anal retraction, which may lead to de novo fecal incontinence.[27–29] To date, one randomized controlled trial of transvaginal versus transanal rectocele repair has been performed.[29] At 1-year follow-up, improved anatomic outcomes were seen in the transvaginal group compared with the transanal group (7% rectocele recurrence compared with 40% rectocele recurrence, respectively). In addition, enteroceles and flatal incontinence were each present in 27% of the transanal repair group, whereas no patients in the transvaginal group had these problems. Improvement in symptoms was also better in the transvaginal group (93% vs 73%).

More recently a newer transanal repair technique has been introduced, the stapled transanal rectal resection (STARR procedure). This technique has the purported advantages of decreased operative time and blood loss while being able to treat rectal intussusception, if present.[30] However, it is limited by increases in patient morbidity.[31,32] In a large registry (n = 379) of patients undergoing the STARR procedure, complications included 3% bleeding requiring reoperation, 2% anal stenosis requiring dilatation, 3% fecal incontinence, and 2 reports of rectal injury and sepsis requiring fecal diversion.[33]

Site-Specific Defect Repair

The rationale for a site-specific rectocele repair is based on the theory that herniation of the rectum into the vagina results from specific tears in the rectovaginal fascia. These injuries may occur as an isolated defect in the lateral, distal, midline, or superior portions of the vaginal wall, or as a combination of defects (**Fig. 2**).[34] During repair of site-specific defects, the posterior vaginal epithelium is incised to the rectocele bulge and the vaginal mucosa is dissected from the underlying Denonvillier fascia all the way to the arcus tendineus on each side. A finger is then placed into the rectum to identify specific fascial defects, which are repaired with interrupted absorbable sutures. Any perineal defects are then corrected in the standard fashion, before skin closure.

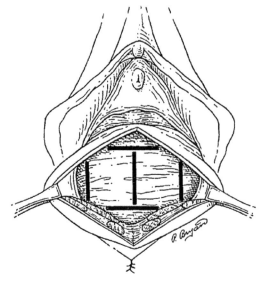

Fig. 2. The various locations of breaks in the rectovaginal septum. (*From* Richardson AC. The rectovaginal septum revisited: its relationship to rectocele and its importance to rectocele repair. Clin Obstet Gynecol 1993;36:980; with permission.)

Posterior Colporrhaphy Versus Site-Specific Defect Repair

Both posterior colporrhaphy and site-specific defect repair have high cure rates. Traditional posterior colporrhaphy has anatomic cure rates of 80% to 96% at 12 months' follow-up or longer.[7,20,35,36] Site-specific defect repair has anatomic cure rates of 82% to 92% at 12 months' follow-up or longer.[3,37–39] In the largest retrospective study, prolapse recurrence rates beyond the hymeneal ring were 4% for traditional colporrhaphy versus 11% for site-specific defect repair, with no differences in postoperative dyspareunia, constipation, or fecal incontinence.[39] To date, only one prospective, randomized controlled trial of traditional colporrhaphy versus site-specific repair has been performed. In the study of Paraiso and colleagues,[5] anatomic cure of prolapse (defined as ≤ Stage 2) was comparable between the posterior colporrhaphy group (86%) and the site-specific group (78%). A follow-up study showed overall improvements in incomplete emptying, straining to defecate, splinting to defecate, and fecal incontinence, regardless of posterior repair type.[40]

Graft Augmentation

Various grafts (including biological, synthetic absorbable, and synthetic nonabsorbable) have been used in an effort to improve the anatomic success rates of posterior compartment repair.

Biological
The use of porcine xenografts has been reported with unsatisfactory anatomic cure rates and persistent bowel-emptying difficulties.[41] In a randomized trial of porcine graft augmentation versus traditional posterior repair, porcine graft repair was associated with a higher failure rate at 1 year (20% with prolapse to or beyond the hymen) compared with the posterior colporrhaphy group (7.1% with prolapse to or beyond the hymen).[5] A more recent randomized trial compared patients treated with a porcine subintestinal submucosal graft-augmented repair with patients undergoing repair with native tissue. After 1 year there was no benefit of graft use, with similar rates of anatomic failure, vaginal bulge symptoms, and defecatory symptoms.[42]

Synthetic absorbable
One prospective randomized study comparing absorbable polyglactin vaginal mesh augmentation with traditional repair in comparison with traditional posterior repair alone has been reported. In this study, the mesh was incorporated as a strip

within the imbricating fold of the endopelvic fascia created during traditional colporrhaphy. The investigators[43] found no difference in recurrence rates when comparing 70 women in the traditional colpoperineorrhaphy arm with 73 women undergoing traditional repair with concomitant polyglactin mesh (10% vs 8%, respectively). Bowel or sexual function was not described.

Synthetic nonabsorbable

Anatomic cure rates with the use of synthetic nonabsorbable mesh are comparable with those for traditional nonmesh repairs. In one descriptive study of 90 patients undergoing loose polyglactin/polypropylene mesh interposition with no primary repair, reported success was 84% at 6-month follow-up.[44] Another study of women who underwent bilateral sacrospinous suspension and polypropylene mesh attachment to the perineal body reported cure of 92.3% (n = 24/25) at 22 months' follow-up.[45] Unfortunately, with mesh use vaginal mesh erosion rates have been reported in up to 12% of patients and de novo dyspareunia has been reported in 3.4% to 7.7% of patients.[44,45] In another study of 31 women who had Prolene mesh interposition for posterior repair, sexual activity decreased by 12% and dyspareunia increased in 63% of patients.[46]

Posterior Vaginal Wall Kit Procedures

"Kit" procedures have been developed by commercial companies to aid in the repair of posterior vaginal wall prolapse. Most of these kits use polypropylene mesh grafts that are anchored to the sacrospinous ligaments or arcus tendineus. Whereas some studies report favorable anatomic outcomes, symptomatic mesh retraction and vaginal mesh exposure have been reported in 8% to 11% of patients, and new-onset dyspareunia has been reported in 11% of the patients.[47,48] While these kits may be useful for a subset of patients, continued research is needed to discover whether the benefits outweigh the risks.

Recommendations on Mesh Use in the Posterior Compartment

At present, The Society of Gynecologic Surgeons Systematic Review Group suggests that native repair remains preferable to graft use for rectocele repair, because there is insufficient evidence to support the use of grafts in posterior compartment repair.[49,50]

In addition to this recommendation, the Food and Drug Administration (FDA) has recently issued some guidance. In October 2008 the FDA released a public health notification warning surgeons and patients about possible complications with the use of mesh in transvaginal prolapse repair. This warning was issued after the FDA received more than 1000 reports from 9 surgical mesh manufacturers of complications including mesh erosion, pain, vaginal scarring, and dyspareunia. The warning was followed up with an updated public health notification in July 2011, in which the FDA noted that mesh complications were more common than previously thought. A systematic review of mesh trials between the years of 1996 and 2011 failed to show evidence that routine mesh use provides added benefit in comparison with native tissue repair, particularly for posterior compartment defects. The FDA continues to recommend specialized training of surgeons for each mesh-placement technique and suggests that every patient be notified of the potential complications of mesh use. All patients should be offered alternatives to mesh repair.[51]

Levatorplasty

High rates of dyspareunia and vaginal pain following colpoperineorrhaphy were first suggested in 1961 by Francis and Jeffcoate.[23] Since then it has been argued that plication of the levator ani increases postoperative vaginal pain and dyspareunia, and also provides a nonanatomic repair.[52] Studies show that high rates of anatomic success can be achieved without the use of levator ani plication as part of a rectocele repair.[7,39] However, whereas some studies suggest minimal de novo dyspareunia following standard colporrhaphy without incorporation of the levator ani,[7,29] others have reported high rates of de novo dyspareunia (up to 27%),[22,36] similar to series of rectocele repair with levator plication.[20,35] Given the equality of repair between the two techniques (with and without levator ani plication) and the historical teaching that levator ani plication increases postsurgical pain, the authors routinely avoid its use. The only exceptions to this rule are in rare cases of very large (Stage 3/4) rectoceles whereby the tissue quality is extremely poor, or during repairs performed concurrently with an Altmeier procedure whereby the Denonvillier fascia has been weakened secondary to rectosigmoidectomy.

COMPLICATIONS

Constipation and pain are common in the perioperative period. Serious complications such as injury to the rectum, hematoma, or the development of a rectovaginal fistula are rare. Long-term defecatory dysfunction, de novo dyspareunia, or sexual dysfunction may occur after surgical repair of posterior compartment defects.[20]

Defecatory Dysfunction

Conflicting data exist about defecatory dysfunction after posterior colporrhaphy. In one retrospective observational study of 244 posterior colporrhaphies with long-term follow-up, prolapse symptoms due to rectocele decreased, but complaints of constipation, incomplete bowel emptying, and fecal incontinence all increased.[36] However, more recent evidence suggests that defecatory dysfunction significantly improves after posterior repair. A randomized controlled trial comparing 3 different surgical techniques showed that bowel symptoms were significantly improved at 1 year regardless of the type of repair. A reduction in bothersome postoperative straining and incomplete emptying were specifically associated with cure (Stage 0 or 1) of posterior vaginal wall prolapse. The development of new-onset bowel dysfunction was uncommon (11%).[5,40] A randomized trial of porcine subintestinal submucosal graft-augmented repair versus native tissue repair reported overall improved symptoms in straining, splinting, and incomplete evacuation; however, almost 45% of subjects had persistent or worsening of one type of defecatory symptom.[42]

Dyspareunia and Sexual Dysfunction

Posterior compartment repair has been associated with de novo dyspareunia in some studies. However, other studies have reported no de novo dyspareunia and improvements in sexual dysfunction.[5,29] In a study of women undergoing prolapse and incontinence surgery, de novo postoperative dyspareunia was significantly lower in the group that did not undergo posterior colporrhaphy.[53] However, both groups reported overall improvements in sexual function based on the pelvic organ prolapse urinary incontinence sexual questionnaire.[53] Another study also found improvements in sexual function 6 months after posterior repair for the sexual domains desire, satisfaction, and pain at 6 months follow-up.[54]

SUMMARY

- A rectocele repair was performed in over one-half of all women undergoing prolapse surgery in 2010.
- The most common presenting symptoms of women with rectoceles are vaginal bulge, constipation, tenesmus, splinting, and fecal incontinence.
- A clinical examination is generally sufficient in the workup of posterior compartment prolapse, and imaging studies should be reserved for cases whereby symptoms do not correlate with the physical examination.
- Transvaginal rectocele repair has better objective and subjective outcomes in comparison with transanal rectocele repair.
- Both traditional and site-specific colporrhaphy have excellent anatomic success rates.
- Defecatory dysfunction, quality of life, and sexual function can significantly improve after either traditional or site-specific colporrhaphy.
- Levator plication is rarely needed during the surgical correction of posterior compartment defects.
- The use of mesh in the posterior compartment should be avoided in most cases of posterior compartment repair.

EDITOR'S COMMENTS

Posterior compartment reconstruction is one of the more difficult aspects of pelvic floor reconstruction. From an evolutionary standpoint, repairs have progressed from plication to site-specific defect and fascial-based reconstructive techniques to the implantation of augmenting meshes and grafts. More recently, there has been a re-emphasis of host tissue. The editors both recommend the site-specific repair as a critical intervention in the appropriately-selected patient. Site-specific repairs are dependent on the presence of fascial segments that can be re-approximated. These segments are very difficult to identify before surgical dissection and therefore, any posterior repair may have to rely on more standard plication procedures or the occasional use of interposition graft.

There has been a trend away from synthetic mesh kit and free graft implantation over the last several years. Both editors still will utilize biologic materials as interposition grafts in those patients who have insufficient native fascia for purposes of adequate reconstruction. Plication repairs, while offering native tissues for reconstructive purposes, are at risk for vaginal constriction and subsequent dyspareunia and therefore should be used with discretion. However, these approaches do provide a reasonable restorative technique.

Of importance during posterior repair is not only the isolated rectocele but recognition of associated high posterior (near the apex) enteroceles, sigmoidoceles, or vault prolapse. As with the anterior compartment, vault stabilization is a critical aspect of surgical success for posterior compartment repairs.

Another important aspect of posterior compartment repair is the distal most aspect of the repair, that being the perineum. Perineorrhaphy is certainly not required in all patients but in those patients with widely splayed transverse perinei muscles, reconstruction should be obtained to stabilize the distal aspect of the vaginal outlet as a foundation for the more proximal remainder of the repair.

As with all prolapse procedures, patient counseling is important to create reasonable expectations for posterior compartment reconstructive repairs. The patient should be aware that some symptoms of bowel dysfunction may persist even after posterior compartment repair, including the bothersome symptoms associated with bowel dysmotility (constipation). It is our practice to prepare the lower intestine, especially in revision repairs where there may be scarification and fibrosis and the possibility of rectal wall disruption. In the circumstance of a prepared bowel, mural injury can be repaired with no consequence and the editors recommend this as a preoperative management component.

Many posterior defects are small and relatively asymptomatic, and certainly neither of the editors recommend posterior compartment repair without the patient experiencing bother and associated symptoms (related to prolapse mass effect and/or bowel dysfunction resulting in the need to splint). Posterior compartment repair may be done as an isolated or combined procedure with other compartments of the vagina at the discretion of the operative surgeon and after informed consent from the patient.

A significant complication associated with posterior compartment repair is vaginal lumenal constriction and resultant lack of distensibility. Therefore, it is incumbent upon any successful repair to maintain as much vaginal distensibility and lack of posterior constriction as possible with whichever of the above techniques is most suited to the individual's presenting anatomy.

Roger R. Dmochowski, MD
Mickey Karram, MD

REFERENCES

1. Wu JM, Kawasaki A, Hundley AF, et al. Predicting the number of women who will undergo incontinence and prolapse surgery, 2010 to 2050. Am J Obstet Gynecol 2011;205(3):230;e1–5.
2. Shah AD, Kohli N, Rajan SS, et al. The age distribution, rates, and types of surgery for pelvic organ prolapse in the USA. Int Urogynecol J Pelvic Floor Dysfunct 2008;19(3):421–8.
3. Cundiff GW, Weidner AC, Visco AG, et al. An anatomic and functional assessment of the discrete defect rectocele repair. Am J Obstet Gynecol 1998;179(6 Pt 1):1451–6 [discussion: 1456–7].
4. Weber AM, Walters MD, Ballard LA, et al. Posterior vaginal prolapse and bowel function. Am J Obstet Gynecol 1998;179(6 Pt 1):1446–9 [discussion: 1449–50].
5. Paraiso MF, Barber MD, Muir TW, et al. Rectocele repair: a randomized trial of three surgical techniques including graft augmentation. Am J Obstet Gynecol 2006;195(6):1762–71.
6. Yamana T, Takahashi T, Iwadare J. Clinical and physiologic outcomes after transvaginal rectocele repair. Dis Colon Rectum 2006;49(5):661–7.
7. Maher CF, Qatawneh AM, Baessler K, et al. Midline rectovaginal fascial plication for repair of rectocele and obstructed defecation. Obstet Gynecol 2004;104(4):685–9.
8. Bump RC, Mattiasson A, Bo K, et al. The standardization of terminology of female pelvic organ prolapse and pelvic floor dysfunction. Am J Obstet Gynecol 1996;175(1):10–7.
9. Haylen BT, de Ridder D, Freeman RM, et al. An International Urogynecological Association (IUGA)/International Continence Society (ICS) joint report on the terminology for female pelvic floor dysfunction. Neurourol Urodyn 2010;29(1):4–20.
10. Mellgren A, Bremmer S, Johansson C, et al. Defecography. Results of investigations in 2,816 patients. Dis Colon Rectum 1994;37(11):1133–41.
11. Bartram C. Dynamic evaluation of the anorectum. Radiol Clin North Am 2003;41(2):425–41.
12. Savoye-Collet C, Koning E, Dacher JN. Radiologic evaluation of pelvic floor disorders. Gastroenterol Clin North Am 2008;37(3):553–67, viii.
13. Dobben AC, Wiersma TG, Janssen LW, et al. Prospective assessment of interobserver agreement for defecography in fecal incontinence. AJR Am J Roentgenol 2005;185(5):1166–72.
14. Savoye-Collet C, Savoye G, Koning E, et al. Defecography in symptomatic older women living at home. Age Ageing 2003;32(3):347–50.
15. Van Laarhoven CJ, Kamm MA, Bartram CI, et al. Relationship between anatomic and symptomatic long-term results after rectocele repair for impaired defecation. Dis Colon Rectum 1999;42(2):204–10 [discussion: 210–1].
16. Fauconnier A, Zareski E, Abichedid J, et al. Dynamic magnetic resonance imaging for grading pelvic organ prolapse according to the International Continence Society classification: which line should be used? Neurourol Urodyn 2008;27(3):191–7.
17. Woodfield CA, Hampton BS, Sung V, et al. Magnetic resonance imaging of pelvic organ prolapse: comparing pubococcygeal and midpubic lines

with clinical staging. Int Urogynecol J Pelvic Floor Dysfunct 2009;20(6):695–701.

18. Sentovich SM, Wong WD, Blatchford GJ. Accuracy and reliability of transanal ultrasound for anterior anal sphincter injury. Dis Colon Rectum 1998;41(8):1000–4.

19. Clemons JL, Aguilar VC, Tillinghast TA, et al. Patient satisfaction and changes in prolapse and urinary symptoms in women who were fitted successfully with a pessary for pelvic organ prolapse. Am J Obstet Gynecol 2004;190(4):1025–9.

20. Arnold MW, Stewart WR, Aguilar PS. Rectocele repair. Four years' experience. Dis Colon Rectum 1990;33(8):684–7.

21. Cespedes RD. The treatment of posterior compartment vaginal defects. Urol Clin North Am 2011;38(1):17–23, v.

22. Weber AM, Walters MD, Piedmonte MR. Sexual function and vaginal anatomy in women before and after surgery for pelvic organ prolapse and urinary incontinence. Am J Obstet Gynecol 2000;182(6):1610–5.

23. Francis WJ, Jeffcoate TN. Dyspareunia following vaginal operations. J Obstet Gynaecol Br Commonw 1961;68:1–10.

24. Sullivan ES, Leaverton GH, Hardwick CE. Transrectal perineal repair: an adjunct to improved function after anorectal surgery. Dis Colon Rectum 1968; 11(2):106–14.

25. Khubchandani IT, Clancy JP 3rd, Rosen L, et al. Endorectal repair of rectocele revisited. Br J Surg 1997;84(1):89–91.

26. Roman H, Michot F. Long-term outcomes of transanal rectocele repair. Dis Colon Rectum 2005;48(3): 510–7.

27. Ho YH, Ang M, Nyam D, et al. Transanal approach to rectocele repair may compromise anal sphincter pressures. Dis Colon Rectum 1998;41(3):354–8.

28. van Dam JH, Huisman WM, Hop WC, et al. Fecal continence after rectocele repair: a prospective study. Int J Colorectal Dis 2000;15(1):54–7.

29. Nieminen K, Hiltunen KM, Laitinen J, et al. Transanal or vaginal approach to rectocele repair: a prospective, randomized pilot study. Dis Colon Rectum 2004;47(10):1636–42.

30. Ommer A, Albrecht K, Wenger F, et al. Stapled transanal rectal resection (STARR): a new option in the treatment of obstructive defecation syndrome. Langenbecks Arch Surg 2006;391(1):32–7.

31. Dodi G, Pietroletti R, Milito G, et al. Bleeding, incontinence, pain and constipation after STARR transanal double stapling rectotomy for obstructed defecation. Tech Coloproctol 2003;7(3):148–53.

32. Pescatori M, Dodi G, Salafia C, et al. Rectovaginal fistula after double-stapled transanal rectotomy (STARR) for obstructed defecation. Int J Colorectal Dis 2005;20(1):83–5.

33. Schwandner O, Furst A. Assessing the safety, effectiveness, and quality of life after the STARR procedure for obstructed defecation: results of the German STARR registry. Langenbecks Arch Surg 2010; 395(5):505–13.

34. Richardson AC. The rectovaginal septum revisited: its relationship to rectocele and its importance in rectocele repair. Clin Obstet Gynecol 1993;36(4): 976–83.

35. Mellgren A, Anzen B, Nilsson BY, et al. Results of rectocele repair. A prospective study. Dis Colon Rectum 1995;38(1):7–13.

36. Kahn MA, Stanton SL. Posterior colporrhaphy: its effects on bowel and sexual function. Br J Obstet Gynaecol 1997;104(1):82–6.

37. Kenton K, Shott S, Brubaker L. Outcome after rectovaginal fascia reattachment for rectocele repair. Am J Obstet Gynecol 1999;181(6):1360–3 [discussion: 1363–4].

38. Singh K, Cortes E, Reid WM. Evaluation of the fascial technique for surgical repair of isolated posterior vaginal wall prolapse. Obstet Gynecol 2003;101(2):320–4.

39. Abramov Y, Gandhi S, Goldberg RP, et al. Site-specific rectocele repair compared with standard posterior colporrhaphy. Obstet Gynecol 2005;105(2):314–8.

40. Gustilo-Ashby AM, Paraiso MF, Jelovsek JE, et al. Bowel symptoms 1 year after surgery for prolapse: further analysis of a randomized trial of rectocele repair. Am J Obstet Gynecol 2007;197(1):76;e1–5.

41. Altman D, Zetterstrom J, Mellgren A, et al. A three-year prospective assessment of rectocele repair using porcine xenograft. Obstet Gynecol 2006;107(1):59–65.

42. Sung VW, Rardin CR, Raker CA, et al. Porcine subintestinal submucosal graft augmentation for rectocele repair: a randomized controlled trial. Obstet Gynecol 2012;119(1):125–33.

43. Sand PK, Koduri S, Lobel RW, et al. Prospective randomized trial of polyglactin 910 mesh to prevent recurrence of cystoceles and rectoceles. Am J Obstet Gynecol 2001;184(7):1357–62 [discussion: 1362–4].

44. Lim YN, Rane A, Muller R. An ambispective observational study in the safety and efficacy of posterior colporrhaphy with composite Vicryl-Prolene mesh. Int Urogynecol J Pelvic Floor Dysfunct 2005;16(2):126–31 [discussion: 131].

45. de Tayrac R, Picone O, Chauveaud-Lambling A, et al. A 2-year anatomical and functional assessment of transvaginal rectocele repair using a polypropylene mesh. Int Urogynecol J Pelvic Floor Dysfunct 2006;17(2):100–5.

46. Milani R, Salvatore S, Soligo M, et al. Functional and anatomical outcome of anterior and posterior vaginal prolapse repair with Prolene mesh. BJOG 2005; 112(1):107–11.

47. Simon M, Debodinance P. Vaginal prolapse repair using the Prolift kit: a registry of 100 successive cases. Eur J Obstet Gynecol Reprod Biol 2011; 158(1):104–9.

48. Elmer C, Altman D, Engh ME, et al. Trocar-guided transvaginal mesh repair of pelvic organ prolapse. Obstet Gynecol 2009;113(1):117–26.

49. Sung VW, Rogers RG, Schaffer JI, et al. Graft use in transvaginal pelvic organ prolapse repair: a systematic review. Obstet Gynecol 2008;112(5):1131–42.

50. Murphy M. Clinical practice guidelines on vaginal graft use from the society of gynecologic surgeons. Obstet Gynecol 2008;112(5):1123–30.

51. FDA safety communication: update on serious complications associated with transvaginal placement of surgical mesh for pelvic organ prolapse. Available at: http://www.fda.gov/medicaldevices/safety/alertsandnotices/ucm262435.htm. Accessed February 14, 2012.

52. Hogston P. Posterior colporrhaphy: its effect on bowel and sexual function. Br J Obstet Gynaecol 1997;104(8):972–3.

53. Komesu YM, Rogers RG, Kammerer-Doak DN, et al. Posterior repair and sexual function. Am J Obstet Gynecol 2007;197(1):101;e1–6.

54. Brandner S, Monga A, Mueller MD, et al. Sexual function after rectocele repair. J Sex Med 2011;8(2):583–8.

Posterior-Compartment Repair
A Urology Perspective

Alex Gomelsky, MD[a],*, Roger R. Dmochowski, MD[b]

KEYWORDS

- Posterior-compartment prolapse • Rectocele • Biological grafts • Rectovaginal fascia plication

KEY POINTS

- The relationship between the degree or severity of anatomic posterior compartment weakness and functional difficulty is not consistent.
- The recurrence rates after most types of posterior compartment repairs are typically low.
- The addition of biologic grafts may not improve the anatomic results of posterior compartment repairs.
- Randomized studies of traditional and graft-augmented repairs are infrequent in the literature.

INTRODUCTION

Whereas the prevalence of all pelvic organ prolapse has been estimated to exceed 11% in several studies,[1] the prevalence of posterior-compartment prolapse (rectocele) specifically is not known. Posterior vaginal wall relaxation is most simply a herniation of the anterior rectal wall that produces a vaginal bulge. The bulge is purely an anatomic finding and can be associated with a wide spectrum of clinical symptoms, ranging from a relative absence of symptoms to significant pain, constipation, and splinting to evacuate the bowels. One of the challenges of treating rectoceles has been that a direct correlation between anatomic findings and clinical symptoms does not always exist.[2] The authors have found that operative repair symptomatically improved a majority of patients with impaired defecation associated with a large rectocele, but this improvement was likely related at least in part to factors other than the size of the rectocele. Multiple surgical techniques are available for rectocele repair, and the literature is not clear regarding indications for each type of surgical intervention. The object of this article is to review the literature regarding various types of posterior-compartment repair, and draw conclusions regarding their absolute efficacy and relative efficacy in comparison with one another. This review is limited to standard repairs and repairs augmented with biological grafts. Repairs using nonabsorbable synthetic mesh, with or without the addition of commercial, transvaginal prolapse kits, are not covered.

ANATOMY OF POSTERIOR-COMPARTMENT LAXITY

DeLancey subdivided the vaginal support of the anterior and posterior compartments into 3 levels.[3] Level I support consists of the cardinal/uterosacral ligament complex, which originates at the cervix and upper vagina and inserts at the sacrum and pelvic side wall. In the posterior compartment, the vagina is separated from the rectum by the trapezoidal rectovaginal septum, with the narrow end located distally.[4] The paravaginal attachments constitute Level II support. While Level II vaginal support in the anterior compartment is provided entirely by the arcus tendineus fasciae pelvis (ATFP), the attachment of the posterior vaginal wall to the pelvic side wall is more complex. The

^a Department of Urology, Louisiana State University Health Sciences Center – Shreveport, 1501 Kings Highway, Shreveport, LA 71130, USA; ^b Department of Urologic Surgery, Vanderbilt University Medical Center, A1302 Medical Center North, Nashville, TN 37232-2765, USA
* Corresponding author.
E-mail address: agomel@lsuhsc.edu

Urol Clin N Am 39 (2012) 371–376
http://dx.doi.org/10.1016/j.ucl.2012.06.010
0094-0143/12/$ – see front matter © 2012 Elsevier Inc. All rights reserved.

distal one-third to one-half of the posterior vaginal wall fuses with the aponeurosis of the levator ani muscle from the perineal body along a line called arcus tendineus rectovaginalis. This line converges with the ATFP approximately halfway between the pubic symphysis and the ischial spine.[5] The rectovaginal septum is fused distally with the urogenital diaphragm and proximal perineal body (Level III support).

Defects of the posterior compartment mirror those found in the anterior compartment in several ways. Loss of Level II support may be central or lateral, and these types of defects have traditionally been repaired with a plication of the rectovaginal fascia in the midline (posterior colporrhaphy). In addition, a site-specific posterior repair that repairs discrete rents in the rectovaginal fascia may be performed instead of a midline plication.[6] Proximal detachment of the rectovaginal septum from the uterosacral ligaments (Level I support) may be associated with an enterocele and repair of concomitant apical prolapse (abdominal sacral colpopexy and uterosacral, sacrospinous, or iliococcygeus suspensions) may be necessary. Loss of Level III support may result in perineal weakness and may be repaired by reapproximating the perineal body (perineorrhaphy).

SUCCESS RATES AFTER STANDARD POSTERIOR-COMPARTMENT REPAIR

Although there are no long-term prospective studies, anatomic cure rates after posterior-compartment repair appear to be high. Maher and colleagues[7] performed a prospective evaluation of 38 consecutive women with symptomatic rectoceles ($\geq$stage II) and obstructed defecation who underwent midline fascial plication of the posterior vaginal wall. The median follow-up was 12.5 months and the subjective success rates were 97% (95% confidence interval [CI] 0.83%–1.00%) at 12 months and 89% (95% CI 0.55%–0.98%) at 24 months. The objective success rates were 87% (95% CI 0.64%–0.96%) at 12 months and 79% (95% CI 0.51%–0.92%) at 24 months. The average points, Ap and Bp, were significantly reduced from preoperative values and the depth of rectocele was also reduced significantly on defecography. The correction of the anatomic defect was associated with improved functional outcome, with 33 women (87%) no longer experiencing obstructed defecation, and there was a significant reduction in postoperative straining to defecate, hard stools, and dyspareunia. The improved anatomic and functional outcomes were reflected in the fact that 97% of the women reported very high satisfaction with their surgery.

The data also support high success after site-specific repairs. Cundiff and colleagues[6] performed site-specific repair without levator plication or perineorrhaphy in 69 women with a median preoperative posterior Pelvic Organ Prolapse Quantitation (POP-Q) stage II. The POP-Q stage had improved for all but 2 women at 6 weeks, and 18% had recurrent rectoceles at 12 months. Mean values for the points describing the posterior vaginal wall improved by greater than 2 cm ($P<.0001$) and functional results mirrored anatomic results, with statistically significant improvement in constipation, splinting, tenesmus, and fecal incontinence. Kenton and colleagues[8] reported on 66 patients with abnormal fluoroscopic results and objective rectocele formation, 46 of whom were objectively assessed at 12 months. Resolution of postoperative symptoms was as follows: protrusion, 90% (35 of 39; $P<.0005$); difficult defecation, 54% (14 of 24; $P<.0005$); constipation, 43% (9 of 21; $P = .02$); dyspareunia, 92% (11 of 12; $P = .01$); and manual evacuation, 36% (4 of 11; $P = .125$). Vaginal topography at 12 months was improved, with a mean Ap point value of -2 cm (range, -3 to 2 cm).

Porter and colleagues[9] performed a retrospective observational study that included 125 women who had undergone site-specific posterior colporrhaphy, either alone or in conjunction with other pelvic procedures. At follow-up examination, surgical correction was achieved in 82% of eligible patients (73 of 89). All daily aspects of living improved significantly ($P<.05$), including ability to do housework (56% improvement or cure), travel (58% improvement or cure), and social activities (60% improvement or cure). Emotional well-being also significantly improved after the operation, as measured by thoughts of embarrassment (57% improvement or cure) or frustration (71% improvement or cure). Sexual function was not affected; however, reports of dyspareunia significantly improved or were cured after the operation in 73% of women (19 of 26), worsened in 19% of women (5 of 26), and arose de novo in 3 women. Results showed no other significant differences in vaginal dryness, orgasm ability, sexual desire, sexual frequency, or sexual satisfaction. Bowel symptoms were assessed subjectively and were noted to improve significantly postoperatively ($P<.008$). The following improvement or cure rates were obtained: defecation difficulties, 55%; pelvic pain or pressure, 73%; vaginal mass, 74%; and splinting, 65%. Singh and colleagues[10] reported on 42 women with symptomatic rectocele ($\geq$stage II) who underwent site-specific repair. Forty of 42 women (95%) were assessed at 6 weeks and 78.5% (33 of 42) followed up at 18 months. At

6 weeks, vaginal protrusion resolved in 87.5% and bowel symptoms in 87%, while at 18 months there was anatomic cure in 92%, improvement in defecation in 81%, and improvement of sexual dysfunction in 35%.

Conversely, Sardeli and colleagues[11] recently reported a case series of 51 women who underwent site-specific rectocele repair under local anesthesia. The mean follow-up period was 26.7 months. Whereas pelvic examination revealed recurrence of posterior prolapse in 31% (16 of 51), improvement in rectal emptying was achieved in only 23% (7 of 30), and 23% (7 of 30) of women experienced relief from constipation. One patient developed de novo dyspareunia. Overall, 92% of the patients (47 of 51) would recommend local anesthesia.

All of these studies are limited by their retrospective nature, relatively brief follow-up periods, variations in patient populations and surgical technique, definitions of success and failure, and indications for repair. These results should thus be interpreted with caution.

AUGMENTATION OF POSTERIOR-COMPARTMENT REPAIR WITH BIOLOGICAL GRAFTS

Augmentation of standard prolapse repair with a graft is appealing because additional material can be used to buttress the native tissue often considered responsible for the initial prolapse. Furthermore, an augmentation graft can be tailored to address both central and lateral Level II defects, and can also repair Level I and III defects simultaneously via attachments to apical landmarks and the perineal body, respectively. Although both biological and synthetic (absorbable and nonabsorbable) grafts have been used for posterior-compartment repairs, only biological grafts are discussed here.

Oster and Astrup[12] were the first to describe a standard posterior colporrhaphy that was reinforced with a submucosal dermis graft. All 15 women were cured of their symptoms at a follow-up of between 1 and 4 years, and a "less perfect" anatomic result was reported in only one woman. Kohli and Miklos[13] used cadaveric dermis anchored to the levator ani to augment site-specific fascial defect repair of the rectovaginal fascia in 43 women, with 30 women achieving a mean follow-up of 12.9 months. The anatomic success rate was 93% and no complications were reported. Kobashi and colleagues[14] used Tutoplast-processed cadaveric fascia lata in 73 women and reported at a mean follow-up of 13.7 months. Their anatomic success rate was 90%, and improvements in stool trapping

(83%), splinting (89.5%), and dyspareunia (64.3%) were reported.

Xenografts have also been described for posterior-compartment graft augmentation. Altman and colleagues[15] reported on 23 women who underwent cross-linked porcine dermis augmentation and were assessed at 3-year follow-up. Preoperatively, all patients had stage II prolapse of the posterior vaginal wall and a rectocele verified at defecography. At the 1-year follow-up, 11 of 29 patients (38%) had rectocele of at least stage II, and 4 patients underwent reoperation. At the 3-year follow-up, 7 of 23 patients (30%) had a rectocele of at least stage II. When including the 4 early anatomic recurrences, a total of 11 of 27 women (41%) had rectocele of at least stage II at 3-year follow-up. There was a significant decrease in rectal emptying difficulties ($P<.01$), sense of incomplete evacuation ($P<.01$), need for splinting ($P<.05$), and symptoms of pelvic heaviness ($P<.001$) at the 3-year follow-up compared with preoperatively. Cure of rectal emptying difficulties was reported by fewer than 50% of patients, and there were no significant changes in anal incontinence scores or symptoms of sexual dysfunction at the 3-year follow-up compared with preoperatively.

Studies by Dell and O'Kelley[16] and Smart and Mercer-Jones[17] also reported the use of cross-linked porcine dermis at short-term follow-up. Both reported encouraging anatomic outcomes and relatively few complications. Daraï and colleagues[18] reported the functional outcomes and quality of life after cross-linked porcine dermis rectocele repair combined with bilateral sacrospinous fixation. The mean follow-up was 38 months in 101 patients with prolapse stage III to IV. Postoperative improvement was noted in the Pelvic Organ Prolapse Distress Inventory-6 ($P<.0001$), Urogenital Distress Inventory-6 ($P = .001$), and Pelvic Floor Distress Inventory scores (PFDI; $P<.0001$) but not in the Colorectal Anal Distress Inventory-8 scores. An improvement was noted in the Urinary Impact Questionnaire-7 ($P<.0001$), Pelvic Organ Prolapse Impact Questionnaire-7 ($P<.0001$), and Pelvic Floor Impact Questionnaire Short Form-7 (PFIQ-7; $P<.0001$) scores, but not in the Colorectal-Anal Impact Questionnaire-7 scores.

COMPARISONS OF POSTERIOR-COMPARTMENT PROCEDURES

There are few comparative studies in the literature, and even fewer Level I studies (ie, randomized controlled trials [RCTs]). Abramov and colleagues[19] retrospectively compared the anatomic and functional outcomes of site-specific rectocele repair and standard posterior colporrhaphy. The study population comprised 124 women following site-specific rectocele repair and 183 consecutive women following standard posterior colporrhaphy without levator ani plication. Recurrence of rectocele beyond the midvaginal plane (33% vs 14%, $P = .001$) and beyond the hymenal ring (11% vs 4%, $P = .02$), recurrence of a symptomatic bulge (11% vs 4%, $P = .02$), and postoperative Bp point (-2.2 vs -2.7 cm, $P = .001$) were significantly higher after the site-specific rectocele repair. Rates of postoperative dyspareunia (16% vs 17%), constipation (37% vs 34%), and fecal incontinence (19% vs 18%) were not significantly different between the 2 study groups.

Novi and colleagues[20] compared preoperative and postoperative sexual function between women undergoing rectocele repair with porcine dermis graft (group 1; n = 50) and women undergoing site-specific repair (group 2; n = 50). The Pelvic Organ Prolapse/Urinary Incontinence Sexual Function Questionnaire (PISQ) was administered to all women before and 6 months after surgery. Preoperative sexual function scores were similar in the 2 groups (group 1: 81.4 ± 7.3; group 2: 83.6 ± 8.2; $P = 1.0$). Six months after surgery, PISQ scores in group 1 significantly increased (score increase 19.9 ± 2.2, $P = .01$), while the mean increase in PISQ scores for group 2 was 6.9 ± 3.1 ($P = .08$). When compared with group 2, subjects undergoing rectocele repair with porcine dermis graft scored significantly higher on the PISQ 6 months after surgery (group 1: 101.3 ± 6.4; group 2: 89.7 ± 7.1; $P = .01$). Biehl and colleagues[21] performed a retrospective chart review comparing 195 women who underwent rectocele repair with either a porcine dermal xenograft or human allogenic cadaveric dermal graft augmentation over a 2-year period. Repair of a site-specific defect was completed before augmentation with the graft. The investigators found that de novo dyspareunia and cure rates for constipation and dyspareunia were not statistically different between the 2 groups.

In an RCT comparing posterior colporrhaphy with biological graft augmentation, Paraiso and colleagues[22] prospectively demonstrated that the addition of porcine small intestinal submucosa does not necessarily improve anatomic outcomes of standard posterior colporrhaphy or site-specific repair. One hundred six women with prolapse of the posterior vaginal wall of stage II or greater were randomly assigned to either posterior colporrhaphy (n = 37), site-specific rectocele repair (n = 37), or site-specific rectocele repair augmented with a porcine small intestinal submucosal graft (Fortagen; Organogenesis, Inc, Canton,

MA, USA; n = 32). After 1 year, those subjects who received graft augmentation had a significantly greater anatomic failure rate (12 of 26; 46%) than those who received site-specific repair alone (6 of 27; 22%) or posterior colporrhaphy (4 of 28; 14%), $P = .02$. There was a significant improvement in prolapse and colorectal scales and overall summary scores of the PFDI-20 and PFIQ-7 after surgery in all groups ($P<.001$ for each) with no differences between groups. The proportion of subjects with functional failures was 15% overall, and not significantly different between groups. There was no significant change in the rate of dyspareunia 1 year after surgery, and there were no differences between groups. Overall sexual function as measured by the PISQ-12 improved significantly in all groups postoperatively ($P<.001$), with no differences between groups.

In an ancillary analysis of the aforementioned study, Gustilo-Ashby and colleagues[23] analyzed the change in bowel function and its relationship to vaginal anatomy 1 year after rectocele repair by 3 techniques. No differences in change in bowel symptoms were noted between treatment groups and, on average, all bowel symptoms evaluated were significantly improved 1 year after surgery. The development of novel "bothersome" bowel symptoms after surgery was uncommon (11%). After controlling for age, treatment group, comorbidities, and preoperative bowel symptoms, corrected postoperative vaginal support (stage 0/1) was associated with a reduced risk of postoperative straining (adjusted odds ratio [OR] 0.17; 95% CI 0.03–0.9) and feeling of incomplete emptying (adjusted OR 0.1; 95% CI 0.01–0.52). Normal support of the posterior vaginal wall (Bp ≤ -2) was associated with a reduced risk of bothersome incomplete emptying (OR 0.08; 95% CI 0.004–0.58) but not with other symptoms.

Finally, a Cochrane systematic review updated in 2010 was unable to draw definitive conclusions regarding the benefit of interposition grafts in the posterior compartment.[24] For prolapse of the posterior vaginal wall, the vaginal repair was associated with a lower rate of recurrent rectocele than was the transanal approach (relative risk 0.24; 95% CI 0.09–0.64), although there was a greater blood loss and postoperative narcotic use. No data exist on efficacy or otherwise of polypropylene mesh in the posterior vaginal compartment.

SUMMARY

Posterior-compartment prolapse is challenging because there is not always a clear relationship between the degree of anatomic defect and functional difficulty. As such, rectocele repair should be aimed at improving functional results while minimizing dyspareunia and vaginal distortion. Several techniques have been described for rectocele repair (midline rectovaginal fascia plication with or without levator plication, site-specific repair, and graft-augmented repair), but the literature is not clearly in favor of any one method. Multiple single-center studies suggest that the recurrence rates after standard rectocele repair are low in the short term and that defecatory symptoms typically improve after anatomic success. Likewise, overall short-term and medium-term anatomic success rates are high for biological graft augmentation with cadaveric allografts and xenografts. Unfortunately, good-quality, prospective RCTs are rare in the rectocele literature and, thus, few conclusions can be drawn. Limited nonrandomized studies suggest that site-specific rectocele repair is associated with higher anatomic recurrence rates, but similar rates of dyspareunia and bowel symptoms, than standard posterior colporrhaphy. Furthermore, the addition of a biological graft may not improve the anatomic success rates over that of a traditional repair. It is clear that well-planned, multi-institutional RCTs are required to answer these questions.

EDITOR'S COMMENTS

Posterior compartment reconstruction is one of the more difficult aspects of pelvic floor reconstruction. From an evolutionary standpoint, repairs have progressed from plication to site-specific defect and fascial-based reconstructive techniques to the implantation of augmenting meshes and grafts. More recently, there has been a re-emphasis of host tissue. The editors both recommend the site-specific repair as a critical intervention in the appropriately-selected patient. Site-specific repairs are dependent on the presence of fascial segments that can be re-approximated. These segments are very difficult to identify before surgical dissection and therefore, any posterior repair may have to rely on more standard plication procedures or the occasional use of interposition graft.

There has been a trend away from synthetic mesh kit and free graft implantation over the last several years. Both editors still will utilize biologic materials as interposition grafts in those patients who have insufficient native fascia for purposes of adequate reconstruction. Plication repairs, while offering native tissues for reconstructive purposes, are at risk for vaginal constriction and subsequent dyspareunia and therefore should be used with discretion. However, these approaches do provide a reasonable restorative technique.

Of importance during posterior repair is not only the isolated rectocele but recognition of associated high posterior (near the apex) enteroceles, sigmoidoceles, or vault prolapse. As with the anterior compartment, vault stabilization is a critical aspect of surgical success for posterior compartment repairs.

Another important aspect of posterior compartment repair is the distal most aspect of the repair, that being the perineum. Perineorrhaphy is certainly not required in all patients but in those patients with widely splayed transverse perinei muscles, reconstruction should be obtained to stabilize the distal aspect of the vaginal outlet as a foundation for the more proximal remainder of the repair.

As with all prolapse procedures, patient counseling is important to create reasonable expectations for posterior compartment reconstructive repairs. The patient should be aware that some symptoms of bowel dysfunction may persist even after posterior compartment repair, including the bothersome symptoms associated with bowel dysmotility (constipation). It is our practice to prepare the lower intestine, especially in revision repairs where there may be scarification and fibrosis and the possibility of rectal wall disruption. In the circumstance of a prepared bowel, mural injury can be repaired with no consequence and the editors recommend this as a preoperative management component.

Many posterior defects are small and relatively asymptomatic, and certainly neither of the editors recommend posterior compartment repair without the patient experiencing bother and associated symptoms (related to prolapse mass effect and/or bowel dysfunction resulting in the need to splint). Posterior compartment repair may be done as an isolated or combined procedure with other compartments of the vagina at the discretion of the operative surgeon and after informed consent from the patient.

A significant complication associated with posterior compartment repair is vaginal lumenal constriction and resultant lack of distensibility. Therefore, it is incumbent upon any successful repair to maintain as much vaginal distensibility and lack of posterior constriction as possible with whichever of the above techniques is most suited to the individual's presenting anatomy.

Roger R. Dmochowski, MD
Mickey Karram, MD

REFERENCES

1. Olsen AL, Smith VJ, Bergstrom JO, et al. Epidemiology of surgically managed pelvic organ prolapse and urinary incontinence. Obstet Gynecol 1997;89:501–6.
2. Van Laarhoven CJ, Kamm MA, Bartram CI, et al. Relationship between anatomic and symptomatic long-term results after rectocele repair for impaired defecation. Dis Colon Rectum 1999;42:204–10.
3. Delancey JO. Anatomic aspects of vaginal eversion after hysterectomy. Am J Obstet Gynecol 1992;166: 1717–24.
4. Zimmerman CW. Pelvic organ prolapse. In: Rock JA, Jones HW, editors. TeLinde's operative gynecology. 9th edition. Philadelphia: Lippincott Williams & Wilkins; 2003. p. 927–48.
5. Lefler KS, Thompson JR, Cundiff GW, et al. Attachment of the rectovaginal septum to the pelvic sidewall. Am J Obstet Gynecol 2001;185:41–3.
6. Cundiff GW, Weidner AC, Visco AG, et al. An anatomic and functional assessment of the discrete defect rectocele repair. Am J Obstet Gynecol 1998;179:1451–6.
7. Maher CF, Qatawneh AM, Baessler K, et al. Midline rectovaginal fascial plication for repair of rectocele and obstructed defecation. Obstet Gynecol 2004; 104:685–9.
8. Kenton K, Shott S, Brubaker L. Outcome after rectovaginal fascia reattachment for rectocele repair. Am J Obstet Gynecol 1999;181:1360–3.
9. Porter WE, Steele A, Walsh P, et al. The anatomic and functional outcomes of defect-specific rectocele repairs. Am J Obstet Gynecol 1999;181:1353–8.
10. Singh K, Cortes E, Reid WM. Evaluation of the fascial technique for surgical repair of isolated posterior vaginal wall prolapse. Obstet Gynecol 2003;101:320–4.
11. Sardeli C, Axelsen SM, Kjaer D, et al. Outcome of site-specific fascia repair for rectocele. Acta Obstet Gynecol Scand 2007;86:973–7.
12. Oster S, Astrup A. A new vaginal operation for recurrent and large rectocele using dermis transplant. Acta Obstet Gynecol Scand 1981;60:493–5.
13. Kohli N, Miklos JR. Dermal graft-augmented rectocele repair. Int Urogynecol J Pelvic Floor Dysfunct 2003;14:146–9.
14. Kobashi KC, Leach GE, Frederick R, et al. Initial experience with rectocele repair using nonfrozen cadaveric fascia lata interposition. Urology 2005; 66:1203–7.
15. Altman D, Zetterström J, Mellgren A, et al. A three-year prospective assessment of rectocele repair using porcine xenograft. Obstet Gynecol 2006;107: 59–65.
16. Dell JR, O'Kelley KR. PelviSoft BioMesh augmentation of rectocele repair: the initial clinical experience in 35 patients. Int Urogynecol J Pelvic Floor Dysfunct 2005;16:44–7.
17. Smart NJ, Mercer-Jones MA. Functional outcome after transperineal rectocele repair with porcine dermal collagen implant. Dis Colon Rectum 2007; 50:1422–7.
18. Daraï E, Coutant C, Rouzier R, et al. Genital prolapse repair using porcine skin implant and: midterm assessment. Urology 2009;73:245–50.
19. Abramov Y, Gandhi S, Goldberg RP, et al. Site-specific rectocele repair compared with standard posterior colporrhaphy. Obstet Gynecol 2005;105: 314–8.
20. Novi JM, Bradley CS, Mahmoud NN, et al. Sexual function in women after rectocele repair with acellular porcine dermis graft vs site-specific rectovaginal fascia repair. Int Urogynecol J Pelvic Floor Dysfunct 2007;18:1163–9.
21. Biehl RC, Moore RD, Miklos JR, et al. Site-specific rectocele repair with dermal graft augmentation: comparison of porcine dermal xenograft (Pelvicol) and human dermal allograft. Surg Technol Int 2008;17:174–80.
22. Paraiso MF, Barber MD, Muir TW, et al. Rectocele repair: a randomized trial of three surgical techniques including graft augmentation. Am J Obstet Gynecol 2006;195:1762–71.
23. Gustilo-Ashby AM, Paraiso MF, Jelovsek JE, et al. Bowel symptoms 1 year after surgery for prolapse: further analysis of a randomized trial of rectocele repair. Am J Obstet Gynecol 2007;197:76. e1–5.
24. Maher C, Feiner B, Baessler K, et al. Surgical management of pelvic organ prolapse in women. Cochrane Database Syst Rev 2010;4:CD004014.

Interstitial Cystitis/Bladder Pain Syndrome
Management of the Pain Disorder: A Urogynecology Perspective

Charles W. Butrick, MD

KEYWORDS

- Interstitial cystitis • Painful bladder syndrome • Pelvic floor hypertonic dysfunction
- Pelvic floor myofascial pain • Vulvodynia • Irritable bowel syndrome • Neuromodulation

KEY POINTS

- IC/BPS is a visceral pain syndrome and therefore central sensitization is key to symptom evolution and typically involves bladder as well as non-bladder pain generators.
- IC/BPS management involves identification of all pain generators and treatment of all pain generators.
- Success of therapy is related to duration of symptoms and number of pain disorders and therefore early identification and treatment of this visceral pain disorder is paramount.
- Multi-modal therapy and patient education is the key to successful management of IC/BPS.

Interstitial cystitis/bladder pain syndrome (IC/BPS) is a poorly defined pain syndrome that is characterized by various pelvic symptoms and urinary storage symptoms. The Society for Urodynamics and Female Urology defined IC/BPS as "an unpleasant sensation (pain, pressure, discomfort) perceived to be related to the urinary bladder, associated with the lower urinary tract symptoms for more than 6 weeks duration, in the absence of infection or other identifiable causes."[1] In the past, we thought this was a rare bladder disorder of unknown cause and difficult to treat. As our understanding of the disorder has evolved, we now realize it is common, with a prevalence between 2.7% and 6.5% of all women[2] and can manifest in many different ways. Although it may involve only bladder symptoms, it typically represents one component of a constellation of symptoms that involve bladder and nonbladder disorders. Its diagnosis is based on symptoms and ruling out other possible causes of those symptoms. Its treatment has also evolved as we

start to manage this disorder as the pain disorder that it is.

Over the past 10 years, we have learned much about the pathophysiology of IC/BPS.[3–5] The treatment of this disorder would be much more successful if we understood the cause of the pain disorder. Although it is likely a heterogeneous disorder with multiple triggers, it is generally agreed that it likely involves some degree of urothelial dysfunction and neuropathic upregulation that includes the process of central sensitization. Recent work also points to the multiple comorbidities[6,7] (ie, nonbladder pain syndromes, such as fibromyalgia, chronic fatigue syndrome, irritable bowel syndrome [IBS], vulvodynia, and voiding dysfunction) that contribute to and may potentiate the bladder symptoms.

The goal of treatment of any pain disorder is to first improve the quality of life of our patients. This goal can best be realized if we, as clinicians, identify each component of our patients' pain experience (pain generators) and treat each of

Disclosures: No relevant disclosures.
The Urogynecology Center, Suite 130, 12200 West 106th Street, Overland Park, KS 66215, USA
E-mail address: cwbutrick@gmail.com

Urol Clin N Am 39 (2012) 377–387
http://dx.doi.org/10.1016/j.ucl.2012.06.007
0094-0143/12/$ – see front matter © 2012 Elsevier Inc. All rights reserved.

these contributing factors. These comorbidities not only add to our patients' suffering but if not treated, then these other pain generators will continue to produce noxious stimuli that are involved in the maintenance of the central sensitization that is key to the persistence of bladder symptoms.

So with this review, the author briefly describes the neuropathology of IC/BPS and explains why patients often develop these nonbladder pain disorders and, therefore, why these are also important to identify and treat. The author then offers a targeted approach to patients with IC/BPS that involves the management of the bladder pain disorder and the management of the other pain generators. This approach has the potential to downregulate the central sensitization that is at the heart of any visceral pain disorder.

CONCEPTUALIZATION OF IC/BPS

As noted in the American Urological Association (AUA) guidelines for the management of IC,[8] it is not known whether IC/BPS is a primary bladder disorder or if the bladder symptoms are secondary to phenomena resulting from another cause. This statement is supported by a large body of evidence concerning visceral pain syndromes. Although IC/BPS is typically described as a disease of the urothelium and there is abundant evidence as to the abnormalities located at this peripheral site, pathologic conditions can occur elsewhere with these urothelial changes developing as a secondary abnormality. In addition to the peripheral abnormalities involving the urothelium, afferent nerve activity, and mast cells, visceral pain disorders can lead to changes within the spinal cord (central sensitization)[9] that can maintain pain long after the removal of the peripheral insult. The changes of central sensitization can be demonstrated in our patients with IC/BPS (startle reflex[10] and diffuse allodynia) and have been described in detail by many investigators. Central sensitization results in the development of multiple neuropathic abnormalities that are thought to trigger the multiple secondary pain disorders and dysfunctions that are so common in patients with IC/BPS. One example of this is the well-understood process of viscero-visceral crosstalk that results in symptoms in neighboring organs in patients with IC/BPS.[11] Classic examples are the development of IBS or increasing dysmenorrhea. This upregulation of the spinal cord (often referred to as wind up) is a major contributor to the development of the nonbladder pain syndromes so common in patients with IC/BPS. Other common nonbladder pain disorders

in our patients with IC/BPS include vulvodynia and pelvic floor hypertonic dysfunction (with its associated voiding dysfunction). We now understand that a plausible explanation for the development of these abnormalities includes the process of viscerosomatic and viscera-muscular–induced hyperalgesia and dysfunction. Both are manifestations of central sensitization.

The key concept to grasp while reviewing the management of IC/BPS is that many of these comorbid pain disorders produce additional noxious input to the sacral cord. This input furthers the upregulation of the dorsal horn and maintenance of the sensitization that results in the perpetuation of chronic pain (**Fig. 1**). Even if the original insult is removed, the persistence of the sensory processing abnormalities and these neuropathic reflexes result in persistent pain. For this reason, multimodal therapy is so important in the treatment of patients with visceral pain disorders, such as IC/BPS and IBS. Therapy directed toward the peripheral pain generator and systemic or centrally directed therapy should provide the highest potential for improved patient quality of life. The clinician ideally uses a careful history and questionnaires to identify the primary pain generator and secondary pain generators (**Fig. 2**) so that therapy directed toward all pain generators will attempt to downregulate the process of central sensitization by decreasing the volume of noxious stimuli impacting the patients' spinal cord. The importance of early identification of patients with visceral pain syndromes and aggressive therapy is exemplified by the finding that the likelihood of successful

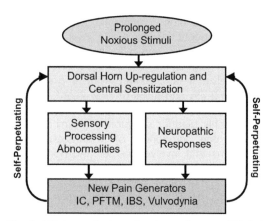

Fig. 1. Etiology of visceral pain syndromes. IBS, irritable bowel syndrome; IC, Interstitial cystitis; PFTM, pelvic floor tension myalgia. (*From* Butrick CW. Pathophysiology of pelvic floor hypertonic disorders. Obstet Gynecol Clin North Am 2009;36(3):702; with permission.)

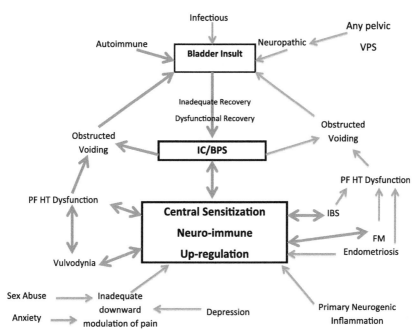

Fig. 2. Proposed neuropathophysiology of IC/BPS and the development of nonbladder pain disorders. The process of central sensitization is important to not only the association of nonbladder pain disorders and IC/BPS but also the self-perpetuation of visceral pain syndromes. FM, fibromyalgia; PFHT, pelvic floor hypertonic; VPS, visceral pain syndromes.

therapy is directly related to the duration of symptoms and the number of associated pain disorders.[12] Multiple studies have shown the benefit of multimodal therapy for chronic pain and recent studies support this concept specifically in patients with IC/BPS.[13,14] This concept of multimodal therapy is noted as a first-line therapeutic approach in the AUA guidelines for the treatment of IC.

TARGETED MANAGEMENT OF IC/BPS
General Patient Care

Patient education is an extremely important early step in patient care. Often patients have been told they have suffered from repeated bladder infections, yeast infections, and overactive bladder. They have been given antibiotics and anticholinergics in an attempt to decrease their bladder symptoms. Teaching patients about IC/BPS as a chronic pain disorder that can be controlled and even placed into remission with therapy is extremely important. Patients must understand that their participation in the management of their symptoms is an important component of successful therapy. The identification of symptom triggers, such as diet, stress, insomnia, depression, and hormone fluctuations, allows patients and clinicians to work together to initiate therapy. Our discussions with patients also

emphasize the importance of managing not only the comorbid pain disorders but also the environmental triggers and potentiators to their pain. This discussion initiates a process of patient empowerment, so they can become involved in what needs to be done to get better. Patients typically have already come to understand that these other pain disorders are somehow linked to their bladder symptoms, so when they learn the importance of managing these other pain disorders, they are typically in full agreement **Table 1**.

BLADDER-TARGETED THERAPIES
Behavior Modification

First-line therapy typically involves behavior modification,[15] which includes fluid management (48–64 oz/d) with the avoidance of bladder irritants, such as acidic foods, alcoholic beverages, caffeine, and so forth. Data are limited concerning the benefits of dietary manipulations on our patients' symptoms but especially in those who report dietary triggers education about the importance of avoidance is important. The use of over-the-counter supplements is poorly studied but calcium glycerophosphate (Prelief) does seem to benefit patients[16] with neutralization of acidic foods for both bladder and bowel symptoms.

Table 1
Associated pain disorders

	History	Findings	Treatment
Vulvodynia	Vulvar/introital pain	Allodynia with examination Negative cultures Variable erythema	Topical down regulation creams Amitriptyline PF relaxation therapy
IBS	Bowel distention with temporally associated pain	No hematochezia (workup needed if present) Tenderness along colon	Treatment based on predominate symptom Daily use of products to normalize pattern of BM
PF hypertonic dysfunction	Pressure Heaviness, aches worse with standing or sitting Postcoital pain	Voiding dysfunction, especially hesitancy Pain with BM or with urination Levator tenderness on examination	PF relaxation therapy Amitriptyline injection therapy Behavioral retraining to stop holding patterns

Abbreviations: BM, bowel movement; PF, pelvic floor.

ORAL THERAPIES
Pentosan Polysulfate

Pentosan polysulfate (PPS) (Elmiron) is the only oral medication that the Food and Drug Administration (FDA) has approved for the management of IC. PPS is the most studied oral medication for IC, with more than 500 patients from 7 randomized trials. These trials are nicely summarized in the AUA guidelines with grade B level evidence concerning efficacy (level of evidence stated are as per the AUA guidelines reference). Results concerning the benefit have been contradictory, but evidence would support 300 mg/d, with the duration of therapy likely a key component to the demonstration of response. The onset of the response seems to be directly associated with the duration of symptoms. Failure to respond after 6 months of therapy is generally thought to be an adequate trial. The mode of action seems to be the replenishment of the glycosaminoglycan (GAG) layer defects and the benefit from the potential antihistaminic effects of this medication on mast cells, which are generally thought to play a role in IC. Adverse event rates are low, with a rate that generally is similar to the placebo groups studied (evidence level B).

Amitriptyline

Amitriptyline (Elavil) is a commonly used medication for various pain disorders. One randomized controlled trial reported efficacy in patients with IC in 63% of patients[17] showing significant improvement in symptoms. Dosage titration is key to the balance of efficacy with drug-induced side effects. The typical starting dose is 12.5 mg at bedtime and increasing the dose as tolerated to 25 to 75 mg. The mode of action is multifactorial, including anticholinergic affects, serotonin-norepinephrine reuptake inhibition, and sedation-induced improvement of sleep disorders. However, this sedation is the most common side effect that makes this drug difficult to tolerate for some patients (evidence level B).

Hydroxyzine

Hydroxyzine (Vistaril) is a commonly used drug for patients with IC, especially if they do not tolerate amitriptyline or if they have a significant history of allergies. Two studies (1 randomized controlled and 1 observational) demonstrate a benefit in patients with minimal side effects other than sedation. The observational study done in patients with significant history of allergies had a 55% response rate.[18] This drug, therefore, is used at bedtime, typically at the dosage of 50 mg each night. Hydroxyzine is an antihistamine with antianxiety and analgesic properties (evidence level C).

Cyclosporine A

This immunosuppressive agent that is used to prevent organ rejection in organ transplant recipients has been used in a selective group of patients with ulcerative and nonulcerative IC unresponsive to traditional therapies. In a randomized trial, compared with PPS, it was found to have a 75% response rate with a decrease in frequency and pain.[19] A response is seen within 6 weeks. Observational studies that involve therapy for up to 5 years demonstrate sustained benefit, with a rapid return of symptoms typically occurring with cessation of therapy. The initial dose is 3 mg/kg/d in 2 divided doses. A slight reduction in dosage (reduced to

1.5 mg/kg after initial response), however, is often nicely tolerated. However, side effects can be serious, and close monitoring of blood pressure and serum creatinine is required during the first few weeks of therapy and every 6 months after that. More commonly seen adverse events of gingival hyperplasia and induction of facial hair growth can be bothersome, especially at higher doses. The long-term safety of this immunosuppressive agent has not been studied in patients with IC and its use is certainly off-label, but in clinical practice with patients who suffer from persistent symptoms, it has provided impressive clinical results. The mode of action involves the modification of the neuroimmune response to inhibit maintenance of inflammation (evidence level C).

INTRAVESICAL THERAPIES
Dimethyl Sulfoxide

Dimethyl sulfoxide (DMSO) is the only intravesical therapy approved by the FDA for the treatment of IC. DMSO is typically associated with postprocedure pain, especially if the solution is held for longer than 20 minutes. Treatment involves 4 to 6 installations at 1-week intervals. Two randomized crossover trials[20,21] and multiple observational studies have shown efficacy rates between 25% and 90%, with various durations of follow-up. If DMSO is used as part of a cocktail, the clinician must be aware of the potential for increased absorption of the other components because of the biologic properties of DMSO. The temporary increase in bladder pain and patient concerns about the garlic odor that is often associated with these treatments makes the acceptance of therapy difficult for some patients (level of evidence C).

Heparin

Heparin is typically used as a component of various bladder cocktails with a proposed mode of action that involves supplementation of a GAG layer deficiency that is often hypothesized to be part of the pathologic conditions seen in patients with IC/BPS. With this as the sole instillation component, 40.0% to 72.5%[22,23] of patients respond with significant improvement in symptoms. There are various cocktails in the literature but most contain lidocaine in combination with heparin. There are a few adverse events reported (level of evidence C).

Lidocaine

Anesthetic therapeutic cocktails are the most frequently used intravesical therapy at this time. A randomized controlled study showed that most patients experienced significant improvement in symptoms compared with placebo 3 days after instillation but not 10 days. Many clinicians use this response to help identify the patients that truly have a bladder source to their bladder symptoms.[24] Because the duration of the benefit is initially short, multiple installations are typically used (1–3 treatments per week for 3–6 weeks), with increasing duration of the benefit often seen. Anesthetic cocktails are often used as a rescue treatment of patients with severe flare. Lidocaine is typically used as a component of cocktails and is often alkalinized to improve penetration of the lidocaine. However, some patients experienced more dysuria when the solution is voided 2 to 3 hours later. Although there are no data to directly compare the benefit of alkalinization of the lidocaine, therapeutic cocktails without buffering agents have been shown to be beneficial. The mode of action likely involves the downregulation of C fibers in the submucos[25] (level of evidence B).

It is important to note that many patients with IC/BPS have such significant urethral allodynia that the placement of a catheter for instillation is simply not tolerated. Procedural techniques to use with all instillation therapies to improve patient tolerance, but especially those with urethral allodynia that is caused by severe hypertonic pelvic muscle dysfunction, include the following: The use of intraurethral viscous lidocaine for 10 to 15 minutes before the instillation and the use of a 8-French pediatric feeding tube for instillation purposes, not a typical 14-French catheter. Self-administration of intravesical therapy is also an option for many patients who can be taught this technique.

CYSTOSCOPY WITH HYDRODISTENTION

This procedure has been used in the past for the diagnosis of IC. Its use solely for the diagnosis of this disorder can no longer be recommended[8,26] but it can still be used for patients who demonstrate a poor response to first- and second-line therapies. If cystoscopy has not previously been done, it also allows the clinician to rule out other possible causes of bladder symptoms. Volume determined at the time of cystoscopy with hydrodistention is also thought to be a prognostic indication of patients who might be at a high risk for poor response to traditional therapies (volume <300 mL). If Hunner ulcers are found, then fulguration using the laser or cautery will rapidly provide symptomatic relief in most patients. Although symptom relief was experienced in 80% to 100% of patients with treatment of these lesions, they often redevelop and additional therapies will be required. If no Hunner lesions are found, then hydrodistention therapy can be done. Low pressure (60–80 cm of water) for 3 to 10 minutes done 1 to 3 times is generally an accepted approach to attempt therapeutic hydrodistention. Efficacy ranges of 30% to 54% at 1 month and 18% to 56% at 2 to 3 months are typical. Less than 10% of patients, however, will have a benefit at the 6-month followup.[27] Patients must be educated about possible immediate postprocedure flare and this low success rate and short-term benefit. The risk of bleeding and bladder rupture should also be discussed with patients. However, these risks are slight following this conservative protocol of hydrodistention (level of evidence C).

SACRAL NERVE STIMULATION

InterStim (Medtronic Inc., Minneapolis, MN, USA) is indicated for the treatment of urgency/frequency syndrome but not pain disorders. It has been used for patients with IC/BPS and has shown to improve symptoms of frequency, urgency, nocturia, and pain. With follow-up, patient satisfaction, however, drops slightly and the revision rate and explant rate is higher in these patients as compared with patients without pain disorders. Efficacy rates ranged between 66% and 91%.[28] Adverse event rates are low and typically involve infection or pain at the implant site. Patients with IC do show a higher rate of reoperation for lack of efficacy or implant site pain than patients with other indications for sacral nerve stimulation.[29] Preliminary work by Peters and colleagues[30] would suggest that pudendal nerve stimulation (another form of sacral nerve stimulation) may provide better efficacy in patients with IC (level evidence C).

Dorsal column stimulation has been found to be beneficial in patients with multiple diffuse visceral pain disorders. Up to 86% of these patients demonstrated a greater than 50% improvement in pain.[31] Various techniques of neuromodulation may play an important role in the treatment of more severe patients in the future.

Botulinum Toxin

Intradetrusor onabotulinumtoxinA (BTX-A) has been shown to benefit patients with IC/BPS based on 6 observational studies. Efficacy rates of 69% to 86% are seen, with duration of the benefit of less than 1 year.[32] The dosage used in the studies varies between 100 and 300 units; retention is still a risk factor to be considered, especially in patients with preexisting voiding dysfunction. Recent case series that involved trigonal injection sites may show improved efficacy.[33] Because of the risk and contradictory results in these observational studies, the use of BTX-A at this time is limited (level of evidence C).

Major Surgical Procedures

Surgical procedures, such as substitutions cystoplasty and urinary diversion, play a small but discrete role in the management of end-stage IC. Patients with small bladder capacity under anesthesia and repeated ulcerative disease who have severe pain that have failed all other therapies are the patients who would be considered for this type of intervention. Even then, persistent pain is frequently seen. Ten of 14 patients in one study had persistent pain, including pouch pain, in 4 patients[34] (level of evidence C).

FLARE MANAGEMENT

The natural history of IC/BPS includes symptom flares. The clinician must first rule out an infectious episode caused by bacterial cystitis. Approximately 31% of the patients with IC will experience a culture-positive urinary tract infection [35] and if recurrent may require episodic or suppressive therapy for this infectious complication. The diagnosis of bacterial cystitis must be based on a positive culture because symptoms of a flare are so similar to the symptoms of bacterial cystitis. If there is no evidence of a urinary tract infection, therapeutic options include increasing fluid intake, bladder analgesics, and anesthetic cocktails. If patients do not receive even temporary benefit from anesthetic cocktails, then the clinician must consider other pain generators, such as pelvic floor tension myalgia and vulvodynia. The occasional patient should consider a very brief course of pulsed steroids[36] (eg, Medrol dose pack) to decrease the inflammatory component seen in some of our patients with bladder flare.

ASSOCIATED PAIN DISORDERS

As noted earlier, most patients with IC/BPS have other pain disorders. With our present understanding of the neuropathology involved in chronic pain disorders and the importance of central sensitization, peripheral sensitization with the associated upregulation and self-perpetuation of pain, it is obvious why successful therapy requires treating all pain generators and pain potentiators. A detailed description of the identification and treatment of each of these associated pain disorders is not possible for this article but a brief review is offered in **Table 2**.

Table 2
Targeted treatment of IC/PBS

	Bladder	Pelvic Floor	Vulvodynia	IBS	FM
First-line therapy	General care to include patient education and behavioral modification (low-acid diet, Prelief supplement, counseling for stress, depression, sexual dysfunction)				
	Amitriptyline PPS or intravesical treatment (especially for severe symptoms)	PT referral for PF rehabilitation with relaxation therapy Elavil	Correction of urogenital atrophy (if present) Amitriptyline	IBS-C Osmotic laxative daily with fiber supplement added as needed IBS-D Reduced-acid diet, Prelief supplement Amitriptyline	Amitriptyline Relaxation therapy
Second-line therapy	Hydroxyzine if positive allergy history Cystoscopy with hydrodistention[a] vs SN stimulation Cyclosporin A	Tizanidine Injections: local anesthesia/Botox	Topical neurolytics[b] 2.5% amitriptyline 2.5% baclofen 2.5% gabapentin	Refer to GI specialist with interest in Tx of IBS	Pregabalin Refer to rheumatology for evaluation

If Hunner ulcer found at any point during evaluation and management, must consider fulguration.
If urethral pain not resolved with intravesical therapy, then this is triggered by the PF hypertonic component.
Abbreviations: GI, gastrointestinal; PF, pelvic floor; PT, physical therapy; SN, sacral nerve; Tx, treatment.
[a] If cystoscopy has not already been done.
[b] Compounded.

Hypertonic Pelvic Floor Dysfunction

The importance of the identification and treatment of this component of IC/BPS cannot be overstated. Hypertonic pelvic floor dysfunction can cause symptoms of frequency and pain. It can induce bladder pain with bladder C-fiber upregulation and urothelial dysfunction because of its affect on voiding. It can also be a secondary pain generator triggered by the bladder pain of IC and by holding urine because of the constant urge to void. Hypertonic pelvic floor dysfunction is present in between 50% and 90%[37-39] of patients with IC/BPS and can be identified by history (especially the history of hesitancy, groin pain worse with increasing bladder volume, and discomfort with the use of tampons). Objective evidence involves a careful pelvic examination to assess relaxation ability and pelvic floor awareness. Urodynamics often demonstrates voiding dysfunction with elevated midurethral pressures. After the identification of hypertonic pelvic floor dysfunction, treatment using physical therapy directed toward relaxation techniques (that often involve reverse Kegel exercises, myofascial release, and therapeutic exercise), the use of various oral muscle relaxers, and trigger point therapy should be initiated.[40] Medications that may provide benefit include amitriptyline, tizanidine, and cyclobenzaprine. These medications are all medications that have been used in patients with fibromyalgia, a diffuse myofascial pain disorder seen in approximately one-third of patients with IC. Evidence to support the management of this component of IC/BPS is extensive[41] and is to be considered one of the first-line therapies as described by the AUA guidelines in patients with IC/BPS but certainly in those who are identified to have pelvic floor hypertonic dysfunction.

Vulvodynia

Vulvar pain disorders affect between 23.4% and 74.5%[42] of women with IC/BPS and are a major contributor to the sexual dysfunction so commonly seen. This underdiagnosed and undertreated disorder is characterized by introital burning that may occur spontaneously (unprovoked or generalized vulvodynia) or may occur only when provoked by pelvic examinations, tampons, or more commonly during or after sexual intercourse. In some patients, this symptom may simply be referred pain from the bladder discomfort (vulvar burning should temporarily resolve with an anesthetic cocktail in this subgroup of patients). In most patients, the vulvar pain is a secondary pain generator induced by the IC/BPS-triggered central sensitization and perpetuated by the commonly associated hypertonic pelvic floor dysfunction. The hypertonic dysfunction not only perpetuates the voiding dysfunction and the bladder pain but also the burning discomfort of vulvodynia. The burning discomfort only perpetuates the hypertonic pelvic floor response. Patients who have IC and vulvodynia symptoms were found to have a much greater degree of levator pain than patients who have IC symptoms without vulvodynia.[43] Therapy involves correcting the peripheral sensitization of the vulvar tissues and correcting the hypertonic dysfunction. Prolong use of oral contraceptives (onset of use before 18 years of age) potentiates the vulvar hyperalgesia[44] and, therefore, should be stopped. If tissues are irritated or erythematous, a brief trial of a topical steroid ointment can be considered. Compounded creams designed to downregulate the neuroimmune upregulation that is present in the peripheral tissues of the introitus have been found to be helpful in most patients with vulvodynia.[45] Amitriptyline/baclofen/gabapentin at a concentration of 2.5% each placed in a pluraderm base applied 2 to 3 times a day has been effective at decreasing the introital burning. As the burning resolves, the relaxation of the pelvic floor through guided pelvic floor rehabilitation will be much more successful. Amitriptyline has been studied as an excellent adjunct to the management of vulvodynia[46] likely through its neurolytic properties at the peripheral tissues and an adjunct to the relaxation of the pelvic floor.

IBS

IBS is defined as a functional bowel disorder in which there is abdominal pain or discomfort associated with defecation or a change in bowel habits.[47] It can involve symptoms of constipation, diarrhea, or mixed symptoms. Just like IC/BPS, IBS involves central sensitization and peripheral sensitization with significant modulation of symptoms as a result of diet and psychological factors. The management is based on the treatment of the predominant symptom. Appropriate dietary changes (basically a cystitis diet) are always the first step. Because of the high prevalence of hypertonic pelvic floor dysfunction in patients with IC/BPS, constipation is commonly seen. Osmotic laxatives and fiber supplements often provide improvement in the symptoms of constipation. If diarrhea is the predominant symptom, fiber supplements and antidiarrheal medicines are indicated. Amitriptyline is commonly used in patients with diarrhea-predominant IBS. Because visceral hyperalgesia is the hallmark of IBS, neuropathic downregulation is often required for more serious dysregulation. There are many drugs that address this component of IBS that are typically only used in patients with more significant symptoms. Pharmacologic therapy for patients with IBS-C includes tegaserod and lubiproston, and alosetron is used for IBS-D. But appropriate referral to a gastroenterologist with interest in the management of IBS, not just the performance of colonoscopy, is typically required for patients that require this more aggressive medical therapy for their IBS.

Psychological Contributors

Using the Research and Development Corporation (RAND) IC Epidemiology Study (RICE) population, a follow-up survey in patients who met the high specificity case definition showed that one-third of this group of patients with IC/BPS had a diagnosis of depression and 52% reported recent panic attacks.[48] The prevalence of these psychological disorders in the general public is estimated at 6.0% and 3.2% respectfully. In the RICE population, if these comorbidities were present, those individuals had worse functioning and increased pain and severity scores related to their IC/BPS. Although there is little evidence that treating the psychological factors improves patients' symptoms of IC, there is considerable evidence concerning the mind-body connection in other functional pain disorders[49] but best studied in patients with IBS. Certainly, addressing these issues will support our patients and our goal of improving their quality of life.

SUMMARY

As clinicians we are starting to realize that IC/BPS is not just an end-organ disease but a visceral pain syndrome. As a visceral pain syndrome, the importance of central sensitization cannot be over emphasized. It is the key to not only understanding the pathophysiology of IC/BPS but it is also the unifying factor in our patients' heterogeneous presentation and the reason they so commonly have multiple nonbladder-related pain syndromes. The therapeutic approach that will benefit our patients the most will likely involve the treatment of all peripheral pain generators and an approach that will allow downregulation of the central dysregulation that occurs in individuals with any chronic pain disorder. This multimodal approach will ideally involve a multidisciplinary team. Although this approach will not be available to all patients with IC/BPS, the concept of the careful identification of all pain generators and potentially treating each must be discussed with patients and used in their management.

Evidence-based medicine supports few of the therapies discussed in this article. As pointed out by Giannantoni and colleagues,[50] studies involving monotherapeutic approaches frequently failed to show significant improvement in symptoms. In clinical practice, we rarely use monotherapy because of this. Additionally, every patient's constellation of symptoms is different. Their predisposing factors (genetic, pelvic floor dysbehaviors, and psychological concerns) and their original trigger that turned on the cascade of events resulting in a chronic pain disorder is always unique to the particular patient. Therapy must, therefore, also be tailored to patients. Being a heterogeneous disorder, there will never be a single therapeutic approach that helps all patients, but as clinicians who are attempting to help their patients with IC/BPS, we must be willing to treat all components of their pain disorder and, therefore, be willing to look beyond the bladder in the management of this bladder pain disorder.

of both patient and practitioner that repetition and subtle additions and deletions of therapy may be required.

There is continued need for additional therapies and for better understanding the causation and persistence of symptoms. Also, the increasing observations that many of these patients have had symptoms dating to childhood, indicates the possible contributions of genetics and developmental contributions to this condition. Perhaps the answer to this puzzling condition will come from recognition of the life-long existence of these symptoms (albeit waxing and waning) and the realization that the condition may be substantially impacted by the central and peripheral nervous system.

Roger R. Dmochowski, MD
Mickey Karram, MD

REFERENCES

1. Hanno P, Dmochowski R. Status of international consensus on interstitial cystitis/bladder pain syndrome/painful bladder syndrome: 2008 snapshot. Neurourol Urodyn 2009;28:274.
2. Konkle KS, Berry SH, Elliott MN, et al. Comparison of an interstitial cystitis/bladder pain syndrome clinical cohort with symptomatic community women from the RAND Interstitial Cystitis Epidemiology study. J Urol 2012;187:508–12.
3. Sengupta JN. Visceral pain: the neurophysiological mechanism. Handb Exp Pharmacol 2009;(194):31–74.
4. Aslam N, Harrison G, Khan K, et al. Visceral hyperalgesia in chronic pelvic pain. BJOG 2009;116:1551–5.
5. Butrick CW. Interstitial cystitis and chronic pelvic pain: new insights in neuropathology, diagnosis, and treatment. Clin Obstet Gynecol 2003;46:811–23.
6. Warren JW, van de Merwe JP, Nickel JC. Interstitial cystitis/bladder pain syndrome and nonbladder syndromes: facts and hypotheses. Urology 2011;78:727–32.
7. Clemens JQ, Meenan RT, O'Keeffe Rosetti MC, et al. Case-control study of medical comorbidities in women with interstitial cystitis. J Urol 2008;179:2222–5.
8. Hanno PM, Burks DA, Clemens JQ, et al. AUA guideline for the diagnosis and treatment of interstitial cystitis/bladder pain syndrome. J Urol 2011;185:2162–70.
9. Woolf CJ. Central sensitization: implications for the diagnosis and treatment of pain. Pain 2011;152:S2–15.
10. Twiss C, Kilpatrick L, Craske M, et al. Increased startle responses in interstitial cystitis: evidence for central hyperresponsiveness to visceral related threat. J Urol 2009;181:2127–33.
11. Giamberardino MA, Costantini R, Affaitati G, et al. Viscero-visceral hyperalgesia: characterization in different clinical models. Pain 2010;151:307–22.
12. Nickel JC, Shoskes D, Irvine-Bird K. Clinical phenotyping of women with interstitial cystitis/painful bladder syndrome: a key to classification and potentially improved management. J Urol 2009;182:155–60.
13. Shoskes DA, Nickel JC, Rackley RR, et al. Clinical phenotyping in chronic prostatitis/chronic pelvic pain syndrome and interstitial cystitis: a management strategy for urologic chronic pelvic pain syndromes. Prostate Cancer Prostatic Dis 2009;12:177–83.
14. Hanley RS, Stoffel JT, Zagha RM. Multimodal therapy for painful bladder syndrome/interstitial cystitis: pilot study combining behavioral, pharmacologic, and endoscopic therapies. Int Braz J Urol 2009;35:467–74.
15. Foster HE Jr, Hanno PM, Nickel JC, et al. Effect of amitriptyline on symptoms in treatment naive patients with interstitial cystitis/painful bladder syndrome. J Urol 2010;183:1853–8.
16. Hill JR, Isom-Batz G, Panagopoulos G, et al. Patient perceived outcomes of treatments used for interstitial cystitis. Urology 2008;71:62–6.
17. van Ophoven A, Pokupic S, Heinecke A, et al. A prospective, randomized, placebo controlled, double-blind study of amitriptyline for the treatment of interstitial cystitis. J Urol 2004;172:533–6.
18. Theoharides TC, Sant GR. Hydroxyzine therapy for interstitial cystitis. Urology 1997;49:108–10.
19. Sairanen J, Tammela TL, Leppilahti M, et al. Cyclosporine A and pentosan polysulfate sodium for the treatment of interstitial cystitis: a randomized comparative study. J Urol 2005;174:2235–8.
20. Peeker R, Haghsheno MA, Holmang S, et al. Intravesical bacillus Calmette-Guerin and dimethyl sulfoxide for treatment of classic and nonulcer interstitial cystitis: a prospective, randomized double-blind study. J Urol 2000;164:1912–5 [discussion: 1915–6].
21. Perez-Marrero R, Emerson LE, Feltis JT. A controlled study of dimethyl sulfoxide in interstitial cystitis. J Urol 1988;140:36–9.
22. Parsons CL, Housley T, Schmidt JD, et al. Treatment of interstitial cystitis with intravesical heparin. Br J Urol 1994;73:504–7.
23. Kuo HC. Urodynamic results of intravesical heparin therapy for women with frequency urgency syndrome and interstitial cystitis. J Formos Med Assoc 2001;100:309–14.

24. Taneja R. Intravesical lignocaine in the diagnosis of bladder pain syndrome. Int Urogynecol J 2010;21: 321–4.

25. Parsons CL. Successful downregulation of bladder sensory nerves with combination of heparin and alkalinized lidocaine in patients with interstitial cystitis. Urology 2005;65:45–8.

26. Erickson DR, Tomaszewski JE, Kunselman AR, et al. Do the National Institute of Diabetes and Digestive and Kidney Diseases cystoscopic criteria associate with other clinical and objective features of interstitial cystitis? J Urol 2005;173:93–7.

27. Ottem DP, Teichman JM. What is the value of cystoscopy with hydrodistension for interstitial cystitis? Urology 2005;66:494–9.

28. Fariello JY, Whitmore K. Sacral neuromodulation stimulation for IC/PBS, chronic pelvic pain, and sexual dysfunction. Int Urogynecol J 2010;21: 1553–8.

29. Powell CR, Kreder KJ. Long-term outcomes of urgency-frequency syndrome due to painful bladder syndrome treated with sacral neuromodulation and analysis of failures. J Urol 2010;183:173–6.

30. Peters KM, Feber KM, Bennett RC. A prospective, single-blind, randomized crossover trial of sacral vs pudendal nerve stimulation for interstitial cystitis. BJU Int 2007;100:835–9.

31. Kapural L, Nagem H, Tlucek H, et al. Spinal cord stimulation for chronic visceral abdominal pain. Pain Med 2010;11:347–55.

32. Giannantoni A, Porena M, Costantini E, et al. Botulinum A toxin intravesical injection in patients with painful bladder syndrome: 1-year follow-up. J Urol 2008;179:1031–4.

33. Pinto R, Lopes T, Frias B, et al. Trigonal injection of botulinum toxin A in patients with refractory bladder pain syndrome/interstitial cystitis. Eur Urol 2010;58: 360–5.

34. Lotenfoe RR, Christie J, Parsons A, et al. Absence of neuropathic pelvic pain and favorable psychological profile in the surgical selection of patients with disabling interstitial cystitis. J Urol 1995;154: 2039–42.

35. Nickel JC, Shoskes DA, Irvine-Bird K. Prevalence and impact of bacteriuria and/or urinary tract infection in interstitial cystitis/painful bladder syndrome. Urology 2010;76:799–803.

36. Taneja R, Jawade KK. A rational combination of intravesical and systemic agents for the treatment of interstitial cystitis. Scand J Urol Nephrol 2007;41: 511–5.

37. Butrick CW. Pathophysiology of pelvic floor hypertonic disorders. Obstet Gynecol Clin North Am 2009;36:699–705.

38. Peters KM, Carrico DJ, Kalinowski SE, et al. Prevalence of pelvic floor dysfunction in patients with interstitial cystitis. Urology 2007;70:16–8.

39. Bassaly R, Tidwell N, Bertolino S, et al. Myofascial pain and pelvic floor dysfunction in patients with interstitial cystitis. Int Urogynecol J 2011;22:413–8.

40. Butrick CW. Pelvic floor hypertonic disorders: identification and management. Obstet Gynecol Clin North Am 2009;36:707–22.

41. Weiss JM. Pelvic floor myofascial trigger points: manual therapy for interstitial cystitis and the urgency-frequency syndrome. J Urol 2001;166: 2226–31.

42. Gardella B, Porru D, Nappi RE, et al. Interstitial cystitis is associated with vulvodynia and sexual dysfunction–a case-control study. J Sex Med 2011; 8:1726–34.

43. Peters K, Girdler B, Carrico D, et al. Painful bladder syndrome/interstitial cystitis and vulvodynia: a clinical correlation. Int Urogynecol J Pelvic Floor Dysfunct 2008;19:665–9.

44. Harlow BL, Vitonis AF, Stewart EG. Influence of oral contraceptive use on the risk of adult-onset vulvodynia. J Reprod Med 2008;53:102–10.

45. Boardman LA, Cooper AS, Blais LR, et al. Topical gabapentin in the treatment of localized and generalized vulvodynia. Obstet Gynecol 2008;112:579–85.

46. Reed BD, Caron AM, Gorenflo DW, et al. Treatment of vulvodynia with tricyclic antidepressants: efficacy and associated factors. J Low Genit Tract Dis 2006; 10:245–51.

47. Chang L, Drossman DA. Irritable bowel syndrome and related functional disorders. In: Meyer EA, Bushnell MC, editors. Functional pain syndromes: presentation and pathophysiology. Seattle (WA): International Association for the Study of Pain Press; 2009.

48. Watkins KE, Eberhart N, Hilton L, et al. Depressive disorders and panic attacks in women with bladder pain syndrome/interstitial cystitis: a population-based sample. Gen Hosp Psychiatry 2011;33:143–9.

49. Porter NS, Jason LA, Boulton A, et al. Alternative medical interventions used in the treatment and management of myalgic encephalomyelitis/chronic fatigue syndrome and fibromyalgia. J Altern Complement Med 2010;16:235–49.

50. Giannantoni A, Bini V, Dmochowski R, et al. Contemporary management of the painful bladder: a systematic review. Eur Urol 2011;61:29–53.

Management of Interstitial Cystitis/Bladder Pain Syndrome
A Urology Perspective

Renee B. Quillin, MD, Deborah R. Erickson, MD*

KEYWORDS

- Interstitial cystitis • Painful bladder syndrome • Guidelines • Therapy

KEY POINTS

- Education and advice on self-care for all patients.
- Fulguration or triamcinolone injection for Hunner lesions.
- For patients without Hunner lesions, many options are available to balance benefits, risks, and burdens.
- Pain management and treatment of comorbid conditions as needed.

INTRODUCTION AND DEFINITIONS

Most experienced clinicians recognize the syndrome originally known as interstitial cystitis (IC). However, a formal clinical definition for IC has never been established. The National Institute of Diabetes, Digestive and Kidney Diseases (NIDDK) established criteria for IC, but these criteria were intended for enrollment of patients into research studies and were not intended for clinical use. In fact, the NIDDK criteria are so restrictive that they exclude approximately half of patients thought by experienced clinicians to have IC.[1]

In addition to the lack of a clinical definition, the term "interstitial cystitis" also suffers from being scientifically inaccurate. The disease may not involve the bladder interstitium, and some patients lack bladder inflammation (cystitis). For all of these reasons, different organizations have proposed new definitions. The International Continence Society published the Painful Bladder Syndrome (PBS) definition in 2002[2]; the European Society for the Study of IC published the Bladder Pain Syndrome definition in 2008,[3] and the Society for Urodynamics and Female Urology published the IC/BPS definition in 2009.[4] The differences between these definitions are summarized in Appendix 1.

For research articles, it is important to specify one of these definitions to allow comparison of study outcomes. In clinical use, the importance of the name depends on the scenario. If a patient is applying for Social Security disability, the name IC should be used because it is a recognized diagnosis for that purpose. It may also be important to use the name IC if prescribing pentosan polysulfate (PPS) or dimethylsulfoxide (DMSO) because they are specifically indicated for IC. On the other hand, the name does not affect one's decision to treat the bladder, after determining that the bladder is the source of pain.

AMERICAN UROLOGICAL ASSOCIATION GUIDELINES

In 2011 the American Urological Association (AUA) completed guidelines on the treatment of IC/BPS, based on a literature review from January 1, 1983 to July 22, 2009. The guidelines are published[5] and

Disclosure: Dr Erickson is a Consultant to Trillium Therapeutics, Inc.
Division of Urology, Department of Surgery, University of Kentucky College of Medicine, 800 Rose Street, MS-275, Lexington, KY 40536-0298, USA
* Corresponding author.
E-mail address: dreric2@email.uky.edu

Urol Clin N Am 39 (2012) 389–396
http://dx.doi.org/10.1016/j.ucl.2012.05.007

are available online (http://www.auanet.org/content/clinical-practice-guidelines/clinical-guidelines/main-reports/ic-bps/diagnosis_and_treatment_ic-bps.pdf). For each treatment, a statement was made based on the available evidence. The different types of statements (eg, standard, recommendation) are summarized in Appendix 2. The guidelines include general clinical principles, followed by 6 specific tiers of treatment.

The general clinical principles were defined as being widely agreed on by urologists or other clinicians, for which there may or may not be evidence in the medical literature. These principles are important for the care of IC/BPS patients and should be kept in mind throughout treatment; they are summarized in Appendix 3. Among these, the authors especially emphasize to stop ineffective treatment after a clinically meaningful interval. Such action is easy to overlook in a busy practice, but is important for 2 reasons. First, it avoids the usual concerns with polypharmacy (expense, drug interactions, and so forth). Also, specific to IC/BPS, many of the usual medicines (and muscle relaxants for comorbid pelvic floor spasm) cause fatigue. If ineffective medicines are stopped, the patient can tolerate higher doses of potentially effective medicines.

Although not specifically discussed in the guidelines, clinicians who care for IC/BPS patients should be aware of the placebo and nocebo effects.[6] The placebo effect refers to real physiologic changes that improve pain and other symptoms. In contrast to common belief, it is not necessary to give an inert substance to elicit the placebo response. In fact, this response can be additive to active drug treatment. Clinicians can elicit the placebo response by explaining the mechanism of symptoms and the mechanisms by which the treatment is expected to relieve the symptoms, thus increasing the patient's expectation of success and giving the patient an increased sense of control. The nocebo effect also is physiologic and refers to the fact that anxiety increases pain perception, something that can be blocked chemically by diazepam or a cholecystokinin receptor antagonist. It follows that clinicians can decrease pain perception through behaviors that decrease anxiety. Not only should the clinician convey that he or she cares, but it is also important to have a reliable person in the office to return phone calls and treat flares promptly. Dedicated urology nurses are very helpful.

The 6 tiers of treatments are listed in Appendix 4 and are discussed in detail in the guidelines.[5] Tier 1 involves education, including IC/BPS knowledge base, risks and burdens of available treatments, the likely need to try multiple treatments, and self-care practices.

It is important to explain clearly the elimination diet trial. The authors' usual practice is to give the patient a list of foods that may possibly exacerbate symptoms. These lists can be found on the International Cystitis Association (ICA) Web site (www.ichelp.org) or in The Interstitial Cystitis Survival Guide.[7] It is explained to the patient that these foods are possible bladder irritants, but that they may not all apply to that individual. It is recommended that the patient avoid all foods on the list for 1 week, after which individual foods can be tried one at a time to evaluate for symptom exacerbation. If a specific food is going to exacerbate symptoms, it will do so within 24 hours.

Stress is well known to exacerbate IC/BPS symptoms; therefore, stress management is an essential aspect of IC/BPS care. Stress management has 2 main components, the first of which is to decrease stress as much as is feasible: working a reduced schedule at work, obtaining help with household chores, psychological help for emotional difficulties, and so forth. However, because some degree of life stress is unavoidable, the second component is to decrease the numerous physiologic effects of stress, which may increase pain in IC/BPS and other pain disorders. Meditation, yoga, mindfulness training, and guided imagery are among methods that may be used to decrease the effects of stress on the body. Future research may reveal specific medical therapies that interrupt the pathways by which stress increases IC/BPS symptoms.

Examples of other self-care practices include: (1) altering the concentration and/or volume of urine, by either fluid restriction or additional hydration; (2) application of local heat or cold over the bladder or perineum; (3) over-the-counter products (eg, neutraceuticals, calcium glycerophosphates, pyridium); (4) bladder training with urge suppression; (5) avoidance of tight-fitting clothing; and (6) avoidance of constipation. Two excellent self-care resources are The Interstitial Cystitis Survival Guide[7] and the ICA Web site www.ichelp.org.

The efficacy of education must not be underestimated. An interesting example comes from two placebo-controlled trials of amitriptyline. In the first trial, the mean decrease in International Cystitis Symptom Index/International Cystitis Problem Index (ICSI/ICPI) scores was 8.4 in the amitriptyline group and 3.5 in the placebo group.[8] In the second trial, mean decrease in ICSI/ICPI scores was 10 in the amitriptyline group and 7.2 in the placebo group.[9] A key difference was that all patients in the second trial received education. Thus, education plus placebo was almost as effective as amitriptyline alone, and much better than placebo alone.

Tier 2 includes several treatments. First, as a clinical principle, appropriate manual physical therapy techniques (eg, maneuvers that resolve pelvic, abdominal, and/or hip muscular trigger points, lengthen muscle contractures, and release painful scars and other connective tissue restrictions), should be offered if appropriately trained clinicians are available. It is important to emphasize that the goal of therapy is muscle or connective tissue relaxation. Pelvic-floor strengthening exercises (eg, Kegel exercises) should be avoided. Second, multimodal pain management approaches (eg, pharmacologic, stress management, manual therapy if available) should be initiated. Third, the guidelines list a variety of oral and intravesical medication options. In brief, these include amitriptyline, cimetidine, hydroxyzine, and PPS; and intravesical DMSO, heparin, and lidocaine.

Tier 3 includes cystoscopic treatments. It is important to recognize Hunner lesions because, if present, the AUA Guidelines recommend going directly to cystoscopic treatment instead of proceeding through the tiers sequentially. In most cases, Hunner lesions can be recognized without bladder distention.[10,11] Descriptions of the appearance of Hunner lesions vary. For example, Peeker and Fall[12] described "a reddened mucosal lesion with small vessels radiating toward a central pale scar, fibrin deposit or coagulum. This site ruptures with increasing bladder distention with petechial oozing of blood from the ulcer and mucosal margins." Parsons[13] described "velvet red patch that looks, for all practical purposes, like carcinoma in situ." They are illustrated in **Fig. 1** and elsewhere.[11,14]

Direct treatment of the Hunner lesion can be fulguration (laser or cautery) or triamcinolone injection. With fulguration, the authors find it useful to first outline the ulcer with the laser or cautery, then fill it in. If one starts from the inside of the ulcer and works out, reactive erythema spreads outward and obscures the original boundaries of the lesion. For either treatment, initial success rates are high but the symptoms (and lesions) usually recur over time. If so, treatment can be repeated.

If Hunner lesions are not present, the Tier 3 option is bladder distention under full general or regional anesthesia, which should be done with low-pressure (60–80 cm water) and duration of less than 10 minutes. The purpose of bladder distention here is to improve symptoms. Distention currently has no role in diagnosis. Symptom relief usually lasts less than 6 months. Partial relief occurs in 50% to 60% of patients, but fewer than 20% achieve excellent improvement.[15–17]

The evidence supporting Tiers 4 and 5 (neuromodulation, cyclosporine A, and botulinum toxin injection) for IC/BPS is limited by many factors including study quality, small sample sizes, and lack of durable follow-up. None of these therapies

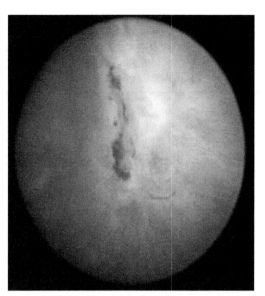

Fig. 1. Hunner lesion, from AUA Guidelines slide presentation. http://www.auanet.org/content/media/IC%20 Slide%20Presentation.2011.ppsx. (*From* Hanno PM, Burks DA, Clemens JQ, et al. Guideline on the diagnosis and treatment of interstitial cystitis/bladder pain syndrome. © 2011, American Urological Association Education and Research, Inc; with permission.)

have been approved by the US Food and Drug Administration (FDA) for this indication. The guidelines state that these interventions are not for generalized use, but rather should be limited to practitioners with experience in managing IC/BPS and willingness to provide long-term care of these patients after intervention.

Tier 6 is substitution cystoplasty or urinary diversion, and should also be limited to experienced providers. Patients with end-stage, structurally small bladders, that is, capacity under anesthesia less than 400 mL, are most likely to have good outcomes.[18,19]

LOCAL ANESTHETIC BLADDER INSTILLATIONS

The guidelines present bladder instillations as a Tier 2 option, but there is not enough evidence in the literature to address the best ingredients, doses, or scheduling.

Regarding ingredients, a key difference is whether or not the instillation contains DMSO. There are no comparative studies to guide this decision. DMSO is FDA-approved for IC, but has disadvantages: it can be painful to instill, some patients have long-term worsening of symptoms after treatment, and all patients have a disagreeable odor after instillation.[20] For these reasons, plus the lack of evidence to demonstrate superiority of

DMSO over non-DMSO cocktails, the authors prefer to start with non-DMSO cocktails.

Published non-DMSO cocktails usually include lidocaine with or without other ingredients including heparin, sodium bicarbonate, PPS, and/or cortico-steroids. Two studies have shown lidocaine-based cocktails to be superior to placebo, but no studies have compared different cocktail formulations or

Table 1
Lidocaine cocktails without DMSO

Source	Formulation	Schedule	Response Definition	Response Rate
Nickel et al[22]	200 mg lidocaine followed by 8.4% Na bicarbonate solution, final volume 10 mL	5 consecutive days, dwell time of 1 h	Moderate or markedly improved GRA	30%
Henry et al[23]	20 mL 8.4% Na bicarbonate with lidocaine concentration 1%–2.5%	2 consecutive days, dwell time 1 h	Response not dichotomized	N/A
Butrick et al[24]	20 mL of 2% lidocaine, 20,000 units of heparin, and 40 mg of triamcinolone	3 weekly treatments	"Helpful"	74%
Taneja[25]	20 mL of 2% lidocaine solution	One instillation	Decrease VAS by 50%	68%
Parsons[26]	40,000 U heparin, 8 mL 1% or 2% lidocaine, 3 mL 8.4% Na bicarbonate	One instillation	PORIS scale at least 50% improvement	1% lidocaine: 75% 2% lidocaine: 94%
Parsons[26]	40,000 U heparin, 8 mL 2% lidocaine, and 3 mL 8.4% Na bicarbonate	3 weekly treatments for 2 wk	PORIS scale at least 50% improvement	80%
Parsons et al[27]	50,000 units heparin, 200 mg lidocaine, 420 mg Na bicarbonate in 15 mL water	One instillation	PORIS scale at least 50% improvement	50%
Davis et al[28,a]	8 mL 1% lidocaine and 3 mL 8.4% Na bicarbonate, followed by 200 mg PPS or 30 mL saline	2 weekly treatments for 6 wk; dwell time 30–60 min	At least moderate on GRA	86% with PPS 90% with saline
Welk and Teichman[29]	8 mL 2% lidocaine, 20,000 U heparin, 4 mL 8.4% Na bicarbonate (first do 10 mL 2% lidocaine jelly in urethra 5 min)	Three times weekly for 3 wk, dwell time up to 60 min	PORIS scale at least 50% improvement	65%

Abbreviations: DMSO, dimethylsulfoxide; GRA, Global Response Assessment; N/A, no data available; PORIS, Patient's Overall Rating of Improvement in Symptoms; PPS, pentosan polysulfate; VAS, Visual Analog Scale.
a All subjects also received oral PPS (200 mg twice a day) for 18 weeks.

dosing schedules. The published trials to date are summarized in **Table 1**. In their practice, the authors usually use bupivacaine instead of lidocaine for reasons both theoretical (more potent, more lipophilic, longer lasting) and practical (no need to add sodium bicarbonate). The authors[21] recently reviewed patients who underwent bupivacaine installation after failing lidocaine-based cocktails. After a single instillation of 20 mL 0.5% bupivacaine, 27% had complete (though transient) pain relief and 53% had partial relief. Much research is still needed to determine the best ingredients and dosing schedules for intravesical instillations in IC/BPS.

SUMMARY

Management of IC/BPS is individualized for each patient. All patients benefit from education and self-care advice. Patients with Hunner lesions usually respond well to fulguration or triamcinolone injection, which can be repeated when the symptoms and lesions recur. For patients without Hunner lesions, numerous treatment options are available. The AUA Guideline tiers present these options in an orderly progression, balancing benefits, risks, and burdens. Along with specific IC/BPS treatments, it is also important to have available resources for stress reduction, pain management, and treatment of comorbid conditions.

EDITOR'S COMMENTS

Interstitial cystitis/painful bladder syndrome is one of the most complicated and least understood syndromes in functional urology. Although consensus statements and guidelines statements have been written (including a recent AUA Guideline), care of the syndrome remains highly variable and only partially (at best) successful. No unifying understanding exists regarding the pathophysiology of this condition, nor any consistent facts which modify the course of the syndrome.

The authors present their hard earned and continuously evolving approaches to the interstitial cystitis/painful bladder syndrome. They emphasize the individualization of therapy and management of patient expectations.

The editors both believe that individualization of therapy and management of expectations are crucial to the management of this chronic condition. Also, the involvement of a multispecialty group of practitioners from other disciplines is critical to managing the sometimes associated bowel, pain, and musculoskeletal conditions. The persistence and flaring of symptoms is a hallmark of this condition and requires the need for intermittent acute plans for symptom management (flare therapy).

Stepwise therapy inclusive of behavioral, physiotherapeutic, pharmacologic and (rarely) surgical interventions can provide some resolution or amelioration of symptoms – with the simultaneous recognition of both patient and practitioner that repetition and subtle additions and deletions of therapy may be required.

There is continued need for additional therapies and for better understanding the causation and persistence of symptoms. Also, the increasing observations that many of these patients have had symptoms dating to childhood, indicates the possible contributions of genetics and developmental contributions to this condition. Perhaps the answer to this puzzling condition will come from recognition of the lifelong existence of these symptoms (albeit waxing and waning) and the realization that the condition may be substantially impacted by the central and peripheral nervous system.

Roger R. Dmochowski, MD
Mickey Karram, MD

APPENDIX 1: DEFINITIONS

Organization	ICS[2]	ESSIC[3]	SUFU[4]
Name	PBS	BPS	IC/BPS
Main symptom	Suprapubic pain	Pelvic pain, pressure, or discomfort	Unpleasant sensation (pain, pressure, discomfort)
Symptom relationship to bladder	Related to bladder filling	Perceived to be related to bladder	Perceived to be related to bladder
Associated symptoms	Other symptoms such as increased daytime and nighttime frequency	At least one other urinary symptom such as persistent urge to void or frequency	Lower urinary tract symptoms
Duration	Not specified	>6 mo	>6 wk
Must exclude	Urine infection or other obvious abnormality	Confusable diseases	Infection or other identifiable causes

APPENDIX 2: TYPES OF STATEMENTS IN AUA GUIDELINES

If sufficient evidence:

- Standard (for or against)
  - Benefits > risks and burdens or vice versa
  - Level A or B evidence
- Recommendation (for or against)
  - Benefits > risks and burdens or vice versa
  - Level C evidence
- Option
  - Benefits = risks or risk/benefit ratio unknown
  - Any level of evidence (A, B, or C)

If insufficient evidence:

- Clinical principle
  - Widely agreed on by urologists or other clinicians
  - May or may not be evidence in the medical literature
- Expert opinion
  - Statement achieved by panel consensus based on members' clinical training, experience, knowledge, and judgment
  - No evidence in the medical literature

APPENDIX 3: GENERAL CLINICAL PRINCIPLES IN AUA GUIDELINES

- Begin with more conservative therapies
- Major surgery only for:
  - End-stage, small fibrotic bladders
  - Conservative measures have been exhausted and quality of life is poor
- Initial choice based on symptom severity, clinician judgment, and patient preference
- Stop ineffective treatment after clinically meaningful interval
- Multiple, simultaneous treatments may be considered if in the best interests of the patient. Reassess to document efficacy
- Continuously assess pain management. If inadequate, consider multidisciplinary approach
- Reconsider diagnosis if no improvement after multiple treatment approaches

APPENDIX 4: TREATMENT TIERS IN AUA GUIDELINES

1. Education, self-care
2. Oral and intravesical medicines, physical therapy, pain management
3. Bladder distention or Hunner lesion treatment
4. Sacral/pudendal nerve stimulation[a]
5. Oral cyclosporine, bladder botulinum toxin injection[a]
6. Substitution cystoplasty or urinary diversion[a]

[a] Only for experienced, committed IC/BPS providers.

REFERENCES

1. Hanno PM, Landis JR, Matthews-Cook Y, et al. The diagnosis of interstitial cystitis revisited: lessons learned from the National Institutes of Health Interstitial Cystitis Database Study. J Urol 1999;161:553.
2. Abrams P, Cardozo L, Fall M, et al. The standardisation of terminology in lower urinary tract function: report from the standardisation sub-committee of the International Continence Society. Neurourol Urodyn 2002;21:167.
3. van de Merwe JP, Nordling J, Bouchelouche P, et al. Diagnostic criteria, classification, and nomenclature for painful bladder syndrome/interstitial cystitis: an ESSIC proposal. Eur Urol 2008;53:60.
4. Hanno P, Dmochowski R. Status of international consensus on interstitial cystitis/bladder pain syndrome/painful bladder syndrome. Neurourol Urodyn 2009;28:274.
5. Hanno PM, Burks DA, Clemens JQ, et al. AUA guideline for the diagnosis and treatment of interstitial cystitis/bladder pain syndrome. J Urol 2011;185:2162.
6. Erickson DR. The placebo response. J Urol 2009;181:945.
7. Moldwin RM. The interstitial cystitis survival guide. Oakland (CA): New Harbinger Publications; 2000.
8. van Ophoven A, Pokupic S, Heinecke A, et al. A prospective, randomized, placebo controlled, double-blind study of amitriptyline for the treatment of interstitial cystitis. J Urol 2004;172:533.
9. Foster HE Jr, Hanno PM, Nickel JC, et al. Effect of amitriptyline on symptoms in treatment naïve patients with interstitial cystitis/painful bladder syndrome. J Urol 2010;183:1853.
10. Braunstein R, Shapiro E, Kaye J, et al. The role of cystoscopy in the diagnosis of Hunner's ulcer disease. J Urol 2008;180:1383.
11. Hanno PM. Bladder pain syndrome (interstitial cystitis) and related disorders. In: Wein AJ, Kavoussi LR, Novick AC, et al, editors. Campbell-Walsh urology. 10th edition. Philadelphia: Saunders; 2012. Chapter 12.
12. Peeker R, Fall M. Toward a precise definition of interstitial cystitis: further evidence of differences in classic and nonulcer disease. J Urol 2002;167:2470.

13. Parsons CL. Interstitial cystitis: clinical manifestations and diagnostic criteria in over 200 cases. Neurourol Urodyn 1990;9:241.

14. Rofeim O, Hom D, Freid RM, et al. Use of the neodymium: YAG laser for interstitial cystitis: a prospective study. J Urol 2001;166:134.

15. Cole EE, Scarpero HM, Dmochowski RR. Are patient symptoms predictive of the diagnostic and/or therapeutic value of hydrodistention? Neurourol Urodyn 2005;24:638.

16. Hanno PM, Wein AJ. Conservative therapy of interstitial cystitis. Semin Urol 1991;9:143.

17. Erickson DR, Kunselman AR, Bentley CM, et al. Changes in urine markers and symptoms after bladder distention for interstitial cystitis. J Urol 2007;177:556.

18. Hohenfeller M, Linn J, Hampel C, et al. Surgical treatment of interstitial cystitis. In: Sant GR, editor. Interstitial cystitis. Philadelphia: Lippincott-Raven; 1997. p. 223–33.

19. Lotenfoe RR, Christie J, Parsons A, et al. Absence of neuropathic pelvic pain and favorable psychological profile in the surgical selection of patients with disabling interstitial cystitis. J Urol 1995;154:2039.

20. Hill JR, Isom-Batz G, Panagopoulos G, et al. Patient perceived outcomes of treatments used for interstitial cystitis. Urology 2008;71:62.

21. Quillin R, Hooper G, Erickson D. Intravesical bupivacaine for lidocaine-refractory patients with painful bladder syndrome/interstitial cystitis. Neurourol Urodyn 2010;29:299.

22. Nickel JC, Moldwin R, Lee S, et al. Intravesical alkalinized lidocaine (PSD597) offers sustained relief from symptoms of interstitial cystitis and painful bladder syndrome. BJU Int 2009;103:910.

23. Henry R, Patterson L, Avery N, et al. Absorption of alkalized intravesical lidocaine in normal and inflamed bladders: a simple method for improving bladder anesthesia. J Urol 2001;165:1900.

24. Butrick CW, Sanford D, Hou Q, et al. Chronic pelvic pain syndromes: clinical, urodynamic, and urothelial observations. Int Urogynecol J Pelvic Floor Dysfunct 2009;20:1047.

25. Taneja R. Intravesical lignocaine in the diagnosis of bladder pain syndrome. Int Urogynecol J 2010;21:321.

26. Parsons CL. Successful downregulation of bladder sensory nerves with combination of heparin and alkalinized lidocaine in patients with interstitial cystitis. Urology 2005;65:45.

27. Parsons CL, Zupkas P, Proctor J, et al. Alkalinized lidocaine and heparin provide immediate relief of pain and urgency in patients with interstitial cystitis. J Sex Med 2012;9:207.

28. Davis EL, El Khoudary SR, Talbott EO, et al. Safety and efficacy of the use of intravesical and oral pentosan polysulfate sodium for interstitial cystitis: a randomized double-blind clinical trial. J Urol 2008;179:177.

29. Welk BK, Teichman JM. Dyspareunia response in patients with interstitial cystitis treated with intravesical lidocaine, bicarbonate, and heparin. Urology 2008;71:67.

Implantable Neuromodulation for Urinary Urge Incontinence and Fecal Incontinence
A Urogynecology Perspective

Paul D.M. Pettit, MD*, Anita Chen, MD

KEYWORDS

- Neuromodulation • Sacral nerve stimulation (SNS) • Urinary urge incontinence • Fecal incontinence
- InterStim

KEY POINTS

- Implantable sacral nerve stimulation is a mainstay of therapy for patients with urinary urge incontinence that have failed conservative therapy.
- Implantable SNS is now part of the treatment algorithm for patients with fecal incontinence, superseding sphincterplasty.
- The best practices and technological advances reviewed in this manuscript have reduced the revision rates, explantation rates and loss of effect.

This article is not certified for *AMA PRA Category 1 Credit*™ because product brand names are included in the educational content. The Accreditation Council for Continuing Medical Education requires the use of generic names and or drug/product classes as the required nomenclature for therapeutic options in continuing medical education.

For more information, please go to www.accme.org and review the Standards of Commercial Support.

INTRODUCTION AND HISTORICAL BACKGROUND

Implantable sacral nerve stimulation (SNS) is now a mainstay of therapy for patients with urinary urge incontinence who fail conservative therapy (**Fig. 1**). Its value for patients with fecal incontinence is now recognized. SNS modulates the neural reflexes, which influence the bladder, urinary and rectal sphincters, and pelvic floor. Neuromodulation is the effect achieved by the SNS, and can result in either stimulation or inhibition. Other modalities of neuromodulation include physical therapy (PT) and medications.

Research has allowed development of an implantable SNS system to treat lower urinary track dysfunction.[1–3] The University of California, Department of Urology in San Francisco, began the clinical program in 1981. A multicenter trial was performed from 1985 to 1992. The SNS approach was Food and Drug Administration (FDA) approved in 1997.[4,5] Medtronic InterStim Therapy System (Medtronic Inc., 710 Medtronic Parkway NE, Minneapolis, MN, USA) is the only SNS system available to clinicians. Before use in the United States, Medtronic received CE (Conformité Européenne) marking for InterStim Therapy in 1994 in Europe to treat pelvic floor disorders.[1] In

---

Disclosures: The authors have no disclosures.
Department of Gynecologic Surgery, Mayo Clinic Florida, 4500 San Pablo Road, Jacksonville, FL 32224, USA
* Corresponding author.
E-mail address: paul.pettit@mayo.edu

urologic.theclinics.com

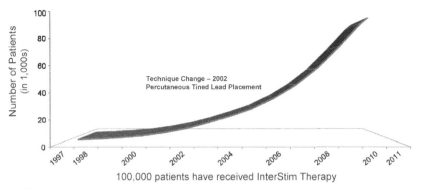

Fig. 1. Number of InterStim implants worldwide.

1999, the InterStim indications were expanded in the United States to include urinary urgency-frequency, and urinary retention. On March 14, 2011, Medtronic received premarket approval for the indication of fecal incontinence.[6]

A unique collaborative atmosphere surrounded the introduction of this therapy. In 2002, a new society was formed, including all who are interested in pelvic floor disorders. The first meeting of The International Society of Pelvic Neuromodulation was held in Ponte Vedra Beach, Florida. The society comprised physicians, researchers, physical therapists, and other care providers with interest in pelvic floor disorders. The group merged with the Society of Urodynamics and Female Urology (SUFU) in 2008. The group continues its mission within the annual SUFU meetings. Interactions of the members of this group with Medtronic have led to significant improvement in the technology and refinements of InterStim technique.[7–10]

This article discusses the topic from the urogynecology perspective. The urologic perspective is discussed by Dr Ken Peters elsewhere in this issue. This article summarizes best practices of implantable neuromodulation (ie, SNS) for urinary urge incontinence and fecal incontinence.

MECHANISM OF ACTION: SNS

The effectiveness of SNS has been established by many publications for urinary and fecal incontinence[11]; however, the mechanism of action that provides beneficial therapeutic effects remains unclear. Amend and colleagues[12] recently highlighted the current understanding of mechanisms of action, and the reader is referred to this comprehensive review. SNS likely exerts its influence by alteration of sacral afferent inflow on storage and emptying reflexes. Therapy likely modulates the

central nervous system at the level where switching between bladder emptying and storage occurs.[13]

Anal rectal function studies have revealed changes in both rectal motor function and rectal sensory function. In particular, balloon distension shows a decrease for the threshold of first urge. The patient is able to sense the presence of rectal contents at lower volumes, which allows the patient more time to respond to the urge to defecate.[14] There seems to be no significant change in the resting pressure of the rectal sphincter, and mixed findings concerning increase in generated squeeze pressure.[15,16] Stimulation of S2 to S4 and the pudendal nerve seems to excite the autonomic and somatic nervous systems, which causes both direct and reflex-mediated responses in the fecal continence mechanism.[17]

RESULTS AND COST-EFFECTIVENESS: URGE INCONTINENCE, FECAL INCONTINENCE

A 2009 Cochran Review (urinary) cited 17 case reports with a 39% cure, and 67% reported an improvement of greater than 50%. The randomized trials reviewed reported 50% cure or improvement of greater than 90%. Greater than 80% had at least a 50% cure. The Cochran review and a review by Brazzelli and colleagues[18] noted that there was no important difference between case study results and randomized studies.[11,18]

A meta-analysis was performed on 34 studies with more than 700 patients treated for fecal incontinence from 2000 to 2008. The report showed improved functional outcomes and quality of life. The effect was prolonged, even in patients with anal sphincter defects.[19] The clinical and cost-effectiveness of SNS for fecal incontinence has been reaffirmed in multiple publications.[20] All reports show effectiveness beyond other surgical options, between 70% and 90%, with far less morbidity.[21,22]

A recent cost analysis was performed in France for patients with urinary and fecal incontinence. They found that the initial cost was similar for urinary and fecal incontinence. The results within the French health system showed that SNS is a cost-effective treatment of both indications, compared with the alternatives. The investigators emphasized the possibility that different heath care systems and countries may have other findings.[23]

An article in 2009 comparing the cost of SNS and medications concluded that SNS should be discussed early with the patients because of poor patient compliance with medications.[24]

PATIENT SELECTION: URINARY URGE INCONTINENCE

Women or men with urinary urge incontinence who do not achieve an adequate quality of life with conservative therapy are candidates for SNS. Each state and insurance carrier can vary in what is meant by a trial of conservative therapy; conservative therapy generally includes the use of medications and some form of pelvic floor PT (**Table 1**).

The basic evaluation should include a bladder diary, focused history, pelvic examination, evaluation for postvoiding residual and urine analysis with culture and sensitivity (**Table 2**). If there is a working diagnosis of urge incontinence, then conservative therapy can be initiated. If a working diagnosis cannot be established, other comorbidities exist (multiple surgeries, endocrine and or neurologic disorders, metabolic syndrome), or, the patient fails conservative therapy, then the clinician should proceed to additional testing. First-line additional testing includes an office cystoscopy and urodynamics. Other evaluations would be added depending on concerns. Consultation from the appropriate specialty helps to identify contributing conditions. When conservative therapy fails, SNS can be trialed.

PATIENT SELECTION: FECAL INCONTINENCE

Patient selection for fecal incontinence is similar to that for urinary dysfunction. First, there is an attempt at conservative therapy. The basic evaluation involves the use of a bowel diary to establish a baseline. The history can help identify conditions that can contribute to the problem. The physical examination can identify other pelvic floor issues, such as genital prolapse and/or rectal prolapse, and provide an assessment of the rectal sphincter function. Based on the findings of the basic examination, the patient may need the surveillance colonoscopy updated, or other gastroenterology, neurologic, or metabolic evaluation. Conservative therapy can be initiated at this point. Conservative therapy includes dietary modification, dietary bulking, medications such as antidiarrheal agents, pelvic floor PT, and biofeedback (**Box 1**). If there is no improvement then SNS can be offered.

Clinical trials have established that an intact sphincter is not necessary for SNS to be successful.[6,25] This finding becomes significant with the recognition that sphincterplasties have poor long-term results of less than 50%.[26] In the past, the sphincter would be evaluated by either an anal ultrasound or, if there were other pelvic floor concerns, by dynamic magnetic resonance imaging. If there was an external sphincter defect and the patient had failed conservative efforts, an overlapping sphincterplasty would have been performed. The finding that an intact sphincter is not a prerequisite to success of SNS has changed the practice algorithm. Regardless of sphincter status, if the patient fails conservative efforts, first-stage InterStim can be trialed.

PROCEDURE: BEST PRACTICES

One of the greatest concerns noted in the literature had been the revision rate and the issue of loss of effectiveness. Since 1997, certain technical advancements and practices have evolved that have allowed both situations to be improved.

Table 1 Conservative therapy for voiding disorders	
Behavioral and PT	**Medications**
Dietary restrictions	Alter medications if opportunity exists
Bowel regulation	Hormone replacement therapy
Fluid management	Antimuscarinic: tolterodine
Bladder drills/timed voiding	Mixed action medications
Kegal (cones) Biofeedback/pelvic floor retraining	Oxybutynin plus direct muscle relaxant and local anesthetic

---

Table 2
Basic evaluation

Focused Medical/Neurologic/ Genitourinary History	Physical Examination
Medication	Abdominal examination
Associated symptoms and factors	Pelvic examination: atrophy, prolapse, levator pain, hypermobility
Duration and characteristics	Rectal sensation, tone, ability to generate a volume contraction
Frequency, timing, and amounts Precipitants and antecedents (ie, surgery) Lower urinary tract symptoms Alterations in bowel	Postvoid residual urinalysis and culture and sensitivity

---

An office percutaneous nerve evaluation (PNE) would initially be performed, which did not last much longer than a week. A successful PNE would lead to the full implant. The greatest downfall of the PNE was that the lead would not stay in position. The other insurmountable problem was the inability to duplicate results when progressing from the PNE to the complete implant. The staged implant became the preferred approach for all bladder indications and now fecal incontinence. In addition to not having to replace the chronic lead, only the staged approach allows a test phase of 3 to 4 weeks, which reduces the risk of confusing a placebo effect with a true clinical response.

The staged procedure has been reviewed in many publications. The most common oversight in managing patients is not reviewing and comparing the pretreatment diary with the post-treatment diary when deciding to progress to the second stage. This is the best safeguard for avoiding placebo effect. The reduction of placebo effect usually requires a longer test phase than 1 to 2 weeks, and we commonly test for 3 to 4 weeks. There is no difference in the technique for either urge urinary incontinence or fecal incontinence.[27]

Following the introduction of the staged implant in the United States, the new lead technology (tined lead) was the next big technical development. Before the tined lead technology, the surgical revision rate was close to 40%. The tined lead technology alone has reduced the surgical revision rate to approximately 10%.[28] We previously reported that the most common reason for explantation at Mayo Clinic Florida is infection, and the most common reasons for surgical revisions is implantable programmable generator (IPG) replacement and loss of effectiveness.[27]

Soon the government will require hospitals to be responsible for many (to be determined) surgical site infections (SSI). The following recommendations are for patients undergoing staged SNS at the Mayo Clinic. Currently all patients having surgery are required to shower from the neck down with Hibiclens (Zenica Pharmaceuticals, Wilmington, DE, USA) the night before and on the morning of surgery. Preoperative antibiotics must be given less than 1 hour before surgery. The skin is prepped with Duraprep or Chloroprep and the skin covered with antimicrobial incision drape. Surgical dressings are allowed to remain in place for 48 hours. The antibiotics that are used should have good skin organism coverage; the most commonly used in our practice is cephazolin 2 g intravenously (IV) (GlaxoSmithKline, Brentford, Middlesex, UK). If an incision will be made 1 to 2 hours after administration of the first dose of cefazolin, cefotaxime, ampicillin, clindamycin, or aztreonam, then we readminister 50% of the dose. If the incision is more than 2 hours from the first dose, we readminister 100% of first dose. Metronidazol, ertapenem, vancomycin, levofloxacin, and gentamicin have significantly longer half-lives and do not require redosing. IV vancomycin (Hospira, Inc., Lake Forest, IL, USA) is used for patients with penicillin allergies. We have found that excising the wound (connection site of tined lead and percutaneous extension lead/future site of

---

Box 1
Conservative treatment of fecal incontinence

Diet advice (avoidance)

Rectal emptying

   Glycerine, bisacodyl, phosphate enema

Biofeedback/pelvic floor retraining

Constipating agents

   Codeine, loperamide, lomotil, bulk agents

IPG) from the first stage has contributed to reduction of SSI. Once the IPG pocket is developed and homeostasis is achieved, we suggest plentiful irrigation. We take it a step further and use a common orthopedic device called a wound irrigation and debridment system for irrigation. The irrigant is 2000 mL of sterile water mixed with 50,000 units of bacitracin (Nycomed US Inc., Melville, NY, USA). If there are any signs of infection, it is best to explant, allow time for healing, and return later for the full implant. Our infection rate (Mayo Clinic Florida) has been reduced to less than 2%.[27]

Treatment of patients with a previous history of infection with methicillin-resistant *Staphylococcus aureus* (MRSA) continues to evolve. The decolonizing efforts begin 7 days before surgery. When we last reviewed this topic, decolonizing efforts began 14 days before surgery. Decolonizing efforts include Bactroban nasal ointment (GlaxoSmithKline, Brentford, Middlesex, UK), applied to the nares twice a day for 7 days. The patient should shower with Hibiclens (Zenica Pharmaceuticals, Wilmington, DE, USA) liquid soap from the neck down once a day for 7 days. Patients receive preoperative antibiotics as outlined earlier (**Table 3**).[29,30]

The transition to the staged implant and the technological advance of the tined lead was made possible by the use of the C-arm.[10] Its use is essential in the short-term and long-term success of SNS. The lead should be placed parallel to the nerve so at least 3 of the electrodes give motor and sensory response. Stimulation should be comfortable between 1 and 2 V. If the stimulation is painful or higher amplitudes are required, the lead needs to be repositioned. Management of loss of effectiveness starts with the proper placement of the chronic lead. Experts do not agree on whether the motor response or

sensory response is more important when determining the ideal placement of the chronic lead. From a practical point of view, placement of a lead with motor responses of the great toe or sacral plexus responses is not tolerated by most patients in the long term. If repositioning of the lead cannot eliminate the undesired motor responses, we default to the S4 level of stimulation as an alternative location.[27]

LOSS OF EFFECTIVENESS

The following outline describes how physicians at Mayo Clinic approach patients with loss of effectiveness, which is the most common reason for return office visits and patient concerns. Our first priority is to rule out a urinary tract infection and confirm that the IPG is on and functioning. If neither of these situations exist, the next step is a program evaluation to check impedances. Lead impedances of less than 50 ohms indicate a short and more than 4000 ohms indicates a break in the electrode wire. The only treatment available is to replace the lead. A temporizing option is to program around the damaged electrode, and then replace the lead when the IPG is exhausted. If the impedances are normal, the sensation of stimulation has often changed. We discovered a quick way to check all combinations of electrodes by completing the impedance testing. Set the amplitude of the impedance testing at a level that is more than the sensory threshold and initiate the test. Patients can alert you when they sense the electrical stimulation in the desired area. Although there is a slight lag in the reading and what is felt, it is usually possible to be within 2 or 3 combinations of settings and quickly resolve the sensory issue. If you still cannot reestablish the desired sensation, select the closest settings

Table 3 Reduction SSIs	
Preoperative Shower	Hibiclens
Preoperative antibiotic within 1 h	Not penicillin allergic: IV cephazolin 2 g. Redose 50% if 1–2 h from first dose, 100% if >2 h from first dose
Penicillin allergic	IV vancomycin
Wound dressing	Remain in place 48 h
Excise the first-stage wound	Future site of the IPG
Irrigation with wound irrigation and debridment system	2000 mL water and 50,000 U bacitracin
MRSA: pretreat 7 d before surgery, day 7 is day of surgery	Bactroban per nares twice a day Hibiclens shower neck down daily Betadine shampoo daily

Table 4
Algorithm for InterStim loss of effect

Rule out urinary tract infection, or IPG is on and not end of life	Treat and/or education
Check impedances to rule out short or fracture of lead	Program around or new lead
Change electrodes or pulse width and or rate to try to recapture desired sensory response	Can be effective with different sensory response
If cannot recapture quality of life, then PA and lateral pelvic radiograph to compare with postoperative images	If lead migration, replace
Fresh look with history, physical exam, urodynamics study and cystoscopy	Treat new problems such as stress urinary incontinence
Appropriate consults	Many patients will develop, or have worsening of, metabolic or neurologic conditions
Restart PT and medications	Antidotal evidence

and modify the pulse width. If you are still unable to recapture the patient's quality of life, the next step is to rule out lead migration. Comparing a new posteroanterior (PA) and lateral pelvic radiograph with the intraoperative films saved at the time of the first stage allows the diagnosis to be made.[27] The only option for migration is lead replacement. If we cannot identify any resolvable issues, we start from the beginning; over time, many patients develop new, treatable lower urinary tract problems such as stress incontinence or other therapies must be explored (**Table 4**).

PUDENDAL IMPLANT ALTERNATIVE

The pudendal nerve is composed of nerve roots that are involved in SNS, with a major advantage. The motor components to the hip, leg, and feet have branched off at this level. The proponents of pudendal nerve stimulation think that they can stimulate more of the sacral nerve roots without any of the unwanted and intolerable motor responses. The development of the tined lead has allowed investigators to carry out a chronic pudendal nerve stimulation using the existing InterStim system. The most popular procedure is a percutaneous approach to the Alcock canal.[2,31,32] The reader is referred to the article by Dr Peters mentioned earlier.

SUMMARY

SNS has been the most significant advance for patients with voiding disorders and fecal incontinence. Since its introduction in 1997, it has become standard of care for urinary disorders and has recently changed the therapeutic algorithm for fecal incontinence. Although understanding of the mechanism of action continues to accrue, the therapy is effective and enduring.

ACKNOWLEDGMENTS

The authors thank Victoria L. Jackson, MLIS (Academic and Research Support, Mayo Clinic Florida) for her editorial assistance in this project.

EDITOR'S COMMENTS

Despite extensive and expanding use of neuromodulation for voiding dysfunction, the exact mechanism of action of this therapy remains undetermined. Possibly be mediating the sacral reflex arc, or direct effect, neuromodulation does provide efficacy for both bladder storage and emptying disorders. Whether by implantation or by less invasive means, neuromodulation is effective in those patients who have failed pharmacologic and behavioral interventions.

Data now exist that support the long term efficacy of this modality; however, efficacy is contingent on ongoing stimulation. Initially thought to require ongoing continuous stimulation, clinical experience suggests that there is some retention of effect after stimulation ceases, which is variable for every individual and which eventually is completely lost.

Neuromodulation requires clinical infrastructure. Patient education is critical prior to embarking on either percutaneous or implantable stimulation. Also important to success, provider and patient commitment to ongoing stimulation monitoring and, when needed, adjustment is essential for ongoing optimization of therapy. With implantable devices, device interrogation and reprogramming provide the avenue to assure optimal stimulation delivery.

Recent FDA labeling changes have removed one barrier to implantable neuromodulation, as device parameter recommendations now formally exist to allow MRI scans to be performed when indicated for other conditions. Also the staged technique (as opposed to the percutaneous testing procedure) is undergoing critical assessment as an improved method to determine responsiveness to stimulation. Both of the editors use the staged technique as their primary mode of implantation.

Continued technical developments almost certainly will change the neuromodulation landscape, with other types of minimally invasive techniques and improved understanding of optimal stimulation delivery and mode of action. However, it is also certain that neuromodulation, as currently practiced, has provided substantial benefit to patients who historically were limited to major surgery as the only option for management of their voiding disorders.

Roger R. Dmochowski, MD
Mickey Karram, MD

REFERENCES

1. Bradley WE, Timm GW, Chou SN. A decade of experience with electronic simulation of the micturition reflex. Urol Int 1971;26(4):283–302.

2. Juenemann KP, Lue TF, Schmidt RA, et al. Clinical significance of sacral and pudendal nerve anatomy. J Urol 1988;139(1):74–80.

3. Tanagho EA, Schmidt RA, de Araujo CG. Urinary striated sphincter: what is its nerve supply? Urology 1982;20(4):415–7.

4. Siegel SW, Catanzaro F, Dijkema HE, et al. Long-term results of a multicenter study on sacral nerve stimulation for treatment of urinary urge incontinence, urgency-frequency, and retention. Urology 2000;56(6 Suppl 1):87–91.

5. Hassouna MM, Siegel SW, Nyeholt AA, et al. Sacral neuromodulation in the treatment of urgency-frequency symptoms: a multicenter study on efficacy and safety. J Urol 2000;163(6):1849–54.

6. Wexner SD, Coller JA, Devroede G, et al. Sacral nerve stimulation for fecal incontinence: results of a 120-patient prospective multicenter study. Ann Surg 2010;251(3):441–9.

7. Janknegt RA, Weil EH, Eerdmans PH. Improving neuromodulation technique for refractory voiding dysfunctions: two-stage implant. Urology 1997; 49(3):358–62.

8. Peters KM. Alternative approaches to sacral nerve stimulation. Int Urogynecol J 2010;21(12): 1559–63.

9. Spinelli M, Weil E, Ostardo E, et al. New tined lead electrode in sacral neuromodulation: experience from a multicentre European study. World J Urol 2005;23(3):225–9.

10. Chai TC, Mamo GJ. Modified techniques of S3 foramen localization and lead implantation in S3 neuromodulation. Urology 2001;58(5):786–90.

11. Herbison GP, Arnold EP. Sacral neuromodulation with implanted devices for urinary storage and voiding dysfunction in adults. Cochrane Database Syst Rev 2009;2:CD004202.

12. Amend B, Matzel KE, Abrams P, et al. How does neuromodulation work. Neurourol Urodyn 2011; 30(5):762–5.

13. Thompson JH, Sutherland SE, Siegel SW. Sacral neuromodulation: therapy evolution. Indian J Urol 2010;26(3):379–84.

14. Uludag O, Morren GL, Dejong CH, et al. Effect of sacral neuromodulation on the rectum. Br J Surg 2005;92(8):1017–23.

15. Matzel KE, Stadelmaier U, Hohenfellner M, et al. Electrical stimulation of sacral spinal nerves for treatment of faecal incontinence. Lancet 1995; 346(8983):1124–7.

16. Altomare DF, Rinaldi M, Petrolino M, et al. Permanent sacral nerve modulation for fecal incontinence and associated urinary disturbances. Int J Colorectal Dis 2004;19(3):203–9.

17. Gourcerol G, Vitton V, Leroi AM, et al. How sacral nerve stimulation works in patients with faecal incontinence. Colorectal Dis 2011;13(8):e203–11.

18. Brazzelli M, Murray A, Fraser C. Efficacy and safety of sacral nerve stimulation for urinary urge incontinence: a systematic review. J Urol 2006;175(3 Pt 1):835–41.

19. Tan E, Ngo NT, Darzi A, et al. Meta-analysis: sacral nerve stimulation versus conservative therapy in the treatment of faecal incontinence. Int J Colorectal Dis 2011;26(3):275–94.

20. Munoz-Duyos A, Navarro-Luna A, Brosa M, et al. Clinical and cost effectiveness of sacral nerve stimulation for faecal incontinence. Br J Surg 2008;95(8): 1037–43.

21. Jarrett ME, Varma JS, Duthie GS, et al. Sacral nerve stimulation for faecal incontinence in the UK. Br J Surg 2004;91(6):755–61.

22. Gourcerol G, Gallas S, Michot F, et al. Sacral nerve stimulation in fecal incontinence: are there factors associated with success? Dis Colon Rectum 2007; 50(1):3–12.

23. Leroi AM, Lenne X, Dervaux B, et al. Outcome and cost analysis of sacral nerve modulation for treating urinary and/or fecal incontinence. Ann Surg 2011; 253(4):720–32.

24. Burks FN, Peters KM. Neuromodulation versus medication for overactive bladder: the case for early intervention. Curr Urol Rep 2009;10(5):342–6.

25. Jarrett ME, Dudding TC, Nicholls RJ, et al. Sacral nerve stimulation for fecal incontinence related to obstetric anal sphincter damage. Dis Colon Rectum 2008;51(5):531–7.

26. Malouf AJ, Norton CS, Engel AF, et al. Long-term results of overlapping anterior anal-sphincter repair for obstetric trauma. Lancet 2000;355(9200):260–5.

27. Pettit P. Current opinion: complications and trouble-shooting of sacral neuromodulation. Int Urogynecol J 2010;21(Suppl 2):S491–6.

28. Spinelli M, Sievert KD. Latest technologic and surgical developments in using InterStim Therapy for sacral neuromodulation: impact on treatment success and safety. Eur Urol 2008;54(6):1287–96.

29. Mangram AJ, Horan TC, Pearson ML, et al; the Hospital Infection Control Practices Advisory Committee. Guideline for the prevention of surgical site infection, 1999. Infect Control Hosp Epidemiol 1999;20(4):247–80.

30. Bode LG, Kluytmans JA, Wertheim HF, et al. Preventing surgical-site infections in nasal carriers of Staphylococcus aureus. N Engl J Med 2010; 362(1):9–17.

31. Peters KM, Feber KM, Bennett RC. Sacral versus pudendal nerve stimulation for voiding dysfunction: a prospective, single-blinded, randomized, cross-over trial. Neurourol Urodyn 2005;24(7):643–7.

32. Reitz A, Gobeaux N, Mozer P, et al. Topographic anatomy of a new posterior approach to the pudendal nerve for stimulation. Eur Urol 2007; 51(5):1350–5 [discussion: 1355–6].

Neuromodulation for Voiding Dysfunction and Fecal Incontinence: A Urology Perspective

Matthew Fulton, MD[a], Kenneth M. Peters, MD[a,b],*

KEYWORDS

- Neuromodulation • Overactive bladder • Fecal incontinence • Sacral nerve • Pudendal nerve
- Tibial nerve

KEY POINTS

- Neuromodulation is an effective, minimally invasive technique for the management of urinary urgency and frequency, urgency incontinence and nonobstructive urinary retention.
- Neuromodulation has recently been approved and shown efficacy in the treatment of fecal incontinence.
- This article reviews the physiology, indications, implantation methods and outcomes of neuromodulation.

INTRODUCTION

Neuromodulation uses electrical or chemical modulation to affect the physiologic response of an organ. Using electrical stimulation to control voiding dysfunction was first described by Tanagho and colleagues[1] in 1989. Those initial reports of success in treating voiding dysfunction refractory to traditional methods have led to significant research over the past 2 decades. This article discusses the physiology, indications, methods, and results of available neuromodulation techniques for the treatment of bladder and bowel dysfunction.

Bladder dysfunction in the form of urinary urge, urinary frequency, and urgency incontinence are commonly described as overactive bladder (OAB). The International Continence Society defines OAB as a symptomatic syndrome suggestive of lower urinary tract dysfunction.[2] It is estimated that 33.3 million adults suffer from OAB in the United States and as the population of aging adults continues

to grow this number is likely to increase.[3] Treatment modalities typically begin with noninvasive measures, like behavioral modification, pelvic floor physical therapy, and pharmacologic therapies. In the past, surgical options, including augmentation enterocystoplasty, detrusor myectomy, bladder denervation, and urinary diversion, were commonly performed.

FI is defined as the involuntary loss of flatus or stool. This experience can be a humiliating and life-altering event for patients. The exact prevalence of this condition is unknown, but published rates have ranged from 1% to 2%[4] to as high as 11% to 15%.[5] The problem is multifactorial, and current treatments result in modest overall success. FI may be secondary to many causes, categorized by having structurally intact but weak anal sphincters (such as rectal prolapse, constipation, neuropathy, and inflammatory bowel disease) or structurally defective sphincters (congenital malformations and obstetric, surgical, and traumatic injury). Traditional nonsurgical

[a] Department of Urology, Oakland University William Beaumont School of Medicine, Royal Oak, MI, USA;
[b] Department of Urology, Beaumont Hospital, Oakland University William Beaumont School of Medicine, 3601 West 13 Mile Road, Street 438, Royal Oak, MI 48073, USA
* Corresponding author. Department of Urology, Beaumont Hospital, Oakland University William Beaumont School of Medicine, 3601 West 13 Mile Road, Street 438, Royal Oak, MI 48073.
E-mail address: kmpeters@beaumont.edu

Urol Clin N Am 39 (2012) 405–412
http://dx.doi.org/10.1016/j.ucl.2012.05.008
0094-0143/12/$ – see front matter © 2012 Elsevier Inc. All rights reserved.

treatment options have included dietary and pharmacologic stool modification, antimotility agents, biofeedback, injectable bulking agents, and radiofrequency application to the anal sphincter, all with results falling short of desired goals.[6–9] The initial surgical management of FI secondary to anal sphincter trauma traditionally has been either direct sphincter repair or, more commonly, overlapping sphincter repair. Long-term success rates are poor, ranging from 35% to 50%.[10] Advanced options have included placement of an artificial bowel sphincter, dynamic gracioplasty, and fecal diversion. These methods are invasive, technically challenging, and fraught with complications, limiting their widespread use.[11,12]

For 15 years, sacral neuromodulation (SNM) has been Food and Drug Administration (FDA) approved for the treatment of urinary urgency and frequency, urgency incontinence, and nonobstructive urinary retention. During that time, many investigators have observed improvement in bowel dysfunction in patients with sacral neuromodulators. These observations and further studies have resulted in the recent FDA approval of SNM for FI. Neuromodulation has gained acceptance as a treatment modality for bladder and bowel dysfunction. It offers a minimally invasive, reversible method with low morbidity when other first-line treatment options have failed.

THE PHYSIOLOGY OF NEUROMODULATION

The exact neural mechanisms responsible for the effects of electrical neuromodulation on the lower urinary tract and bowel are unknown. Prior to discussing how neuromodulation works, the normal micturition pathway is reviewed briefly. Normal detrusor function relies on a balance between excitatory and inhibitory pathways to maintain continence and the ability to volitionally void. Baseline activity of the sympathetic system provides storage and continence by inhibiting detrusor contractions and maintaining sphincter tone. Parasympathetic activation stimulates detrusor contraction, sphincter relaxation, and ultimately micturition. This balance between sympathetic and parasympathetic nervous systems is under suprasacral control. Bladder afferent signaling relays information about fullness, pressure, stretch, and pain, initiating voiding through multiple reflex pathways. Supraspinal input from the pontine micturition center and cerebral cortex on these sacral reflex pathways control voiding in a voluntary manner. The pontine micturition center provides negative feedback to inhibit voiding and promote continued storage and positive input leading to the induction of voiding. This complex system to maintain control

of voiding can be altered by loss of supraspinal inhibitory control or increased sensitization to bladder afferent signals, both contributing to involuntary voiding.[13]

The control of sensory input to the central nervous system (CNS) is thought to work through a gate-control mechanism.[14] The gate-control theory states that noxious stimuli perception does not entirely depend on the A-delta and C-fiber sensory nerves transmitting information to the CNS but on the pattern of peripheral nerve activity.[15] A-delta bladder afferent nerve fibers project to the pontine nuclei to provide inhibitory and excitatory input to reflexes controlling bladder and sphincter function. Afferent C-fibers within the bladder are normally thought to be mechano-insensitive and unresponsive and are thus referred to as silent C-fibers. These normally inactive C-fibers may be sensitized by neurologic diseases, inflammation, infection, or normal bladder functions, such as distention, thus causing activation of involuntary micturition reflexes and OAB.[16] Sensory input from large myelinated pudendal nerve fibers may modulate erroneous bladder input conveyed by A-delta or C-fiber afferents at the gate control level of the spinal cord. OAB may then be attributed to a deficiency of the inhibitory control systems involving pudendal afferent nerves.

A significant amount of research has focused on the effect of SNM on afferent sensory nerve fibers with the dominant theory that electrical stimulation of these somatic afferent fibers modulates voiding and continence reflex pathways in the CNS.[14] The success of electrical neuromodulation for OAB may result from the restoration of the balance between bladder inhibitory and excitatory control systems.[17] Electrical stimulation modulates the afferent sensory input of the bladder on the pontine center, thereby inhibiting involuntary contractions. Neuromodulation may also remedy OAB by the alteration of afferent signals delivered to the spinal cord that effect activity and basal tone of the pelvic floor.[18]

SACRAL NEUROMODULATION

The InterStim Therapy System (Medtronic, Minneapolis, MN, USA) is the only FDA-approved device for sacral nerve stimulation as a means to treat refractory urinary urgency, frequency, incontinence, and nonobstructive urinary retention. The device has also received recent FDA approval for treatment of FI. This device consists of a tined quadripolar lead that is inserted percutaneously through the S3 sacral foramen and attached to a permanent implantable pulse generator (IPG).

Electrical stimulation is transmitted through the IPG to the lead in proximity to the sacral nerve roots at S3, thereby modulating bladder function. The device has several parameters that can be adjusted, including pulse width, frequency, and energy level. Transcutaneous programming can be used to adjust which leads are positive and negative, giving physicians the ability to trial several settings and adjust parameters to optimize patient outcomes. Patients are equipped with a handheld remote that allows 4 different programs with different stimulation settings to be used.

INDICATIONS FOR BLADDER DYSFUNCTION

Patient selection for SNM is a process in evolution and parameters to predict patient successes derived from prospective trials are limited. Patients undergoing initial test stimulation generally have symptoms that are refractory to behavioral modification and medical therapy for OAB. In the authors' experience, failure to have relief of symptoms after a trial of behavioral therapy and 2 anticholinergic medications is sufficient to consider offering patients SNM therapy. It is also important to consider the high rate of medication discontinuation with medical therapy for OAB, thus patients who cannot tolerate anticholinergic medications should be given consideration for SNM therapy.[19]

Preoperative evaluation often includes a careful history and physical examination with pelvic examination, including assessment of pelvic floor musculature and support. It is important to evaluate these patients for infectious, malignant, or anatomic conditions that might be the root cause of their symptoms. Thus, urine culture, cytology, and cystoscopy may aid in making an accurate diagnosis. Urodynamics may assist in the diagnosis of detrusor overactivity when the clinical symptoms are unclear. Urodynamics are not required for every patient prior to SNM, especially if patients have a clear history of urge incontinence. There is limited data to support which patients urodynamics will provide predictive value about the potential benefit from neuromodulation. Groenendijk and colleagues[20] demonstrated that patients with urinary urge incontinence without detrusor overactivity had as much or more success with SNM therapy as those patients who had urinary urge incontinence and urodynamic findings of detrusor overactivity. A voiding diary chronicling voiding frequency, voided volumes, associated urgency, and incontinence episodes per day is important part of the evaluation to adequately assess improvement after the test stimulation.

IMPLANTATION METHODS

Prior to permanent generator implantation, patients undergo a temporary trial to determine if they benefit from stimulation. During the test period, patients repeat a voiding diary, with emphasis on voiding frequency, voided volumes, and episodes of incontinence. Patients are considered to have a positive response to therapy if they have a 50% or better improvement in their symptoms, such as a decrease in incontinent episodes per day or an increase in voided volumes. Patients who have at least a 50% improvement are candidates for IPG placement.

There are 2 trial stimulation techniques commonly used, a monopolar percutaneous nerve evaluation (PNE) or staged placement of a quadripolar lead. PNE is performed in the office under local anesthesia, usually without fluoroscopic guidance, inserting a fine monopolar wire through the third sacral foramen. Correct lead placement is determined by a levator ani motor response, plantar flexion of the ipsilateral great toe, and induction of perineal sensory activation. The temporary lead is fixed to the skin with an adhesive dressing and stimulation is delivered through an external device for 3 to 5 days. Advantages to this approach include avoiding multiple trips to the operating room, associated anesthetic risks, and cost. The reliability of the PNE at predicting long-term success has been questioned. The temporary lead with its single stimulation point can be easily dislodged from its position in the sacral foramen, leading to an inaccurate test period. If a patient has a successful PNE test, it may not predict robust long-term outcomes with a permanent implant. Bosch and Groen[21] reported that 28% of patients who started with a percutaneous lead and went on to receive a permanent tined lead and IPG did not experience the same efficacy that was experienced during the test period, suggesting that the placement of the tined lead after PNE did not replicate the exact anatomic position of the PNE or that the short test period may not accurately reflect the clinical response.

Staging SNM using a permanent quadripolar lead and IPG was first described by Janknegt and colleagues[22] in 1997. The patient is positioned prone in the operating room under sedation with a local anesthetic injected in the overlying skin of the insertion site. The quadripolar tined lead is placed through a small incision into the S3 foramen with fluoroscopic guidance. Anterior to posterior fluoroscopic images as well as cross-table lateral images of the lead should be taken and saved. These confirm accurate positioning and serves as reference at a later date if a patient should lose efficacy of the therapy and lead migration is suspected. Placement in the S3 foramen is confirmed by several indictors, including fluoroscopic position and motor and sensory response. A typical motor response is identification of a levator bellow and/or greater toe flexion with stimulation. Sensory response is typically perceived as a tapping or pulsation in the rectal, perineal, scrotal or vaginal region. Obtaining an accurate sensory response while patients are under sedation is not always easy and a recent study demonstrated that sensory response is not necessary when placing a sacral lead.[23] A test period of 2 weeks using a staged approach is ideal to assess whether there is an adequate response to therapy.

Literature on the efficacy of the 2-stage procedure suggests that this technique is more dependable in identifying responders to therapy than the PNE technique.[21,24,25] Borawski and colleagues[26] evaluated 30 patients aged 55 years and older with refractory urge incontinence randomized to either PNE or a staged technique. The likelihood of progressing to IPG was significantly greater in the staged cohort (15 of 17 patients; 88%) compared with the PNE group (6 of 13 patients; 46%). A formal cost analysis comparing PNE to staged implantation has not been performed. Baxter and Kim[25] reported on Medicare physician reimbursement rates in California in 2009. Unilateral staged implantation performed in the operating room reimbursed $742.73 with subsequent IPG paying $1055.85 for a total compensation of $1798.58. Unilateral office-based PNE trial reimbursed $1792.62 and, if successful, an additional $1055.85 for the IPG placement for a total of $2848.47, perhaps providing a financial incentive for physicians to perform this less-sensitive measure for a trial period.[25]

OUTCOMES

Many studies have shown that SNM is efficacious for its approved indications of urinary frequency, urgency, and urinary incontinence. van Kerrebroeck and colleagues[27] published a 5-year, prospective, multicenter trial that evaluated the long-term safety and efficacy of SNM in patients with refractory urinary urge incontinence and urinary urgency and frequency. This trial collected voiding diaries annually for 5 years and clinical success was defined as 50% or greater improvement from baseline in primary voiding diary variables. The study found that clinical success was achieved in 58% of patients with regards to the number of leaks per day and a 68% clinical success rate in the number of heavy leaks per day. The study also reported a 61% clinical success rate in the

number of pads used per day. With regards to urgency and frequency, a clinical success rate of 40% was observed in decreasing the number of voids per day and a 56% success rate in decreasing the degree of urinary urgency per day at 5 years after implantation.

Common complications were pain at the implant or lead site in 25% of patients; lead-related problems, such as lead migration, in 16%; replacement and repositioning of the IPG in 15%; wound problems in 7%; adverse effects on bowel function in 6%; infection in 5%; and generator problems in 5%. Permanent removal of the electrodes was reported in 9% of patients. Technical changes with time have been associated with decreased complication rates. Overall the reoperation rate in implanted cases was 33%. The most common reason for surgical revision was relocation of the generator because of pain and infection.[28]

SACRAL NEUROMODULATION FOR NONOBSTRUCTIVE URINARY RETENTION

Shaker and Hassouna[29] reported the use of SNM for nonobstructive urinary retention in 1998. Since then, several clinical trials have shown that SNM is effective for nonobstructive urinary retention.[30,31] van Kerrebroeck and colleagues[27] also evaluated patients with retention receiving SNM in their 5-year prospective study. They found that the average number of catheterizations per day decreased for by 50% for 58% of patients at 5 years after implantation. The average catheterized volume also decreased with a clinical success rate of 71%. The exact mechanism of action is unknown, but SNM may work by activating areas of the micturition centers of the brain and reducing high-tone pelvic floor dysfunction.

PUDENDAL NEUROMODULATION

Subsets of patients have severe refractory urgency, frequency, and incontinence despite maximal therapy, including SNM. Neuromodulation of the pudendal nerve may be an alternative treatment option that has shown success at controlling bladder dysfunction. Pudendal neuromodulation is not FDA approved. The pudendal nerve is a major contributor to bladder afferent regulation and bladder function. It is a peripheral nerve that is mainly composed of afferent sensory fibers from sacral nerve roots S1, S2, and S3. The bulk of afferent sensory fibers are contributed by S2 (60.5%) and S3 (35.5%) according to afferent activity mapping procedures.[32] These bladder afferent fibers act on sacral reflex arcs, activating storage through sphincter activation via the pudendal nerve. Direct pudendal nerve stimulation activates more afferents than SNS and may do so without the side effects of off-target stimulation of leg and buttock muscles. Pudendal nerve entrapment often leads to significant pelvic and perineal pain along with voiding dysfunction, including urinary incontinence and OAB.[33,34] Modulating the pudendal nerve may help relief the symptoms of pudendal neuropathy.

Chronic stimulation of the pudendal nerve has been described using the InterStim device. The nerve is accessed via a posterior approach through the ischiorectal fossa or transgluteal under flouroscopic guidance. Electrophysiologic monitoring is required to confirm stimulation of the pudendal nerve. A 2-week staged procedure is typically performed and if a greater than 50% improvement in symptoms is identified, an IPG is placed.

Spinelli and colleagues[35] evaluated 15 treatment refractory patients with neurogenic bladder after chronic pudendal nerve stimulation with a tined lead placed under neurophysiologic guidance. Statistically significant reductions in incontinent episodes ($P<.02$) and improvements in maximum cystometric capacity and pressure on urodynamics studies were seen. Constipation and FI also improved. Several studies at the authors' institution have compared pudendal nerve stimulation with standard sacral nerve stimulation. In a prospective, single-blind, randomized trial, patients had both sacral and pudendal quadripolar tined leads placed in the first stage of their operation (**Fig. 1**). Patients were randomized to begin either sacral or pudendal stimulation and each was tested for 7 days. While still blinded, patients rated symptoms on each lead and chose the preferred site for stimulation. Pudendal stimulation resulted in a 63% improvement in symptoms

versus a 46% improvement in symptoms with sacral stimulation. The pudendal lead was chosen as the superior lead by 79.2% of patients.[36] Analysis from a prospective database of 55 patients with chronic pudendal neuromodulation (median follow-up 24.1 months) demonstrated significant improvements in frequency ($P<.0001$), voided volume ($P<.0001$), incontinence ($P<.0001$), and urgency ($P = .0019$).[37] Almost all patients (93.2%) who had previously failed SNM responded to pudendal stimulation.

Chronic pudendal neuromodulation is an excellent alternative for patients who have failed SNM for voiding dysfunction. In addition, many patients suffer from chronic pelvic pain due to pudendal nerve entrapment syndrome. The authors have successfully treated many of these patients with pudendal neuromodulation, often performing a series of pudendal nerve blocks with a local anesthetic and steroid solution to assess short-term improvement in symptoms. If relief is obtained, but not sustained, a trial of pudendal neuromodulation is considered. This minimally invasive approach has spared many patients from open surgical decompression of the pudendal nerve.

SACRAL NEUROMODULATION FOR BOWEL DISORDERS

In addition to affecting bladder function, stimulating the sacral nerves seems to modulate the function of the rectum and anal sphincter.[38] The InterStim device received FDA approval for treatment of FI in 2011. Wexner and colleagues[10] reported on a prospective multicenter trial of 133 patients with FI who underwent test stimulation with a 90% success rate. A permanent implant was placed in 120 patients with a mean age of 60.5 years and mean duration of FI of 6.8 years. At 12 months, 83% of subjects achieved therapeutic success ($P<.0001$), and 41% achieved 100% continence. Therapeutic success was 85% at 24 months. Incontinent episodes decreased from a mean of 9.4 per week at baseline to 1.9 at 12 months and 2.9 at 2 years. Several recent randomized studies have compared SNM in patients with severe FI to a control group receiving optimal medical therapy, demonstrating significant benefit of SNM.[39,40] SNM is a new and effective technique for the management of FI. Given the low morbidity and good efficacy of SNM compared with the poor long-term results and significant morbidity of traditional surgical treatments, SNM deserves consideration as a first-line surgical treatment of FI.

In addition to treatment of FI, SNM is emerging as a therapy for refractory constipation. Although

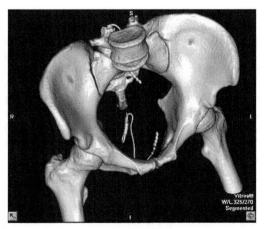

Fig. 1. CT scan demonstrating patient with sacral lead passing through S3 sacral foramina, and additional lead running in proximity to the pudendal nerve.

there are no large randomized trials, available evidence suggests that for selected patients with idiopathic slow or normal transit constipation and obstructive defecation, SNM therapy may provide beneficial results. A significant increase in bowel movements and a reduction in episodes with abdominal pain and bloating have been reported.[41–43]

NEUROMODULATION OF THE TIBIAL NERVE

The tibial nerve is a peripheral mixed sensory-motor nerve that originates from spinal roots L4 through S3, which also contribute directly to sensory and motor control of the urinary bladder, bowel, and pelvic floor. Percutaneous tibial nerve stimulation (PTNS) is typically performed with patients in the supine position with the knees abducted and the soles of the feet together. A 34-gauge needle is inserted 3 cm into the skin at level 3 fingerbreadths cephalad to the medial malleolus. A grounding pad is placed on the arch of the ipsilateral foot. The amplitude of the stimulation is increased until the large toe curls or the toes fan. Patients typically undergo 10 to 12 weekly treatment sessions, with each session lasting approximately 30 minutes. The lure of the tibial nerve is that it is easily accessible and minimally invasive, without requiring an operating room, an anesthetic, or any device implantation.

Several studies have demonstrated that PTNS shows efficacy in treating symptoms of OAB[44] and altering urodynamic findings in patients with OAB.[45] A recently published randomized, multicenter, controlled study compared the effectiveness of PTNS to extended-release tolterodine. A total of 100 adults with urinary frequency were randomized 1:1 to 12 weekly treatments of PTNS or to daily extended-release tolterodine (4 mg). Assessment of OAB symptoms compared with baseline demonstrated a statistically significant improvement in the PTNS arm with 79.5% reporting cure or improvement compared with 54.8% of subjects on tolterodine.[46] The second phase of this trial demonstrated sustained therapeutic efficacy of PTNS in subjects with OAB during 1 year of continued treatment.[46] A validated sham for tibial nerve stimulation was developed.[47] This sham used a placebo needle and active transcutaneous nerve stimulation to simulate the sensations of active PTNS. This validated sham was used in the SUmiT trial, a randomized controlled trial of 220 patients demonstrating PTNS in urinary incontinence to be significantly more effective than sham stimulation (54.5% vs 20.9% improvement).[48] The efficacy of PTNS demonstrated in these studies supports the use of peripheral neuromodulation therapy for overactive bladder.

PTNS is commonly used in Europe for FI. The evidence supporting its effectiveness is limited but suggests a benefit over conservative treatment options. Findlay and Armstrong[49] recently reviewed the available literature on PTNS for FI. A total of 8 published studies, all from Europe, have included 129 patients with FI (with variable etiologies), all of whom had failed conservative management. The studies demonstrated significant heterogeneity in population, methodology, and outcome measures. Short-term primary endpoint success ranged from 30.0% to 83.3%, but 6 of 8 studies attained short-term success. Their review concluded that at this point there is insufficient evidence to determine if PTNS is an efficacious treatment option for FI. It is expected that this question will be answered soon. Three separate randomized, controlled, double-blind studies evaluating PTNS for FI and are currently being conducted in Europe. If proved effective, PTNS would provide another minimally invasive novel for the management of this complex problem.

SUMMARY

The continued development of novel neuromodulation techniques over the past decade has changed the treatment paradigm for patients with refractory voiding and fecal dysfunction. In the past, patients who failed conservative behavioral or pharmacologic measures were confined to live with their symptoms or undergo invasive and often ineffective procedures. Now with the ability to modulate the nerves innervating the bowel and bladder, physicians can offer a minimally invasive, reversible, safe, and effective treatment alternative. Utilization of alternative stimulation methods and the ability to apply this to different nerves has expanded treatment options for patients suffering from bowel and bladder disorders.

EDITOR'S COMMENTS

Despite extensive and expanding use of neuromodulation for voiding dysfunction, the exact mechanism of action of this therapy remains undetermined. Possibly be mediating the sacral reflex arc, or direct effect, neuromodulation does provide efficacy for both bladder storage and emptying disorders. Whether by implantation or by less invasive means, neuromodulation is effective in those patients who have failed pharmacologic and behavioral interventions.

Data now exist that support the long term efficacy of this modality; however, efficacy is contingent on ongoing stimulation. Initially thought to require ongoing continuous stimulation, clinical experience suggests that there is some retention of effect after stimulation ceases, which is variable for every individual and which eventually is completely lost.

Neuromodulation requires clinical infrastructure. Patient education is critical prior to embarking on either percutaneous or implantable stimulation. Also important to success, provider and patient commitment to ongoing stimulation monitoring and, when needed, adjustment is essential for ongoing optimization of therapy. With implantable devices, device interrogation and reprogramming provide the avenue to assure optimal stimulation delivery.

Recent FDA labeling changes have removed one barrier to implantable neuromodulation, as device parameter recommendations now formally exist to allow MRI scans to be performed when indicated for other conditions. Also the staged technique (as opposed to the percutaneous testing procedure) is undergoing critical assessment as an improved method to determine responsiveness to stimulation. Both of the editors use the staged technique as their primary mode of implantation.

Continued technical developments almost certainly will change the neuromodulation landscape, with other types of minimally invasive techniques and improved understanding of optimal stimulation delivery and mode of action. However, it is also certain that neuromodulation, as currently practiced, has provided substantial benefit to patients who historically were limited to major surgery as the only option for management of their voiding disorders.

Roger R. Dmochowski, MD
Mickey Karram, MD

REFERENCES

1. Tanagho EA, Schmidt RA, Orvis BR. Neural stimulation for control of voiding dysfunction: a preliminary report in 22 patients with serious neuropathic voiding disorders. J Urol 1989;142:340–5.
2. Wein AJ, Rovner ES. Definition and epidemiology of overactive bladder. Urology 2002;60(5 Suppl 1): 7–12.
3. Tyagi S, Thomas CA, Hayashi Y, et al. The overactive bladder: epidemiology and morbidity. Urol Clin North Am 2006;33:433–8.
4. Nelson R, Norton N, Cautley E, et al. Community-based prevalence of anal incontinence. JAMA 1995;274:559–61.
5. Macmillan AK, Merrie AE, Marshall RJ, et al. The prevalence of fecal incontinence in community-dwelling adults: a systematic review of the literature. Dis Colon Rectum 2004;47:1341–9.
6. Heymen S, Jones KR, Ringel Y, et al. Biofeedback treatment of fecal incontinence: a critical review. Dis Colon Rectum 2001;44:728–36.
7. Malouf AJ, Vaizey CJ, Norton CS, et al. Internal anal sphincter augmentation for fecal incontinence using injectable silicone biomaterial. Dis Colon Rectum 2001;44:595–600.
8. Cheetham M, Brazzelli M, Norton C, et al. Drug treatment for fecal incontinence in adults review. Cochrane Database Syst Rev 2003;3:CD002116.
9. Norton C, Chelvanayagam S, Wilson-Barnett J, et al. Randomized controlled trial of biofeedback for fecal incontinence. Gastroenterology 2003;125:1320–9.
10. Wexner SD, Coller JA, Devroede G, et al. Sacral nerve stimulation for fecal incontinence: results of a 120-patient prospective multicenter study. Ann Surg 2010;251(3):441–9.
11. Carmona R, Company RA, Vila JR, et al. Long-term results of artificial bowel sphincter for the treatment of severe fecal incontinence. Are they what we hoped? Colorectal Dis 2009;11:831–7.
12. O'Brien PE, Dixon JB, Skinner S, et al. A prospective, randomized, controlled clinical trial of placement of the artificial bowel sphincter (Acticon neosphincter) for the control of fecal incontinence. Dis Colon Rectum 2004;47:1852–60.
13. Vasavada S, Rackley RR. Electrical stimulation and neuromodulation in storage and emptying failure. In: McDougal WS, Wein AJ, Kavoussi LR, et al, editors. Campbell-Walsh urology, vol. 3. 10th edition. Philadelphia (PA): Elsevier; 2012. p. 2026–2047. Chapter 70.
14. Leng WW, Chancellor MB. How sacral nerve stimulation neuromodulation works. Urol Clin North Am 2005;23:11–8.
15. Melzack R, Wall PD. Pain mechanisms: a new theory. Science 1965;150:971–9.
16. Cheng CI, Ma CP, de Groat WC. Effect of capsaicin on micturition and associated reflexes in rats. Am J Physiol 1993;34:132–8.
17. van der Pal F, Heesakkers J. Current opinion on the working mechanisms of neuromodulation in the treatment of lower urinary tract dysfunction. Curr Opin Urol 2006;16:261–7.
18. Schmidt RA, Jonas U, Oleson KA, et al. Sacral nerve stimulation for treatment of refractory urinary urge incontinence. J Urol 1999;62:352–7.
19. Basra RK, Wagg A, Chapple C, et al. A review of adherence to drug therapy in patients with overactive bladder. BJU Int 2008;102:774.

20. Groenendijk PM, Lycklama à Nyeholt AA, Heesakkers J, et al. Urodynamic evaluation of sacral neuromodulation for urge urinary incontinence. BJU Int 2007;101:325–9.

21. Bosch JL, Groen J. Sacral nerve neuromodulation in the treatment of patients with refractory motor urge incontinence: long term results of a prospective longitudinal study. J Urol 2000;163:1219–22.

22. Janknegt RA, Weil EH, Eerdmans PH. Improving neuromodulation for refractory voiding dysfunctions: two stage implant. Urology 1997;49:358–62.

23. Peters KM, Killinger KA, Boura JA. Is sensory testing during lead placement crucial for achieving positive outcomes after sacral neuromodulation? Neurourol Urodyn 2011;30(8):1489–92.

24. Everaert K, Kerckhaert W, Caluwaerts H, et al. A prospective randomized trial comparing the 1-stage with the 2-stage implantation of a pulse generator in patients with pelvic floor dysfunction selected for sacral nerve stimulation. Eur Urol 2004;45:649–54.

25. Baxter C, Kim JH. Contrasting the percutaneous nerve evaluation versus staged implantation in sacral neuromodulation. Curr Urol Rep 2010;11(5):310–4.

26. Borawski K, Foster RT, Webster GD, et al. Predicting implantation with a neuromodulator, using two different test stimulation techniques: a prospective randomized study in urge incontinence women. Neurourol Urodyn 2007;26:14–8.

27. van Kerrebroeck PE, van Voskuilen AC, Heesakkers J, et al. Results of sacral neuromodulation therapy for urinary voiding dysfunction: outcomes of a proscective, worldwide clinical study. J Urol 2007;178:2029–34.

28. Brazzelli M, Murray A, Fraser C. Efficacy and safety of sacral nerve stimulation for urinary urge incontinence: a systematic review. J Urol 2006;175:835–41.

29. Shaker HS, Hassouna M. Sacral neuromodulation in idiopathic nonobstructive chronic urinary retention. J Urol 1998;159:1476–8.

30. Jonas U, Fowler CJ, Chancellor MB, et al. Efficacy of sacral nerve stimulation for urinary retention: results of 18 months after implantation. J Urol 2001;165:15–9.

31. Aboseif S, Tamaddon K, Chalfin S, et al. Sacral neuromodulation in functional urinary retention: an effective way to restore voiding. BJU Int 2002;90:662–5.

32. Huang JC, Deletis V, Vodusek DB, et al. Preservation of pudendal afferents in sacral rhizotomies. Neurosurgery 1997;41:411–5.

33. Beco J, Climov D, Bex M. Pudendal nerve decompression in perineology: a case series. BMC Surg 2004;4:15.

34. Popeney C, Ansell V, Renney K. Pudendal entrapment as an etiology of chronic perineal pain: dianosis and treatment. Neurourol Urodyn 2007;26:820–7.

35. Spinelli M, Malgut S, Giardiello G, et al. A new minimally invasive procedure for pudendal nerve stimulation to treat neurogenic bladder: description of method and preliminary data. Neurourol Urodyn 2005;24:226–30.

36. Peters KM, Feber KM, Bennett RC. Sacral versus pudendal nerve stimulation for voiding dysfunction: a prospective, single-blinded, randomized, crossover trial. Neurourol Urodyn 2005;24:643–7.

37. Peters KM, Killinger KA, Boguslawski BM, et al. Chronic pudendal neuromodulation: expanding available treatment options for refractory urologic symptoms. Neurourol Urodyn 2010;29(7):1267–71.

38. Matzel KE, Stadelmaier U, Hohenfellner M, et al. Electrical stimulation of sacral spinal nerves for treatment of fecal incontinence. Lancet 1995;346:1124–7.

39. Tjandra JJ, Chan MK, Yeh CH, et al. Sacral nerve stimulation is more effective than optimal medical therapy for severe fecal incontinence: a randomized controlled study. Dis Colon Rectum 2008;51:494–502.

40. Leroi A, Parc Y, Lehur P, et al. Efficacy of sacral nerve stimulation for fecal incontinence: results of a multicenter double-blind crossover study. Ann Surg 2005;242:662–9.

41. Kenefick NJ, Vaizey CJ, Cohen CR, et al. Double-blind placebo-controlled crossover study of sacral nerve stimulation for idiopathic constipation. Br J Surg 2002;89(12):1570–1.

42. Masin A, Ratto C, Ganio E, et al. Effect of sacral nerve modulation in chronic constipation. Ital J Public Health 2005;2:305.

43. Kamm MA, Dudding TC, Melenhorst J, et al. Sacral nerve stimulation for intractable constipation. Gut 2010;59(3):333–40.

44. Govier F, Litwiller S, Nitti V, et al. Percutaneous afferent modulation for the refractory over active bladder: results of a multicenter study. J Urol 2001; 165:1193–6.

45. Van Balken MR, Vandoninck V, Gisolf K, et al. Posterior tibial nerve stimulation as neuromodulatory treatment of lower urinary tract dysfunction. J Urol 2001; 166:914–49.

46. Macdiarmid SA, Peters KM, Wooldridge LS, et al. Randomized trial of percutaneous tibial nerve stimulation versus extended-release tolterodine: results from the overactive bladder innovative therapy trial. J Urol 2009;182(3):1055–61.

47. Peters KM, Carrico D, Burks F. Validation of a sham for percutaneous tibial nerve stimulation (PTNS). Neurourol Urodyn 2009;28(1):58–61.

48. Peters KM, Carrico DJ, Perez-Marrero RA, et al. Randomized trial of percutaneous tibial nerve stimulation versus Sham efficacy in the treatment of overactive bladder syndrome: results from the SUmiT trial. J Urol 2010;183(4):1438–43.

49. Findlay JM, Armstrong CM. Posterior tibial nerve stimulation and faecal incontinence: a review. Int J Colorectal Dis 2011;26:265–73.

Management of Mesh Complications and Vaginal Constriction

A Urogynecology Perspective

Dani Zoorob, MD[a], Mickey Karram, MD[a,b],*

KEYWORDS

- Synthetic mesh augmentation • Incontinence • Prolapse • Sling

KEY POINTS

- Mesh complications related to synthetic slings are relatively rare and can usually be managed in a fairly straight forward fashion.
- Complications reported from mesh kits for prolapse repair significantly increased between 2008 & 2010, resulting in an FDA warning and in changing the classification of these kits to class III devices.
- Vaginal constriction and pain remain the most challenging of all mesh complications to manage.

INTRODUCTION

Once thought of as a long-term solution to pelvic organ prolapse, currently synthetic mesh augmentation is regarded as a dark area that is being critically assessed by surgeons, hospitals, industry, and most importantly the Food and Drug Administration (FDA). With industry integrated so deeply in the medical field, more and more products have been produced in the hope of accommodating the needs of physicians. For the last 15 years, industry has made a big financial commitment in the field of pelvic floor surgery, initially developing slings for incontinence and then later investing in prolapse mesh kits.

The development of midurethral sling kits has revolutionized the surgical treatment of stress incontinence. Retropubic and transobturator (TOT) slings have excellent long-term efficacy with acceptable complication rates.

Mesh used to augment a prolapse repair ideally should be durable, carry no carcinogenic potential, be unlikely to get infected or inflamed, have lifelong durablity, and carry no risk of erosion. Despite all of the research, this ultimate material is yet to exist. Grafts of various materials were developed, some of a synthetic nature and others of biologic origin. Kits also varied in their shape and insertion technique.

These systems, however, were not rigorously tested but instead marketed after being cleared by the FDA through a simple 510 K regulatory process using a previously approved predescent material. An FDA safety net, known as the "Maude database," allows self-reporting of complications by surgeons and requires mandatory reporting of all complications reported to the manufacturer of the device or material. A significant increase in reported complications of mesh between 2008 and 2010 prompted a series of actions by the FDA that resulted in reclassifying mesh kits to class III devices and requiring the manufacturers of these devices to pursue research studies specific to their device (522 studies) if they desire to continue to market and sell their devices.

[a] Department of Obstetrics and Gynecology, Division of Female Pelvic Medicine and Reconstructive Surgery, The Christ Hospital/University of Cincinnati, 231 Albert Sabin Way, Cincinnati, OH 45267, USA; [b] The Christ Hospital, 2123 Auburn Avenue, Suite 307, Cincinnati, OH 45219, USA
* Corresponding author. The Christ Hospital, 2123 Auburn Avenue, Suite 307, Cincinnati, OH 45219.
E-mail address: mickey.karram@thechristhospital.com

Urol Clin N Am 39 (2012) 413–418
http://dx.doi.org/10.1016/j.ucl.2012.06.011

This article reviews the management of mesh complications resulting from synthetic slings and mesh used to augment prolapse repair.

DEFINITIONS

Terms used to describe mesh complications include erosion, extrusion, contraction, vaginal constrictions, paraurethral banding, dyspareunia, and diffuse pelvic and groin pain. Mesh extrusion refers to the mesh pushing itself out of the tissue and producing a protrusion, whereas mesh erosion refers to the absence or destruction of the vaginal layer theoretically covering the mesh, which then migrates usually into the vaginal lumen. Erosion into a neighboring viscus (bowel bladder or urethra) has also been reported.[1–3] Erosion seems to be a more chronic issue depending on the graft nature and the interaction between the local tissue and the implant.[4]

Mesh contraction refers to the graft shrinking over time, typically unequally, with up to 75% shrinkage possible.[5] Because of the reduced vaginal wall conformity and subsequent wall stiffness, the repercussions can be severe, impacting sexual, defecatory, and urinary function of the patient. Dyspareunia refers to pain with intercourse associated with penetration and is very commonly present in any woman who develops postoperative pelvic pain after mesh placement. The frequency of pelvic pain is believed to increase significantly as more mesh is implanted in the vagina; however, this is difficult to prove because very few randomized trials comparing mesh augmentation with native tissue repair exist.

Synthetic slings, have been associated with a significant positive impact on sexual function secondary to the high success of correcting incontinence. However, in some patients this positive sexual outcome may be offset by paraurethral banding, the pain generated by penile manipulation of the mucosa underneath the sling. This complication is specific to TOT slings where a band is palpable at the midurethral region, perpendicular to the axis of the urethra, along the tract of the entire sling to the vaginal sidewalls. Tenderness is typically reproducible on manipulation of the band. This is associated with vaginal pain and dyspareunia. In a retrospective study by Cholhan and coworkers,[6] 52% of women developed some banding after having a TOT sling placed with up to 24% of these patients developing dyspareunia and subsequent deterioration in their sexual life. The same study assessed patients who had undergone retropubic synthetic slings and could not identify banding in any of these patients.

MANAGEMENT OF COMPLICATIONS OF SYNTHETIC MIDURETHRAL SLINGS
Vaginal Erosion or Extrusion

When mesh is exposed in the lumen of the vagina (should occur in <3% of cases) it only needs to be treated if it becomes symptomatic. Common symptoms include penile pain during intercourse or what has been termed "hisparunia," and vaginal discharge and spotting. The goal in managing such patients is to remove the exposed mesh and cover the defect with healthy well-vascularized vaginal tissue. Up to 30% of the time women may develop recurrent stress urinary incontinence (SUI) after such procedures.

Urethral and Bladder Erosion

Treatment of urethral and bladder erosion usually involves complete excision of all sling material from the urethra or bladder, with mobilization of healthy tissue to close the defect in layers. Timing from initial surgery is crucial. If urethral erosion is identified within the first 2 weeks postoperative, it may be possible to simply remove the sling by grasping it vaginally and applying continuous traction to pull it out. In the authors' experience complete tissue ingrowth occurs somewhere between 14 and 21 days postoperative, after which such a maneuver is impossible. Urethral closure in layers in a tension-free fashion is mandatory to prevent tissue breakdown and subsequent fistula formation. If a bladder or urethral erosion is detected after this timeframe, alternative techniques may be used. Transurethral or cystoscopic techniques have been described whereby the edges of the sling are resected with a Holmium laser. In 2005, Giri and coworkers[7] reported on excisions after intravesical sling erosions occurred. In 2011, Doumouchtsis also reported transurethral laser excisions that were noted to require further resection at a later stage.[8] The laser is used to trim the edges of the sling tape once identified. If traversing the urethra, ensuring resection deep to the urethral mucosa is important to prevent stone formation at the resected edge and to ensure adequate healing at that site. If a stone is already present on the mesh, it is advisable to break it down mechanically, and then proceed with the tape resection cystoscopically.

If excision is initiated vaginally for urethral erosion or bladder erosion that can be addressed vaginally, a midline or inverted U-shaped vaginal incision is performed. The rationale for use of the U incision is to avoid having the vaginal suture line covering the urethral incision. After resection of the mesh is done and the urethra or bladder is repaired primarily, it is important to drain the bladder with a catheter for a prolonged period of time (10–14 days of continuous drainage).

Paraurethral Banding

In cases where slings are removed because of paraurethral banding, it may be advisable to excise as much of the TOT sling as possible. If recurrent SUI occurs, a pubovaginal or retropubic synthetic sling should be performed. Excision is preferably performed under general anesthesia to allow for more extensive access to the sling ends. The routine vaginal preparation is placed and the urethra catheterized with a Foley catheter. Then, the band is identified, followed by infiltrating a solution of local anesthetic and epinephrine along the entire accessible tract of the TOT, followed by incising the skin in the midline down to the sling. A gritty feeling typically indicates proximity to the sling and the appropriate dissection depth. Release of the sling from the underlying tissue is then performed. Inserting a right-angle clamp can facilitate this process as long as the posterior urethral wall is protected. Opening the right angle clamp releases the sling further. Then, the sling is incised in the midline and the edges are held with clamps, and careful dissection of the overlying mucosa and underlying tissues is performed all the way to the obturator membrane if accessible. Deng and coworkers[9] reported the technique of extensive excision and urethrolysis with subsequent urethral reinforcement with a second layer of paraurethral tissue after the sling was mobilized. The need for extensive excision and not simple midline release is to prevent future erosion and banding which may occur along the sidewalls.

MESH AUGMENTATION FOR REPAIR OF PROLAPSE

Initially, the concept of augmenting the prolapse repair with mesh made a lot of sense because the gold standard for prolapse repair is believed by many to be sacrocolpopexy, which involves attaching mesh to the vagina. It made sense to think of alternative routes to facilitate insertion and fixation of the mesh, such as through vaginal delivery systems in a standardized fashion. Thus, mesh kits were developed and initially very well received. However, over time a variety of complications, some of which were very difficult to treat, were described. These included mesh erosion in approximately 15%–20% of cases and a variety of pain syndromes as well as alterations in bladder and bowel function.

In some situations the vaginal walls may become less pliable and less responsive to pressure,

and the rigidity causes intercourse to become uncomfortable. In a prospective observational study, Milani and coworkers[10] reported a 69% dyspareunia rate after either anterior or posterior mesh augmentation procedures. Furthermore, vaginal mesh has been reported to be associated with contractures, resulting in pain and tightening of the vagina. In a retrospective study, Blandon and coworkers[11] showed that 48% of patients referred for pain after a vaginal mesh kit had reduction in vaginal caliber, defined as either a decrease in girth or length. In a retrospective study involving 684 patients, Caquant and coworkers[12] reported a 3.4%, 5%, and 17.6% contracture rate in total, posterior, and anterior mesh inlay procedures, respectively. They also reported uterine conservation to have a protective effect at time of mesh inlay placement. Collinet and coworkers[13] reported increased rates of mesh exposure in patients who had concurrent hysterectomies and vaginal kits placed (odds ratio, 5.17) and inverted-T colpotomies (odds ratio, 6.06). However, de Landsheere and coworkers[14] did not find any correlation with hysterectomies in their study, which involved 524 patients who were followed for 3 years. Trocar-based systems involve passage of trocars blindly through the obturator membrane and inner groin (anterior kits) or pararectally through the levator muscle (posterior kits). Accordingly, erroneous tracts may be created with subsequent development of bowel perforations and pararectal and rectal abscesses noted postoperatively.[15] Fistulas with abscess formation have also been reported.[15–17] A systematic review by Feiner and coworkers[18] assessed the Apogee mesh kit (American Medical Systems, Minnetonka, MN, USA) was associated with erosion in 11% and dyspareunia in 1% of the patients in eight studies. Other complications were perineal, buttock, and groin pain in 1% of the patients. In the same report, 6% of patients had grade III Dindo classification, thus requiring definite surgical intervention. Dindo grade III indicates a surgical intervention is necessary, whereas grade IV indicates a life-threatening status frequently requiring intensive care unit admission.

Fistulas (specifically vesicovaginal) also have been reported with anterior mesh kits. They are more likely to occur if an unrecognized bladder perforation is encountered intraoperatively and not repaired immediately. Bekker and coworkers[19] reported combining a transurethral and suprapubic excision technique to repair such defects. In cases where the bladder is traversed with either inlay mesh or sling mesh, open excision may be performed either vaginally if accessible or abdominally. Such erosions may even require partial cystectomies if extensive mesh adhesion into the bladder occurs.

The most common complication of prolapse repair using synthetic mesh has been vaginal erosion. In a randomized controlled trial by Nieminen and coworkers,[20] 19% mesh exposure rates were identified within 36 months. In a case series by Gauruder-Burmester and coworkers,[21] 8% of patients with the Perigee system (American Medical Systems, Minnetonka, MN, USA) had mesh exposures with 3% requiring excisions. Feiner and coworkers'[18] systematic review involved the Prolift system (Ethicon Women's Health and Urology, Somerville, NJ, USA). Eight studies, involving around 1300 patients, assessed posterior and total Prolifts. The review showed a 16% mesh complication rate, with 7% related to erosion and 2% to dyspareunia. Vaginal and buttock pain occurred in 2%, whereas mesh contracture occurred in 1.5%. Up to 6% of complications were considered Dindo grade III and one case as Dindo grade IV because of necrotizing fasciitis.

MANAGEMENT OF COMPLICATIONS OF KITS FOR PROLAPSE

Typically, treatment of any mesh complication is individualized based on the case.

Vaginal Mesh Erosion

In patients with mesh that is exposed vaginally, conservative therapy may be initiated by instructing the patient to abstain from intercourse and to apply vaginal estrogen cream to the area of erosion. If the outcomes are not satisfactory, minimally invasive measures can usually be used, which involve simple resection of the exposed mesh. The dissection should ensure enough resection away from the free edge of the mucosa followed by a tension-free closure of the vaginal wall. The release of the mucosa off the graft is highly advisable so as to avoid having denuded areas, which may require biologic or skin grafts. Mucosa may be released off the mesh graft in a plane parallel to the graft by holding its edge firmly with an Allis or Kocher clamp and using sharp dissection with the tips of Metzenbaum scissors aiming toward the mesh and away from any viscus in the vicinity. If exposure has recurred after prior resections, a more aggressive attempt at graft resection must be undertaken after informing the patient that this is associated with higher morbidity and increased risk of prolapse recurrence.

Pain Caused by Mesh Contracture

If contractures are present, it is important to anatomically identify the exact areas of pain while the patient is awake. In the operating room these areas are marked with the goal of releasing as much tension off surrounding tissues as possible. The vaginal mucosa over the painful areas is opened and the band is released by incising completely through the full thickness of the mesh. This is performed by placing a clamp on the band that is palpable and exposing its edges to undermine the rest of the graft and allow resection as far lateral as possible. Simple release of a contracture in the mesh by incising or excising a small part of the band is not a definitive treatment for such a complication. It is crucial that the resection go as far lateral as possible while ensuring anatomic orientation and being aware of the potential to enter the bladder or bowel, which are commonly in very close proximity. Ensuring that the mesh can be freed off the bladder or rectum is in the authors' opinion crucial.

Mesh Erosion into Bladder or Bowel

If erosion into any of these structures occurs, the mesh must be completely excised followed by a tension-free closure of the bladder or bowel. Ureteral stenting is advisable particularly if the erosion into the bladder is close to the trigone. Mesh in the gastrointestinal tract may require diversion of bowel contents before surgical removal. The approach for excision of vaginal mesh kits is usually vaginally, with the rare need for laparoscopy or laparotomy.[22]

Other Complications

Other rare complications have included significant vaginal constriction, perirectal or inner groin pain, and recurrent perirectal abscesses. These types of complications challenge even the most skilled surgeons. Each of these types of cases must be individualized and surgical correction is often done in a staged fashion.

MANAGEMENT OF MESH COMPLICATIONS ASSOCIATED WITH SACROCOLPOPEXY

The most common mesh complication after sacrocolpopexy is vaginal erosion of the mesh, which occurs in 3% to 8% of cases. Rarely, this may be associated with concurrent sinus formation connecting the vagina to the mesh deeply attached to the sacrum. South and coworkers[23] reported the use of endoscopic-assisted transvaginal mesh resection to excise sinus tracts along the mesh between the apex and the sacrum. Kohli and coworkers[24] reported a technique where they simply excised the exposed granulated mesh/tissue and after mobilizing the defect covered it with vaginal mucosa. The goal is to resect the mesh high up into the vagina after applying significant traction on the mesh. This allows a tension-free closure of healthy vagina with the mesh retracted well away from the vaginal incision. At times aggressive resections result in recurrent prolapse and thus a simple suture repair of an enterocele or apical prolapse may also be required. The excision is tremendously simplified if the peritoneum is entered. One-year follow-up showed no erosion recurrences or change in vaginal support.[24] The procedure is done while the patient is under general anesthesia and after adequate preparation. The erosion site is identified and held with a Kocker clamp under significant continuous traction, followed by the release of the vaginal mucosa off the mesh edge if possible. This is done using a Mayo-type scissors. The further the mucosal release, the deeper the mesh mobilization, the higher the likelihood of deeper excision. Coring of the visualized mesh as high and deep as possible is performed, which then retracts up toward the sacrum after traction is discontinued, followed by the closure of the vaginal mucosa.

SUMMARY

Unfortunately a significant number of mesh complications are still being managed at many referral centers and outcomes remain unpredictable. It is hoped that future studies on indications and techniques for mesh use will reduce these complication rates.

EDITOR'S COMMENTS

Complications related to the use of mesh for pelvic floor indications are increasingly being noted in clinical practice. Many factors have contributed to this increasing incidence. Clearly, the increased use of mesh for both midurethral slings and pelvic floor repair has increased the numbers of patients at risk for complications. Importantly, however, subtle differences between devices (regarding technique and insertion) may add additional variables to procedural outcome. Technical familiarity with these variations is critical for the implanting surgeon. Moreover, variations and modifications in device design have occurred rather rapidly, possibly impacting the individual surgeon's ability to have as robust a familiarity as possible with the most recent devices.

Another contributing factor to mesh complications is the patient comorbidity. Vaginal atrophy, chronic steroid use, prior surgery, and other local vaginal variables all conspire to increase the risk of mesh complication. In patients with either autoimmune or other wound-healing deficits, a further impact may be noted.

Management of mesh complications is individualized and somewhat predicated by the presenting scenario. Mesh exposure may occur in small or large volume and may or may not be complicated by vaginal constriction and damage to underlying viscera. Mesh erosion into underlying viscera (bladder, bowel, or rectum) further complicates presentation in that mesh in these circumstances leads to the potential of stone formation, recurrent urinary tract infection, hematuria, and altered bladder or bowel function dependent upon the organ involved. Another commonly encountered complication is pain at the site of mesh implantation. Pain may be related to mesh exposure alone, impacting sexual function. However, in some patients, mesh constriction may place undo tension both on underlying structures and also surrounding musculo-fascial supportive structures, resulting in chronic discomfort which may be extremely problematic for the patient.

Any comprehensive management plan should take into account the underlying symptoms, the degree to which resection of mesh should occur (partial versus total), and the need for simultaneous reconstruction of bladder and/or bowel wall. It is critical to prepare the woman for the likelihood that not all presenting symptoms will resolve and that there may be persistence of some aspect of the bothersome complaints that she is currently experiencing. These may include persistence of pain, return or exacerbation of incontinence, and impact upon bowel function. Additionally, long-term fibrosis may affect vaginal caliber and even without mesh being present, chronically may restrict vaginal distensibility and impact sexual function. The key to successful mesh complication management is a thoughtful, structured approach with an informed and aware patient. All due effort should be paid to optimizing the surgical field (treatment of infection, use of topical vaginal estrogens, and complete and thorough assessment of all potential mesh areas of exposure or erosion).

Although the majority of patients who have had mesh implanted have not had consequences of this implantation, those who have, are faced with a daunting burden. It is incumbent upon the pelvic floor medicine proceduralist to be aware of the potential ramifications of these complications and acute and chronic management thereof.

Roger R. Dmochowski, MD
Mickey Karram, MD

REFERENCES

1. Leboeuf L, Miles RA, Kim SS, et al. Grade 4 cystocele repair using four-defect repair and porcine xenograft acellular matrix (Pelvicol) outcome measures using SEAPI. Urology 2004;64(2):282–6.
2. David-Montefiore E, Barranger E, Dubernard G, et al. Treatment of genital prolapse by hammock using porcine skin collagen implant Pelvicol. Urology 2005;66(6):1314–8.
3. Achtari C, Hiscock R, O'Reilly BA, et al. Risk factors for mesh erosion after transvaginal surgery using polypropylene (Atrium) or composite polypropylene/polyglactin 910 (Vypro II) mesh. Int Urogynecol J Pelvic Floor Dysfunct 2005;16(5):389–94.
4. Mistrangelo E, Mancuso S, Nadalini C, et al. Rising use of synthetic mesh in transvaginal pelvic reconstructive surgery: a review of the risk of vaginal erosion. J Minim Invasive Gynecol 2007;14(5):564–9.
5. Cosson M, Debodinance P, Boukerrou M, et al. Mechanical properties of synthetic implants used in the repair of prolapse and urinary incontinence in women: which is the ideal material? Int Urogynecol J Pelvic Floor Dysfunct 2003;14(3):169–78 [discussion: 178].
6. Cholhan HJ, Hutchings TB, Rooney KE. Dyspareunia associated with paraurethral banding in the transobturator sling. Am J Obstet Gynecol 2010; 202(5):481.e1–5.
7. Giri SK, Drumm J, Flood HD. Endoscopic holmium laser excision of intravesical tension-free vaginal tape and polypropylene suture after anti-incontinence procedures. J Urol 2005;174(4 Pt 1):1306–7.
8. Doumouchtsis SK, Lee FY, Bramwell D, et al. Evaluation of holmium laser for managing mesh/suture complications of continence surgery. BJU Int 2011; 108(9):1472–8.
9. Deng DY, Rutman M, Raz S, et al. Presentation and management of major complications of midurethral slings: are complications under-reported? Neurourol Urodyn 2007;26(1):46–52.
10. Milani R, Salvatore S, Soligo M, et al. Functional and anatomical outcome of anterior and posterior vaginal prolapse repair with prolene mesh. BJOG 2005;112(1):107–11.
11. Blandon RE, Gebhart JB, Trabuco EC, et al. Complications from vaginally placed mesh in pelvic reconstructive surgery. Int Urogynecol J Pelvic Floor Dysfunct 2009;20(5):523.
12. Caquant F, Collinet P, Debodinance P, et al. Safety of transvaginal mesh procedure: retrospective study of 684 patients. J Obstet Gynaecol Res 2008;34(4): 449–56.
13. Collinet P, Belot F, Debodinance P, et al. Transvaginal mesh technique for pelvic organ prolapse repair: mesh exposure management and risk factors. Int Urogynecol J Pelvic Floor Dysfunct 2006;17(4): 315–20.
14. de Landsheere L, Ismail S, Lucot JP, et al. Surgical intervention after transvaginal Prolift mesh repair: retrospective single-center study including 524 patients with 3 years' median follow-up. Am J Obstet Gynecol 2012;206(1):83.e1–7.
15. Hilger WS, Cornella JL. Rectovaginal fistula after posterior intravaginal slingplasty and polypropylene mesh augmented rectocele repair. Int Urogynecol J Pelvic Floor Dysfunct 2006;17(1):89–92.
16. Chen HW, Guess MK, Connell KA, et al. Ischiorectal abscess and ischiorectal-vaginal fistula as delayed complications of posterior intravaginal slingplasty: a case report. J Reprod Med 2009;54(10):645–8.
17. Grynberg M, Teyssedre J, Staerman F. Gluteovaginal fistula after posterior intravaginal slingplasty: a case report. Int Urogynecol J Pelvic Floor Dysfunct 2009;20(7):877–9.
18. Feiner B, Jelovsek JE, Maher C. Efficacy and safety of transvaginal mesh kits in the treatment of prolapse of the vaginal apex: a systematic review [review]. BJOG 2009;116(1):15–24.
19. Bekker MD, Bevers RF, Elzevier HW. Transurethral and suprapubic mesh resection after Prolift bladder perforation: a case report. Int Urogynecol J 2010; 21(10):1301–3.
20. Nieminen K, Hiltunen R, Takala T, et al. Outcomes after anterior vaginal wall repair with mesh: a randomized, controlled trial with a 3 year follow-up. Am J Obstet Gynecol 2010;203(3):235.e1–8.
21. Gauruder-Burmester A, Koutouzidou P, Rohne J, et al. Follow-up after polypropylene mesh repair of anterior and posterior compartments in patients with recurrent prolapse. Int Urogynecol J Pelvic Floor Dysfunct 2007;18:1059–64.
22. Baessler K, Hewson AD, Tunn R, et al. Severe mesh complications following intravaginal slingplasty. Obstet Gynecol 2005;106(4):713–6.
23. South MM, Foster RT, Webster GD, et al. Surgical excision of eroded mesh after prior abdominal sacrocolpopexy. Am J Obstet Gynecol 2007;197(6): 615.e1–5.
24. Kohli N, Walsh PM, Roat TW, et al. Mesh erosion after abdominal sacrocolpopexy. Obstet Gynecol 1998;92(6):999–1004.

Controversies in the Management of Mesh-Based Complications: A Urology Perspective

Brian K. Marks, MD*, Howard B. Goldman, MD

KEYWORDS

- Pelvic organ prolapse • Dyspareunia • Urinary incontinence, stress • Complication • Postoperative

KEY POINTS

- Multiple options for managing mesh complications after pelvic reconstructive surgery are described in the literature, but the paucity of supportive data creates a challenge for the patient and pelvic surgeon electing a treatment.
- Expectant management or topical estrogen therapy for vaginal mesh extrusion has reported success in 37% to 42% of patients.
- Mesh in the bladder or urethra can be managed endoscopically using various tools; however, success is often less than 50%.
- If conservative measures or endoscopic approaches fail, timely definitive management with open suprapubic, transvaginal, or laparoscopic techniques is appropriate.
- Pure transvaginal techniques for extrusions and urethral and bladder perforations have been described with good outcomes and earlier convalescence than major abdominal operations.

INTRODUCTION

Unsatisfactory success rates and relative morbidity of native tissue repair for stress urinary incontinence and pelvic organ prolapse encouraged innovative investigation into augmenting repair with synthetic and biologic grafts. The success of the tension-free transvaginal tape introduced by Ulmsten and Petros[1] in 1995 spurred widespread development of transvaginal synthetic mesh delivery systems to treat incontinence and pelvic organ prolapse. The first synthetic mesh repair system for pelvic organ prolapse was approved for use by the U.S. Food and Drug Administration in 2001, and since then many of these "kits" have been marketed.[2] Use of these novel methods by pelvic surgeons opened an unsuspected Pandora's box of mesh-specific complications to the field. Management of these sequelae varies between surgeons, and most published data are limited to case reports and small retrospective series. This article focuses on the differing management options for treating synthetic mesh complications after incontinence and prolapse surgery.

TYPES OF MESH-BASED COMPLICATIONS AND REPORTED INCIDENCE

A variety of adverse events associated with the use of synthetic mesh in female reconstructive surgery have been reported in the literature. This article focuses on mesh-specific complications after mid-urethral slings, transvaginal mesh delivery systems for pelvic organ prolapse, and sacrocolpopexy.

Center for Female Pelvic Medicine and Reconstructive Surgery, Glickman Urological and Kidney Institute, Cleveland Clinic, Lerner College of Medicine, 9500 Euclid Avenue, Cleveland, OH 44195, USA
* Corresponding author. Center for Female Pelvic Medicine and Reconstructive Surgery, Glickman Urological and Kidney Institute, Cleveland Clinic, 9500 Euclid Avenue, Q10-1, Cleveland, OH 44195.
E-mail address: marksb@ccf.org

Urol Clin N Am 39 (2012) 419–428
http://dx.doi.org/10.1016/j.ucl.2012.05.009
0094-0143/12/$ – see front matter © 2012 Elsevier Inc. All rights reserved.

The discussion is limited to complications in which the "correct" treatment choice is controversial, and focuses on terminology established by the International Continence Society and International Urogynecological Association, highlighting alternatives in management of mesh exposure, extrusion, prominence, perforation, contraction, pelvic pain, and dyspareunia.[3]

Synthetic midurethral slings have an overall re-operation rate of 1.8% to 5.4%,[4] partly because of complications such as mesh extrusion, pelvic pain, dyspareunia, and urethral and bladder perforations. Bladder perforation rates have been reported as high as 12%, occurring in 2.7% to 3.9% of cases in randomized controlled trials.[4,5] Bladder perforations were identified in 4.7% of bottom-to-top retropubic slings compared with 8.5% of top-down approaches and in only 0.3% of transobturator slings.[6] In a contemporary review of a large insurance-based cohort, trocar bladder perforation occurred in 1.4% of cases, although these results may be limited by underreporting.[7] The number of missed trocar perforations that present with delayed complications is more difficult to define. Mesh has been identified in 14% to 27% of symptomatic patients presenting with delayed complications after synthetic midurethral slings.[8,9] Intraoperative urethral perforations occur rarely and are reported in fewer than 1% of sling operations.[7] Delayed presentation of urethral extrusion or missed perforation is reported in 0.3% to 1.0% of patients.[5,10] Vaginal extrusion of mesh occurs in approximately 3% of cases.[5,11] The reoperation rate for vaginal mesh extrusion after synthetic midurethral sling is reported to be 0.8%.[7]

Similar types of mesh complications occur after prolapse repair. Vaginal mesh extrusion rates range from 2.7% to 11.3% after transvaginal mesh delivery systems according to large retrospective cohorts.[12,13] Randomized controlled trials comparing mesh repair and native tissue repair report extrusion in 11.7% to 16.9% of patients.[2,14,15] The rate of bladder perforation, either dissection-related or trocar-related, is between 0.6% to 0.73%.[12-14] Bowel and rectal perforations occur less commonly, and postoperative vesicovaginal fistulas occur in 0.29% of cases.[13]

In randomized controlled trials, the rate of de novo dyspareunia was found to be 8.0% to 9.1% in patients receiving mesh, although no statistical difference was found compared with native tissue repair.[14,15] An observational cohort of 294 women found de novo pelvic pain in 5% and de novo dyspareunia in 26% of patients after transvaginal mesh.[16] In this study, pain and dyspareunia before surgery were independent risk factors for postoperative symptoms.[16] Several studies report lower rates of dyspareunia in patients with mesh repair than in those with traditional repairs.[15,17] Symptomatic mesh contraction varies greatly between studies, reported as low as 0.4% and as high as 11.7%.[12,13]

MANAGEMENT OF MESH COMPLICATIONS AFTER SYNTHETIC MIDURETHRAL SLINGS
Vaginal Extrusion

Differing treatment options for the management of vaginal mesh extrusion are described in the literature, and most outcomes data are derived from small case reports with varying success. Thus, a dilemma is created for the surgeon managing these complications. Described methods range from observation alone, use of topical estrogen or antiseptics, systemic or topical antibiotics, office-based trimming of the extruded material, and operative excision. Adding to the conundrum, the duration and frequency of medical therapy are not proven, the appropriate time to intervene for treatment failure is not known, and the amount of mesh to excise has not been standardized.

Outcomes for expectant management and treatment with topical therapies such as estrogen differ among studies. Four patients with vaginal mesh extrusion in a cohort of 90 retropubic slings were all treated expectantly without any topical estrogen or antibiotics.[18] The area of extrusion was 0.5 to 1.0 cm and all resolved spontaneously with epithelialization after 6 weeks.[18] In a series involving both prolapse and sling mesh, failure with conservative methods was reported in 63%.[19] Success has not been reproducible and definitive treatment with mesh excision is often recommended.[20]

Office-based trimming and operative excision with approximation of the vaginal epithelium are preferred management options, particularly if conservative therapies have failed. The questions to answer are the timing of intervention and the amount of mesh to excise. One should ensure adequate tissue quality before reconstruction, and any evidence of infection, inflammation, or atrophy must be addressed. Addition of vaginal estrogen cream before surgical reconstruction may enhance tissue quality. Once the decision has been made to surgically intervene, the choice of office-based excision or surgical exploration depends on the amount and location of the mesh extrusion and its accessibility to the surgeon; involvement of adjacent organs; and patient comfort. The amount of mesh to excise also depends on the size and location of the extrusion, involvement of adjacent structures, and symptoms. In managing asymptomatic extrusion or focally symptomatic extrusion, excision of enough material to allow tension-free approximation of vaginal epithelium is necessary to prevent dehiscence or recurrence. Leaving protruding edges of mesh may increase this risk. Care must be taken to not excise more than necessary, because maintenance of continence is key. Tijdink and colleagues[19] report a 36% recurrent stress incontinence rate after excision for mesh extrusion. This finding approximates published incontinence rates after sling incision for obstruction, reported at 21%.[21]

Surgical excision is often an ambulatory procedure well tolerated by most patients, and has shown good outcomes. Marcus-Braun and colleagues[22] report on 104 mesh removal operations, of which 44 were for vaginal extrusion. After 6 months' follow-up, only five patients underwent intervention for recurrence, yielding an 88% success rate. This series, however, includes both synthetic mesh slings and mesh prolapse repair.[22] High success with these techniques applies to type I mesh, such as lightweight large-pore polypropylene. Earlier series involving different classes of synthetics have lower success and higher complication rates.[8,23] Sometimes, infection is present and the entire foreign body must be removed for healing to occur. With type I polypropylene, this is less likely and partial excision is highly successful.[22]

The authors' experience with expectant management and topical estrogen therapy often yields less-than-satisfactory results. However, use of vaginal estrogen cream before planned resection of extruded mesh may improve the vaginal tissue quality if atrophic vaginitis is present. Referrals to the authors' tertiary practice have often yielded failed conservative measures and their preferred management is operative excision in an ambulatory surgical center. After proper surgical preparation, exposure is obtained with a weighted speculum and elastic hooks with or without a ring retractor. The surrounding vaginal epithelium is injected with 0.5% lidocaine with 1:200,000 epinephrine to facilitate dissection.

Vaginal epithelial flaps are created by incising the epithelium adjacent to the extrusion site in a direction perpendicular to the mesh. However, the incision is tailored on a case-by-case basis, and horizontal, inverted-U–shaped, or circumferential incisions may be used. Using a combination of sharp dissection with Metzenbaum scissors and blunt dissection with a Kittner, vaginal flaps 1 to 2 cm in length are created on both sides of the extrusion. A blunt-tipped instrument such as a Kelly clamp or Mixter right angle forceps is passed between the mesh and underlying fascia adjacent to the urethra. The clamp is carefully opened to raise the synthetic mesh off the underlying fascia and the sling is incised. Each cut edge is grasped with an Allis clamp for traction and dissected free from the underlying fascia with a combination of sharp and blunt dissection. Care is taken to keep the dissection on the mesh and not wander into deeper tissue. Pointing the tips of the Metzenbaum scissors toward the mesh helps avoid inadvertent urethral or bladder injury. The mesh is transected with a curved Mayo scissor once it has been dissected free from the underlying fascia. Enough mesh is excised to provide at least a 1-cm margin from the edge of the extrusion. The edges of vaginal epithelium are then approximated with a running 2-0 polyglycolic acid suture after copious irrigation.

Urethral Perforation or Extrusion

Urethral extrusions or perforation have been managed with transvaginal excision, endoscopic, and combined techniques. The controversy arises in determining which technique to use and what outcomes are expected. Several studies report on varying management strategies, but are limited to small retrospective case series. Pure transvaginal techniques are similar to transvaginal approaches for vaginal extrusion.

In the transvaginal technique, vaginal flaps are created over the urethra after injection of lidocaine with epinephrine. Midline and inverted-U incisions have been reported.[23,24] The authors' preference is to use an inverted-U–shaped incision to avoid overlapping suture lines in an attempt to prevent urethrovaginal fistulas. The vaginal flap dissection was described in the previous section. The mesh is isolated, a blunt instrument such as a Mixter right angle forceps is placed behind, and the mesh is incised adjacent to the urethra. When the mesh is free floating within the urethra it can be approached by incising the urethra circumferentially around the mesh on both sides where it perforates the urethra. Sharp dissection and gentle spreading of the Metzenbaum scissors will often release the mesh from the urethra so it can be pulled through for removal. Placing a small hemostat into the urethra to grasp the synthetic material may help with dissection.[25] When the mesh is adherent to or only partially visible within the urethra, one will likely have to incise into the urethra for the length of the perforation. Once the mesh is excised, the urethra is closed and other layers of tissue are closed over it.

Another author described an innovative means of using a lighted nasal speculum within the urethra to improve exposure and sharply dissect the sling from the urethral side wall.[26] In that series, none of the three patients required repeat excision, but all developed recurrent stress incontinence.[26] After the mesh is removed, the urethra is debrided and closed with interrupted 4-0 or 5-0 polyglycolic acid sutures to form a water-tight closure. Additional layers of periurethral or pubocervical fascia are developed sharply and closed over the urethra. The vaginal epithelium can then be approximated with a running 2-0 polyglycolic acid suture. A urethral Foley, 14 to 16 French, is left as a drain for 7 to 14 days.

The use of an additional graft or flap in this situation, such as a Martius flap, is debated.[9,23,25] If the patient presents with a urethrovaginal fistula, then extirpation of the mesh along with reconstruction and Martius flap interposition is often recommended.[9] Potential adverse sequelae include recurrent stress incontinence and urethrovaginal fistula. In one series, the rate of incontinence after transvaginal excision was 83%, although others report no incidence of de novo stress urinary incontinence after surgery to correct urethral perforations.[8,23] Deng and colleagues[9] report three postoperative urinary vaginal fistulas that required a second reconstructive procedure with Martius flap interposition. If recurrent stress urinary incontinence occurs, expert opinion recommends an autologous fascia pubovaginal sling after adequate time for tissue healing.[8,23]

Controversy exists regarding the use of endoscopic methods to remove mesh from the urethra. Velemir and colleagues[24] report on a technique of pure endoscopic excision in four patients. A forceps is introduced alongside a cystoscope and used to grasp the mesh for traction.[24] Endoscopic scissors are introduced through the cystoscope and the mesh fibers are sharply incised.[24] In follow-up, two of these patients needed at least one additional endoscopic procedure to remove remaining mesh, yielding a 50% failure rate.[24] Another series also reported a 50% failure rate with endoscopic management, and these patients ultimately required transvaginal removal.[25] Doumouchtsis and colleagues[27] applied a Holmium laser fiber to the mesh as close to the mucosa as possible. Failure in this series was high and only one of four patients was symptom-free and without endoscopic evidence of recurrence at 2 years.[27] One patient underwent repeat laser excision, and the remaining two continued to have residual fiber extrusion at the end of follow-up.[27] Comparison of data from each series are presented in **Table 1**. Based on the available data and the authors' experience, transvaginal excision is their preferred management for most patients presenting to their center.

Bladder Perforation or Extrusion

Extirpation of intravesical mesh after complications from synthetic midurethral slings requires a tailored management plan based on the extent and location of the mesh perforation. The location of mesh depends on the type of sling: retropubic versus transobturator. Perforation with retropubic slings will often be at the dome in a 10 to 2 o'clock location; however, mesh can be identified along the lateral walls and near the bladder neck. After a transobturator approach, the expected location will be along the bladder base or bladder neck in a 4 to 8 o'clock location. Location dictates management strategies. As with urethral perforation, options include open or endoscopic techniques. Pure transvaginal and pure laparoscopic methods have also been described.[28–30]

Techniques for endoscopic management include cystoscopic resection with endoscopic scissors, the use of Holmium laser, and transurethral resection using diathermy, and results are highlighted in **Table 1**. Often, urolithiasis develops on the mesh and concomitant litholapaxy or lithotripsy is the first step. Using monopolar diathermy, significant thermal energy is generated when the element contacts adjacent bladder tissue and the mesh can be cut.[26] Of the nine patients who underwent transurethral resection with monopolar diathermy, one required a repeat transurethral resection and two required retropubic extraperitoneal exploration to remove the remaining mesh.[26] Bipolar elements do not require contact with bladder tissue and may reduce the risk of inadvertent injury or fistula. Holmium laser resection is similar to that described for managing urethral mesh extrusion.[25,27] The laser fiber is applied to the mesh along the bladder mucosa and an attempt is made to transect the material deep to the urothelium. Reported energy levels used to attain success are in the range of 2.5 kW.[27] Traction on the mesh using endoscopic instruments introduced along the cystoscope may aid removal.

Bekker and colleagues[31] described placing the mesh under tension with a laparoscopic grasper advanced through a 5-mm laparoscopic trocar inserted via suprapubic cystotomy. Doumouchtsis and colleagues[27] report on two cases managed with Holmium laser resection, both of whom required repeat procedures. One underwent laparotomy for complete excision at 1 year and the second underwent repeat laser excision at 2 years. In another series, 14 patients underwent mesh resection using a 26 French resectoscope with a loop electrode.[32] The mesh was resected deep beyond the detrusor muscle and into underlying perivesical adipose.[32] The bladder was left to catheter drainage and resolution occurred in 13 of 14 patients after a mean follow-up of 18 months.[32]

If endoscopic methods are not elected or have failed, a retropubic extraperitoneal exploration is often used for intravesical mesh located at or near the dome. Access is obtained via either

Table 1
Endoscopic management of mesh complications

Series	Patients	Technique	Mesh Type	Location	Success	Sequelae
Bekker et al,[31] 2010	1	Combined bipolar diathermy and suprapubic trocar	Transvaginal prolapse kit	Bladder	1/1	None reported
Doumouchtsis et al,[27] 2011	5	Holmium laser	4 RP slings 1 TOT sling 1 colposuspension	Bladder (2) Urethra (4)	0/2 (1 repeat laser; 1 open surgery) 1/4 (2 repeat laser; 1 residual mesh)	1 recurrent SUI
Foley et al,[26] 2010	9	Monopolar TUR Nasal speculum	8 RP slings 1 TOT	Bladder (9) Urethra (3)	6/9 (1 re-TUR, 1 open) 3/3	3 recurrent SUI
Frenkl et al,[25] 2008	11	Endoscopic scissor (4), Holmium laser (4), TUR (2)	Suture in 9 Sling mesh in 11 Sacrocolpopexy in 1	Bladder and urethra	50%	Not available
Oh & Ryu,[32] 2009	14	TUR	11 RP slings 3 TOT	Bladder	92.9% (1 re-TUR)	1 recurrent SUI, 1 VVF
Velemir et al,[24] 2008	4	Endoscopic scissors	3 RP slings 1 TOT	Bladder and urethra	2/4	3 recurrent SUI

Abbreviations: RP, retropubic; SUI, stress urinary incontinence; TOT, transobturator tape; TUR, transurethral resection; VVF, vesicovaginal fistula.

a Pfannenstiel or a low midline incision. A cystotomy is created and the mesh is identified within the bladder. Through placing traction on the intravesical mesh, one can usually identify both portions of mesh outside the bladder. Both of those are cut, after which one can incise through the bladder wall at both points of perforation and remove all of the mesh passing through the bladder. Each "puncture" site can then be closed with a figure-of-eight full-thickness stitch. A large-caliber urethral catheter is left for at least 7 days and a cystogram may be obtained to ensure healing before its removal. An additional suprapubic catheter is usually unnecessary.

Misrai and colleagues[30] describes a laparoscopic extraperitoneal approach for sling removal using three port sites: two 5-mm ports medial to the anterior superior iliac spine and a 10-mm telescope port midway between the pubis and umbilicus. The retropubic space is developed and the two arms of the tape are identified along the pubis, grasped, and sharply dissected free from the rectus muscle and fascia.[30] Each side of the sling is released from the surrounding tissue and dissected medially to the urethra.[30] The sling is transected and removed in two halves without additional transvaginal exploration when possible.[30]

The authors' group described a pure transvaginal method for excising mesh perforation within the bladder.[28,29] The authors prefer this approach for the removal of synthetic mesh located between 4 and 8 o'clock at the bladder base. A 0.5% lidocaine with 1:200,000 epinephrine solution is used for hydrodissection of the vaginal epithelium from the underlying fibromuscular fascia. A U-shaped incision is elected to avoid potential overlapping suture lines, and the vaginal flap is created using sharp dissection. The mesh is identified and traced to its point of perforation into the bladder. A blunt instrument such as a Kelly clamp or Mixter right angle forceps is passed between the mesh and bladder adjacent to the urethra to facilitate transection of the mesh. Each cut edge is grasped with an Allis clamp and a combination of sharp dissection with Metzenbaum scissors and blunt dissection with a Kittner is used to free the mesh from the underling pubocervical fascia. Care is taken to point the tips of the Metzenbaum scissors toward the mesh to avoid injury to the bladder or urethra.

Once the point of entry into the bladder is identified, a cystotomy is made sharply alongside the mesh. The portion of the mesh within the bladder is sharply debrided. Enough mesh is removed to avoid protruding edges that may extrude into the bladder or through the vaginal epithelium. At this time, the cystotomy is closed in three layers. Urothelium is approximated with interrupted 3-0 polyglycolic sutures followed by a two-layer closure of the

detrusor using interrupted 2-0 polyglycolic acid sutures. Additional layers of pubocervical fascia can be developed and closed over the bladder. The vaginal flap is then approximated using a running 2-0 polyglycolic acid suture. A large-bore urethral catheter is left in place for approximately 2 weeks and removed after a cystogram shows no leak. The authors have previously published a case series of patients that underwent transvaginal mesh excision for mesh perforation after prolapse repair using a transvaginal mesh delivery system.[28] No complications occurred and all patients showed normal cystograms with resolution of symptoms postoperatively.[28]

Pain and Dyspareunia

Another controversial topic is the management of chronic pain after mesh placement. The origin of pain is not always clear. Isolated pain secondary to vaginal extrusion may be managed with transvaginal excision. Other causes of pain include protrusion of sling material or banding in the lateral fornices.[33] In these cases, regional extirpation of the mesh is recommended. When multiple sites or generalized pain is the presenting symptom, complete synthetic removal has been advocated. Open suprapubic, transvaginal, laparoscopic, and combined extirpation have been described.[30] In any method, care must be taken to remove only what is safe and necessary to treat symptoms, because intraoperative complications such as vascular injury, bleeding, and visceral perforation are possible. With suspected nerve entrapment or injury, one must use caution when promising pain alleviation. Misrai and colleagues[30] report that all patients experienced a decrease in total pain after either complete extirpation through laparoscopy or transvaginal partial resection, but quantified metrics were not used as part of the assessment.

MANAGEMENT OF MESH COMPLICATIONS AFTER PROLAPSE REPAIR USING SYNTHETIC MESH
Vaginal Mesh Extrusion

Management strategies for extrusion after implantation of transvaginal mesh delivery systems or sacrocolpopexy for pelvic organ prolapse are similar to those used for managing sling complications. Options include expectant management, topical estrogens, and trimming or surgical excision of mesh. The dilemma again arises in timing of the intervention and determining the appropriate amount of mesh to excise; the latter is important because recurrent pelvic organ prolapse is a risk. In a retrospective series of 684 patients who underwent transvaginal mesh prolapse repair, vaginal extrusion occurred in 11.3%, and 42% of extrusions resolved with medical treatment alone.[13] Medical management included antibiotics, vaginal antiseptics, and estrogen creams, but a standard protocol was not used.[13] A recent retrospective study of 524 patients, however, showed much lower success for medical management, and 13 of 14 mesh extrusions required surgical intervention after a median of 3 years' follow-up.[12]

Akin to the authors' experience managing vaginal sling extrusion, success with medical management alone is limited and most patients proceed to surgery. Choice of technique depends on the accessibility, location and amount of mesh extrusion. Transvaginal excision is preferred and the technique is similar to the management of sling mesh extrusion. After injection of lidocaine with epinephrine, a circumscribing incision is made at the junction of the extrusion and vaginal flaps are created with sharp dissection.[19,34] Enough mesh is excised to allow a tension-free closure of the vaginal epithelium.

Varying success for transvaginal mesh excision is reported in the literature. The authors' group has showed that in a cohort of 12 patients undergoing mesh excision for extrusion, no patient underwent a repeat operation for extrusion; however, only 79% of the entire cohort presented for follow-up at a median of 33 weeks.[34] No major intraoperative complications were reported, but one patient required a postoperative transfusion secondary to a rectovaginal hematoma. Of those presenting for follow-up, 20% reported a recurrent vaginal bulge. In a large series of 73 patients undergoing mesh excision, 8% of those undergoing partial excision for mesh extrusion required a repeat excision.[19] These extrusions included those following prolapse mesh, sacrocolpopexy, and synthetic midurethral slings.[19] Recurrence of pelvic organ prolapse occurred in 5% of partial excisions and 29% of complete excisions.[19] Intraoperative complications occurred in 5% and included bowel injuries and major bleeding. Postoperative complications occurred in 16% and included bleeding, hematomas, ileus, and infection.[19] One patient had a ureteral obstruction.[19] Most adverse events occurred during management of mesh complications following sacrocolpopexy.[19]

Management of vaginal extrusions following sacrocolpopexy can be challenging given the location of the mesh and its attachment to the sacrum with surrounding major vascular structures and bowel. South and colleagues[35] showed a 53.3% success rate for transvaginal management of sacrocolpopexy mesh extrusion. Significantly more adverse events occurred in the seven patients who proceeded on to open abdominal exploration after transvaginal surgery failed.[35]

Bladder Perforation or Extrusion

Open abdominal, laparoscopic, pure transvaginal and combination approaches have been described for removing mesh from the bladder.[19,25,28,36] Either a transvaginal or open abdominal approach provides access for removal of bladder mesh and closure of a concomitant vesicovaginal fistula.[19,34,36] Bekker and colleagues[31] report a case of endoscopic management in a patient with bladder mesh and a vesicovaginal fistula. In this case, a 5-mm laparoscopic trocar was placed in the bladder via a suprapubic cystotomy and used to aid in retraction.[31] The mesh was cut using bipolar diathermy down to the mucosa and a suprapubic catheter was left as a drain for 2 weeks.[31] They report that the bladder wall was healed after 6 weeks without need for additional intervention.[31]

Others have reported endoscopic management of bladder mesh after mesh-based prolapse repair with varying results (see **Table 1**). Frenkl and colleagues[25] showed a 50% success rate for endoscopic management of intravesical foreign bodies following pelvic floor reconstruction, including attempted removal of sutures or mesh following sacrocolpopexy. The authors' preferred method of management in these cases is a transvaginal approach as previously described, which is best suited for mesh located along the bladder base or bladder neck between 4 and 8 o'clock. In other locations, an open extraperitoneal retropubic technique provides appropriate access and definitive management of the mesh perforation.

Pain, Dyspareunia, and Mesh Contraction

Mesh contraction is a topic greatly debated. It is commonly applied to symptomatic complications following transvaginal mesh for pelvic organ prolapse. Not only does controversy exist over the management of the symptoms and findings of mesh contraction, but the existence of the entity itself has come into question. In a study of 40 women undergoing four-dimensional translabial ultrasound after transvaginal anterior prolapse repair with mesh, no radiographic evidence for mesh contraction was identified over an observation period of almost 60 woman-years.[37] This study actually found a statistically significant increase in mesh length after a mean 18 months' follow-up.[37] Multiple randomized controlled trials comparing transvaginal mesh kits for pelvic organ prolapse with native tissue repair have shown no significant difference in total vaginal length between groups, providing another set of data questioning the phenomena of mesh contraction.[2,14,15] In one of these studies, Sokol and colleagues[14] found that a significant change in vaginal diameter, vaginal volume, and total vaginal length occurred after both native tissue repair and transvaginal mesh implantation, but no difference was seen between the cohorts. A series of 17 women underwent mesh excision secondary to symptomatic vaginal mesh contraction.[38] Presenting symptoms included severe vaginal pain exacerbated by movement, dyspareunia, focal tenderness on examination, and findings of vaginal tightness and shortening.[38] The approach described is similar to transvaginal excision for mesh extrusion. The difference is that the mesh arms are dissected as lateral as possible and then transected in attempt to remove most of the mesh.[38] Substantial reduction in vaginal pain was achieved in 88% of patients, and 64% had reduction of dyspareunia.[38] Three patients had persistent symptoms and underwent a repeat procedure for complete excision of the mesh with subsequent alleviation of symptoms.[38] In some cases pain is related to excessive tension on the mesh arms and simple incision of the arm, similar to sling incision, can be useful to alleviate the symptoms.

SUMMARY

Introduction of synthetic mesh for pelvic floor reconstruction has created new challenges for the pelvic surgeon. Management of mesh-based complications is wrought with dilemmas, and electing the best strategy is often individualized. Asymptomatic small mesh exposures or extrusions can be managed with medical therapy initially, but definitive surgical options should be sought if timely spontaneous resolution does not occur. The authors' preference is transvaginal excision when feasible, because earlier convalescence is expected. Endoscopic techniques yield variable results in the literature and are an option for patients who do not wish to undergo open surgery or have comorbidities that preclude a more involved operation. Randomized prospective data with long-term follow-up is needed to better quantify the efficacy of each management strategy.

EDITOR'S COMMENTS

Complications related to the use of mesh for pelvic floor indications are increasingly being noted in clinical practice. Many factors have contributed to this increasing incidence. Clearly, the increased use of mesh for both midurethral slings and pelvic floor repair has increased the numbers of patients at risk for complications. Importantly, however, subtle differences between devices (regarding technique and insertion) may add additional variables to procedural outcome. Technical familiarity with these variations is critical for the implanting surgeon. Moreover, variations and modifications in device design have occurred rather rapidly, possibly impacting the individual surgeon's ability to have as robust a familiarity as possible with the most recent devices.

Another contributing factor to mesh complications is the patient comorbidity. Vaginal atrophy, chronic steroid use, prior surgery, and other local vaginal variables all conspire to increase the risk of mesh complication. In patients with either autoimmune or other wound-healing deficits, a further impact may be noted.

Management of mesh complications is individualized and somewhat predicated by the presenting scenario. Mesh exposure may occur in small or large volume and may or may not be complicated by vaginal constriction and damage to underlying viscera. Mesh erosion into underlying viscera (bladder, bowel, or rectum) further complicates presentation in that mesh in these circumstances leads to the potential of stone formation, recurrent urinary tract infection, hematuria, and altered bladder or bowel function dependent upon the organ involved. Another commonly encountered complication is pain at the site of mesh implantation. Pain may be related to mesh exposure alone, impacting sexual function. However, in some patients, mesh constriction may place undo tension both on underlying structures and also surrounding musculo-fascial supportive structures, resulting in chronic discomfort which may be extremely problematic for the patient.

Any comprehensive management plan should take into account the underlying symptoms, the degree to which resection of mesh should occur (partial versus total), and the need for simultaneous reconstruction of bladder and/or bowel wall. It is critical to prepare the woman for the likelihood that not all presenting symptoms will resolve and that there may be persistence of some aspect of the bothersome complaints that she is currently experiencing. These may include persistence of pain, return or exacerbation of incontinence, and impact upon bowel function. Additionally, long-term fibrosis may affect vaginal caliber and even without mesh being present, chronically may restrict vaginal distensibility and impact sexual function. The key to successful mesh complication management is a thoughtful, structured approach with an informed and aware patient. All due effort should be paid to optimizing the surgical field (treatment of infection, use of topical vaginal estrogens, and complete and thorough assessment of all potential mesh areas of exposure or erosion).

Although the majority of patients who have had mesh implanted have not had consequences of this implantation, those who have, are faced with a daunting burden. It is incumbent upon the pelvic floor medicine proceduralist to be aware of the potential ramifications of these complications and acute and chronic management thereof.

Roger R. Dmochowski, MD
Mickey Karram, MD

REFERENCES

1. Ulmsten U, Petros P. Intravaginal slingplasty (IVS): an ambulatory surgical procedure for treatment of female urinary incontinence. Scand J Urol Nephrol 1995;29(1):75–82.

2. Culligan PJ, Littman PM, Salamon CG, et al. Evaluation of a transvaginal mesh delivery system for the correction of pelvic organ prolapse: subjective and objective findings at least 1 year after surgery. Am J Obstet Gynecol 2010;203(5):506.e1–6.

3. Haylen BT, Freeman RM, Swift SE, et al. An International Urogynecological Association (IUGA)/International Continence Society (ICS) joint terminology and classification of the complications related directly to the insertion of prostheses (meshes, implants, tapes) and grafts in female pelvic floor surgery. Neurourol Urodyn 2011;30(1):2–12.

4. Novara G, Galfano A, Boscolo-Berto R, et al. Complication rates of tension-free midurethral slings in the treatment of female stress urinary incontinence: a systematic review and meta-analysis of randomized controlled trials comparing tension-free midurethral tapes to other surgical procedures and different devices. Eur Urol 2008; 53(2):288–308.

5. Ogah J, Cody DJ, Rogerson L. Minimally invasive synthetic suburethral sling operations for stress urinary incontinence in women: a short version Cochrane review. Neurourol Urodyn 2011;30(3):284–91.

6. Ogah J, Cody JD, Rogerson L. Minimally invasive synthetic suburethral sling operations for stress urinary incontinence in women. Cochrane Database Syst Rev 2009;4:CD006375.

7. Nguyen JN, Jakus-Waldman SM, Walter AJ, et al. Perioperative complications and reoperations after incontinence and prolapse surgeries using prosthetic implants. Obstet Gynecol 2012;119(3):539–46.

8. Clemens JQ, DeLancey JO, Faerber GJ, et al. Urinary tract erosions after synthetic pubovaginal slings: diagnosis and management strategy. Urology 2000;56(4):589–94.

9. Deng DY, Rutman M, Raz S, et al. Presentation and management of major complications of midurethral slings: are complications under-reported? Neurourol Urodyn 2007;26(1):46–52.

10. Karram MM, Segal JL, Vassallo BJ, et al. Complications and untoward effects of the tension-free vaginal tape procedure. Obstet Gynecol 2003; 101(5 Pt 1):929–32.

11. Richter HE, Albo ME, Zyczynski HM, et al. Retropubic versus transobturator midurethral slings for stress incontinence. N Engl J Med 2010;362(22):2066–76.

12. de Landsheere L, Ismail S, Lucot JP, et al. Surgical intervention after transvaginal Prolift mesh repair: retrospective single-center study including 524 patients with 3 years' median follow-up. Am J Obstet Gynecol 2012;206(1):83.e1–7.

13. Caquant F, Collinet P, Debodinance P, et al. Safety of trans vaginal mesh procedure: retrospective study of 684 patients. J Obstet Gynaecol Res 2008; 34(4):449–56.

14. Sokol AI, Iglesia CB, Kudish BI, et al. One-year objective and functional outcomes of a randomized clinical trial of vaginal mesh for prolapse. Am J Obstet Gynecol 2012;206(1):86.e1–9.

15. Withagen MI, Milani AL, den Boon J, et al. Trocar-guided mesh compared with conventional vaginal repair in recurrent prolapse: a randomized controlled trial. Obstet Gynecol 2011;117(2 Pt 1):242–50.

16. Withagen MI, Vierhout ME, Hendriks JC, et al. Risk factors for exposure, pain, and dyspareunia after tension-free vaginal mesh procedure. Obstet Gynecol 2011;118(3):629–36.

17. Nguyen JN, Burchette RJ. Outcome after anterior vaginal prolapse repair: a randomized controlled trial. Obstet Gynecol 2008;111(4):891–8.

18. Kobashi KC, Govier FE. Management of vaginal erosion of polypropylene mesh slings. J Urol 2003; 169(6):2242–3.

19. Tijdink MM, Vierhout ME, Heesakkers JP, et al. Surgical management of mesh-related complications after prior pelvic floor reconstructive surgery with mesh. Int Urogynecol J 2011;22(11):1395–404.

20. Huang KH, Kung FT, Liang HM, et al. Management of polypropylene mesh erosion after intravaginal midurethral sling operation for female stress urinary incontinence. Int Urogynecol J Pelvic Floor Dysfunct 2005;16(6):437–40.

21. Goldman HB. Simple sling incision for the treatment of iatrogenic urethral obstruction. Urology 2003; 62(4):714–8.

22. Marcus-Braun N, von Theobald P. Mesh removal following transvaginal mesh placement: a case series of 104 operations. Int Urogynecol J 2010; 21(4):423–30.

23. Amundsen CL, Flynn BJ, Webster GD. Urethral erosion after synthetic and nonsynthetic pubovaginal slings: differences in management and continence outcome. J Urol 2003;170(1):134–7 [discussion: 137].

24. Velemir L, Amblard J, Jacquetin B, et al. Urethral erosion after suburethral synthetic slings: risk factors, diagnosis, and functional outcome after surgical management. Int Urogynecol J Pelvic Floor Dysfunct 2008;19(7):999–1006.

25. Frenkl TL, Rackley RR, Vasavada SP, et al. Management of iatrogenic foreign bodies of the bladder and urethra following pelvic floor surgery. Neurourol Urodyn 2008;27(6):491–5.

26. Foley C, Patki P, Boustead G. Unrecognized bladder perforation with mid-urethral slings. BJU Int 2010; 106(10):1514–8.

27. Doumouchtsis SK, Lee FY, Bramwell D, et al. Evaluation of holmium laser for managing mesh/suture complications of continence surgery. BJU Int 2011; 108(9):1472–8.

28. Firoozi F, Goldman HB. Transvaginal excision of mesh erosion involving the bladder after mesh placement using a prolapse kit: a novel technique. Urology 2010;75(1):203–6.

29. Firoozi F, Ingber MS, Goldman HB. Pure transvaginal removal of eroded mesh and retained foreign body in the bladder. Int Urogynecol J 2010;21(6): 757–60.

30. Misrai V, Roupret M, Xylinas E, et al. Surgical resection for suburethral sling complications after treatment for stress urinary incontinence. J Urol 2009; 181(5):2198–202 [discussion: 2203].

31. Bekker MD, Bevers RF, Elzevier HW. Transurethral and suprapubic mesh resection after Prolift bladder perforation: a case report. Int Urogynecol J 2010; 21(10):1301–3.

32. Oh TH, Ryu DS. Transurethral resection of intravesical mesh after midurethral sling procedures. J Endourol 2009;23(8):1333–7.

33. Cholhan HJ, Hutchings TB, Rooney KE. Dyspareunia associated with paraurethral banding in the transobturator sling. Am J Obstet Gynecol 2010; 202(5):481.e1–5.

34. Ridgeway B, Walters MD, Paraiso MF, et al. Early experience with mesh excision for adverse outcomes after transvaginal mesh placement using prolapse kits. Am J Obstet Gynecol 2008;199(6):703.e1–7.

35. South MM, Foster RT, Webster GD, et al. Surgical excision of eroded mesh after prior abdominal sacrocolpopexy. Am J Obstet Gynecol 2007;197(6):615.e1–5.

36. Yamada BS, Govier FE, Stefanovic KB, et al. Vesicovaginal fistula and mesh erosion after Perigee (transobturator polypropylene mesh anterior repair). Urology 2006;68(5):1121.e5–7.

37. Dietz HP, Erdmann M, Shek KL. Mesh contraction: myth or reality? Am J Obstet Gynecol 2011;204(2): 173.e1–4.

38. Feiner B, Maher C. Vaginal mesh contraction: definition, clinical presentation, and management. Obstet Gynecol 2010;115(2 Pt 1):325–30.

Index

Note: Page numbers of article titles are in **boldface** type.

http://dx.doi.org/10.1016/S0094-0143(12)00068-7
0094-0143/12/$ – see front matter © 2012 Elsevier Inc. All rights reserved.

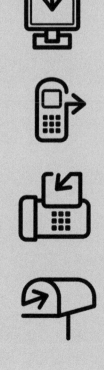

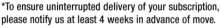

Printed and bound by CPI Group (UK) Ltd, Croydon, CR0 4YY

03/10/2024

01040344-0013